dIFIORE'S ATLAS OF HISTOLOGY WITH FUNCTIONAL CORRELATIONS TENTH EDITION

Victor P. Eroschenko, PhD
Professor of Anatomy
WWAMI Medical Program
University of Idaho
Moscow, Idaho

LIPPINCOTT WILLIAMS & WILKINS
A **Wolters Kluwer** Company

Philadelphia · Baltimore · New York · London
Buenos Aires · Hong Kong · Sydney · Tokyo

Executive Acquisitions Editor: Betty Sun
Developmental Editor: Kathleen Scogna
Marketing Manager: Joseph Schott
Production Editor: Jennifer Ajello
Designer: Risa Clow
Compositor: Graphic World
Printer: R.R. Donnelley & Sons (Willard)

351 West Camden Street
Baltimore, MD 21201

530 Walnut Street
Philadelphia, PA 19106

Printed in the United States of America

Library of Congress Cataloging-in-Publication Data is available: ISBN 13: 978-0-7817-5021-9
ISBN 10: 0-7817-5021-0

To purchase additional copies of this book, call our customer service department at **(800) 638-3030** or fax orders to **(301) 824-7390.** International customers should call **(301) 714-2324.**

Visit Lippincott Williams & Wilkins on the Internet: http://www.LWW.com. Lippincott Williams & Wilkins customer service representatives are available from 8:30 am to 6:00 pm, EST.

07 08
3 4 5 6 7 8 9 10

dIFIORE'S ATLAS OF HISTOLOGY WITH FUNCTIONAL CORRELATIONS TENTH EDITION

To those who matter so much

Ian
McKenzie
Sarah
Shannon

      and
      Diane
      Kathryn
      Tatiana
      Sharon

            and
            Todd
            Shaun
            Jacob

                  and most especially and always
                        Elke

PREFACE

Recent research in cell and molecular biology has added a vast amount of new information to science. Histology has become essential to understanding and interpreting the significance of this new knowledge. At the same time, major changes are taking place in the manner in which histology is taught and studied. Much less time is now devoted to the use of the microscope in the laboratory. Instead, more and more students are using computer-generated and electronic media to view histology images. Modern histology texts and atlases must recognize these changes and offer students tools that will allow them to master the necessary information.

Basic approach

The 10th edition of *diFiore's Atlas of Histology* continues its vaunted tradition of providing realistic, full-color composite and idealized illustrations of histology slides. Over the years, this approach has served the needs of undergraduate and graduate students of histology and biology, allied health students, and medical and veterinary students. Countless professors and students have testified to the usefulness of this approach. Idealized views of cells and tissues are not only an excellent learning resource, but they also provide a comprehensive means of review for both written and practical examinations.

In the last edition of the atlas, photomicrographs were introduced to serve as comparisons to the idealized illustrations. We continue to include photomicrographs in the present edition, offering the right balance between the photographic and the idealized images.

Changes in the 10th edition

Several significant changes in design have been instituted in this edition. However, the changes are more than cosmetic. A comprehensive summary of all of the changes is as follows:

- The format of the atlas has been completely redesigned to make it more open and modern. Color is used to highlight chapter headings and functional correlations.
- All introductory sections and figure descriptions for each chapter have been completely rewritten, and all structural/functional correlations have been updated and expanded to reflect new scientific findings and interpretations.
- Old illustrations have been replaced with 115 new, original, and digitized color illustrations.
- A new chapter on the cell and basic cytology has been added. This chapter includes 10 transmission electron micrographs, as well as a description of the functional correlations of the major cytoplasmic organelles.
- The photomicrographs that were in the back of each chapter have now been incorporated with the rest of the illustrations in the chapter for easier comparison and interpretation of structures.
- The chapter on the nervous system has been subdivided into two sections, the central nervous system and the peripheral nervous system.
- A new section on staining has been added to the Introduction that explains each technique's specific staining characteristics.

Electronic atlas

Perhaps the most exciting change in the 10th edition is the inclusion of an interactive electronic atlas with each copy of the book. This ancillary allows students to test their knowledge of structure and function on each of the images in the book. Features of the electronic atlas include a labels on/labels off feature, rollover "hot spots," and rollover labels. A self-testing feature lets students practice identifying features on the illustrations and photomicrographs. An instructor version of the electronic ancillary contains 677 additional digitized photomicrographs, organized by chapter. Each image can be exported into Power Point to provide visual information during lectures and/or laboratory exercises.

Acknowledgments

I have been very fortunate to be associated with numerous individuals who were very instrumental in assisting me in preparing and improving the new edition of the histology atlas.

Dr. E. Roland Brown, owner of drbrown.us and an auxiliary faculty member at the University of Utah, prepared all of the new histology illustrations. His talent in this endeavor is unprecedented, as the new illustrations demonstrate.

Sonja L. Gerard of Oei Graphics, Bellevue, Washington, prepared the beautiful lead-in art for the cell and cytoplasm chapter and improved the colors in the rest of the lead-in art of the atlas.

Dr. Mark E. DeSantis, a long-time colleague and professor at the WWAMI Medical Education Program and Department of Biology, University of Idaho, Moscow, Idaho, provided constructive suggestions for improving the chapters on the muscle and nervous systems.

Dr. Rex A. Hess, a long-time colleague and professor of Reproductive Biology and Toxicology, Department of Veterinary Biosciences, University of Illinois, Urbana, Illinois, graciously provided the high-quality transmission electron micrographs for the new cell and cytoplasm chapter.

Betty Sun, Executive Editor at Lippincott Wilkins & Williams, initiated the revision process and prepared the contractual agreements with the artists.

Jennifer Ajello, Production Editor at Lippincott Wilkins & Williams, corrected the final version of the proofs.

Kathleen H. Scogna, Developmental Editor at Lippincott Wilkins & Williams, was instrumental in initiating the major changes in the format and style of the present edition of the atlas. In addition, she read, corrected, and edited every page of the text and art. Moreover, her suggestions for improving the text were especially valuable because she represented the position of the student. Kathleen's editorial efforts and inquiries have vastly improved this edition of the atlas, and I want to express my special appreciation to her.

In addition, I express sincere appreciation to all of the highly talented and professional individuals with whom I had the pleasure of collaborating during the preparation of this atlas.

Victor P. Eroschenko, PhD
Moscow, Idaho
November, 2003

CONTENTS

CHAPTER 7   Nervous Tissue 121

PART II   ■   ORGANS   151

CHAPTER 8   Circulatory System 153

PART I

TISSUES

Interpretation of Histologic Sections

Histologic sections are thin, flat slices of fixed and stained tissues and/or organs that are mounted on glass slides. Such sections are normally composed of cellular, fibrous, and tubular structures. The cells exhibit a variety of shapes, sizes, and layers. The fibrous structures are solid and are found in the connective, nervous, and muscle tissues. The tubular structures are hollow and represent various types of blood vessels, ducts, and glands.

In the tissue or organ, the cells, fibers, and tubes have a random orientation in space and are a part of a three-dimensional structure. During the preparation of histology slides, the thin sections do not have depth. In addition, the plane of section does not always cut these structures exactly in the transverse or cross section. This produces variation in the appearance of the cells, fibers, and tubes, depending on the angle of the plane of section. As a result, it is difficult to perceive correctly on a flat slide the three-dimensional structure from which the sections were prepared. Therefore, correct visualization and interpretation of these sections in their proper three-dimensional perspective on the slide become important criteria for mastering histology.

For better orientation and interpretation of the three-dimensional composition of tissues and organs on the histology slide, the first two figures of the atlas have been especially prepared to illustrate how the appearance of cells and tubes changes with the plane of section.

FIGURE I.1 ■ Planes of Section of a Round Object

To illustrate how the shape of a three-dimensional cell can be altered in a histologic section, a hard-boiled egg has been sectioned in longitudinal and transverse (cross) planes. The composition of a hard-boiled egg serves as a good example of a cell, with the yellow yolk representing the nucleus and the surrounding egg white representing the cytoplasm. Enclosing these structures are the soft egg-shell membrane and a hard egg shell (yellow). At the rounded end of the egg is the air space (blue).

The **midline** sections of the egg in the **longitudinal plane** (a) and in the **transverse plane** (d) disclose its correct shape and size, because they appear in these planes of section. In addition, these two planes of section reveal the correct appearance, size, and distribution of the internal contents within the egg.

Similar but more **peripheral** sections of the egg in the **longitudinal plane** (b) and in the **transverse plane** (e) still show the external shape of the egg. However, because the sections were cut peripheral to the midline, the internal contents of the egg are not seen in their correct size or distribution within the egg white. In addition, the size of the egg appears smaller.

The **tangential planes** (c, f) of section graze or only pass through the outermost periphery of the egg. These sections reveal that the egg is an oval (c) or a small, round (f) object. The egg yolk is not seen in either section, because it was not located in the plane of section. As a result, such tangential sections do not reveal sufficient detail for correct interpretation of the egg size, its contents, or their distribution within the internal membrane.

FIGURE I.2 ■ Planes of Section of a Tube

Tubular structures are often seen in histologic sections. Tubes are most easily recognized when they are cut in transverse (cross) sections. However, if the tubes are sectioned in other planes, they must first be visualized as three-dimensional structures to be recognized as tubes. To illustrate how a blood vessel, duct, or glandular structure may appear in a histologic section, a curved tube with a simple (single) epithelial cell layer is sectioned in the longitudinal, transverse, and oblique planes.

A **longitudinal** (a) plane of section that cuts the tube in the midline produces a U-shaped structure. The sides of the tube are lined by a single row of cuboidal (round) cells around an empty lumen except at the bottom, where the tube begins to curve; in this region, the cells appear multilayered.

Transverse (d, e) planes of section of the same tube produce round structures that are lined by a single layer of cells. The variations that are seen in the cytoplasm of different cells result from the planes of section through the individual cells, as explained earlier. A transverse section of a straight tube can produce a single image (e). The double image (d) of the same structure can represent either two tubes running parallel to each other or a single tube that has curved in the space of the tissue or organ that is sectioned.

A **tangential** (b) plane of section through the tube produces a solid, multicellular, oval structure that does not resemble a tube. The reason is that the plane of section grazed the outermost periphery of the tube as it made a turn in space; the lumen was not present in the plane of section. An **oblique** (c) plane of section through the tube and its cells produces an oval structure that includes an oval lumen in the center and multiple cell layers at the periphery.

A **transverse** (f) section in the region of a sharp curve in the tube grazes the innermost cell layer and produces two oval structures that are connected by a multiple, solid layer of cells (f). These sections of the tube also contain an oval lumen, indicating that the plane of section passed at an angle to the structure.

Thus, in a histologic section, the shape and size of an individual structure may vary, depending on the plane of section. Some cells may exhibit full cross-sections of their nuclei, which appear prominent in the cells. Other cells may exhibit only a fraction of the nucleus, and the cytoplasm appears large. Still other cells may appear only as clear cytoplasm without any nuclei. All these variations result from different planes of section through the nuclei. Understanding these variations in cell and tube morphology will result in better interpretation of the histologic sections.

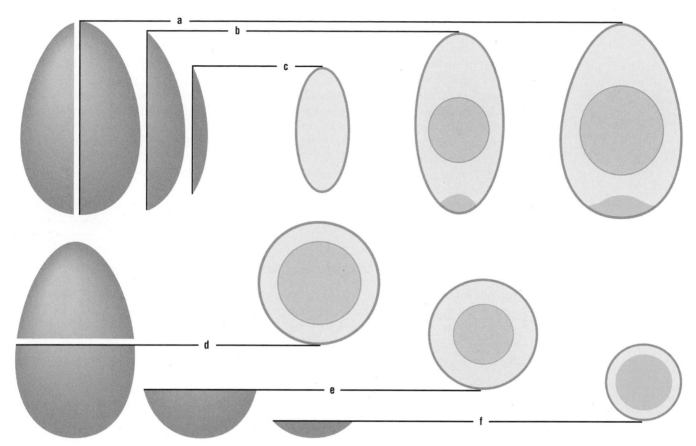

FIGURE I.1 ■ Planes of Section of a Round Object.

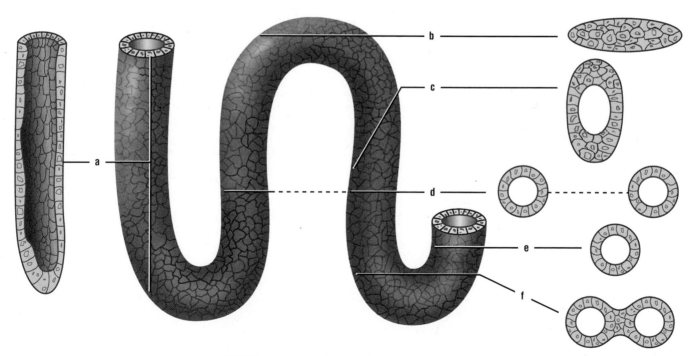

FIGURE I.2 ■ Planes of section of a tube.

FIGURE I.3 ■ Tubules of the Testis in Different Planes of Section

Organs such as testes and kidneys consist primarily of highly twisted or convoluted tubules. When flat sections of such organs are seen on histology slides, the cut tubules exhibit a variety of shapes because of the plane of section. To show how twisted tubules appear in a histology slide, a portion of a testis was prepared for examination. Each testis consists of numerous, highly twisted seminiferous tubules that are lined by multilayered or stratified germinal epithelium.

A **longitudinal plane (1)** through a seminiferous tubule produces an elongated tubule with a long lumen. A **transverse plane (2)** through a single seminiferous tubule produces a round tubule. Similarly, a **transverse plane through a curve (3, 5)** of a seminiferous tubule produces two oval structures that are connected by solid layers of cells. An **oblique plane (4)** through a tubule produces an oval structure with an oval lumen in the center and multiple cell layers at the periphery. A **tangential plane (6)** of a seminiferous tubule passes through its periphery. As a result, this plane produces a solid, multicellular, oval structure that does not resemble a tube, because the lumen is not seen.

Interpretation of Structures Prepared Using Different Type of Stains

Interpretation of histologic sections is greatly aided by the use of different stains, which stain certain specific properties in different cells, tissues, and organs. The most prevalent stain that is used for the preparation of histology slides is hematoxylin and eosin (H&E) stain. Most of the images prepared for this atlas were taken from slides stained with H&E. To show other and more specific features characteristic of different cells, tissues, and organs, other stains are used.

Listed below are the different stains that were used to prepare the slides and their specific staining characteristics.

H&E Stain

- Nuclei stain blue.
- Cytoplasm stains pink or red.
- Collagen fibers stain pink.
- Muscles stain pink.

Masson's Trichrome Stain

- Nuclei stain black or blue black.
- Muscles stain red.
- Collagen and mucus stain green or blue.
- Cytoplasm of most cells stains pink.

Periodic Acid-Schiff (PAS) Reaction

- Glycogen stains deep red or magenta.
- Contents of goblet cells in digestive organs and respiratory epithelia stain magenta or deep red.
- Basement membranes and brush borders in kidney tubules stain positive, or pink.

Verhoeff's Stain for Elastic Tissue

- Elastic fibers stain jet black.
- Nuclei stain gray.
- Remaining structures stain pink.

Mallory-Azan Stain

- Fibrous connective tissue, mucus, and hyaline cartilage stain deep blue.
- Erythrocytes stain red-orange.
- Cytoplasm of liver and kidney stain pink.
- Nuclei stain red.

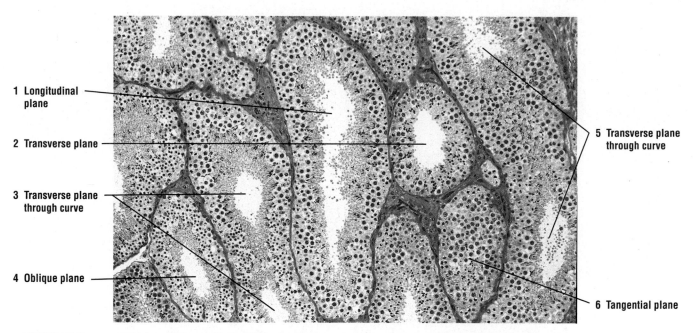

1 Longitudinal plane

2 Transverse plane

3 Transverse plane through curve

4 Oblique plane

5 Transverse plane through curve

6 Tangential plane

FIGURE I.3 ▪ Tubules of the testis in different planes of section. Stain: hematoxylin and eosin (plastic section). 30×

Wright's or Giemsa's Stain

- Erythrocyte cytoplasm stains pink.
- Lymphocyte nuclei stain dark purple-blue, with pale blue cytoplasm.
- Monocyte cytoplasm stains pale blue, and nucleus stains medium blue.
- Neutrophil nuclei stain dark blue.
- Eosinophil nuclei stain dark blue, and granules stain bright pink.
- Basophil nuclei stain dark blue or purple, cytoplasm pale blue, and granules deep purple.
- Platelets stain light blue.

Cajal's and Del Rio Hortega's Methods (Silver and Gold Impregnation Methods)

- Myelinated and unmyelinated fibers and neurofibrils stain blue-black.
- General background is nearly colorless.
- Astrocytes stain black.
- Depending on the methods used, the end product can stain black, brown, or gold.

Osmic Acid (Osmium Tetroxide) Stain

- Lipids in general stain black.
- Lipids in the myelin sheath of nerves stain black.

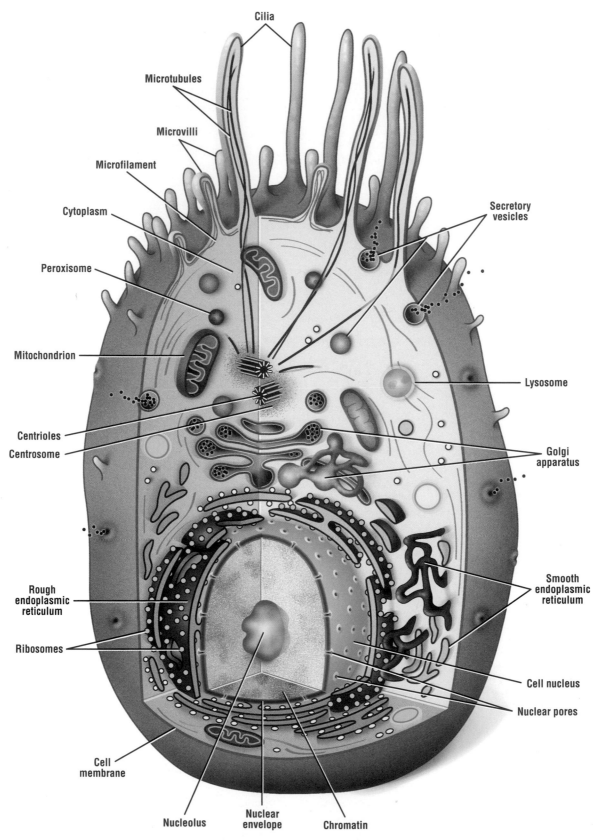

Cilia

Microtubules

Microvilli

Microfilament

Cytoplasm

Peroxisome

Mitochondrion

Centrioles

Centrosome

Rough
endoplasmic
reticulum

Ribosomes

Cell
membrane

Nucleolus

Nuclear
envelope

Chromatin

Secretory
vesicles

Lysosome

Golgi
apparatus

Smooth
endoplasmic
reticulum

Cell nucleus

Nuclear pores

OVERVIEW FIGURE ■ Composite illustration of a cell and its cytoplasmic organelles.

CHAPTER 1

The Cell and Cytoplasm

Introduction—Light and Electron Microscopy

Histology or microscopic anatomy is a visual, colorful science. For many years, microscopists relied on compound microscopes to study the characteristics of cells, tissues, and organs. The light source for the early microscopes was the sun. For modern microscopes, an electric light bulb with tungsten filaments serves as the main source of light.

Much initial information in histology was gained by examining tissue slides with a light microscope, but its resolving power was too limited. Additional resolution was needed. Even with the primitive microscopes, however, most mammalian cells exhibited a nucleus and a cytoplasm surrounded by some sort of a border or a cell membrane. With the use of various histochemical, immunocytochemical, and staining techniques, the cytoplasm of different cells was shown to contain numerous subcellular elements called organelles.

Only with the advent of transmission electron microscopy did more superior resolution and higher magnification of cells and their cytoplasm become possible. Histologists were now able to examine the ultrastructure of the cell, its membrane, and its numerous cytoplasmic organelles.

The Cell

All living organisms contain a multitude of different cell types, the main function of which is to maintain a proper homeostasis in the body. To perform this task, the cells possess certain structural elements in their cytoplasm that are common to all cell types. As a result, it is possible to illustrate a cell in a more generalized, composite form with various organelles. It is essential to remember, however, that the quantity, appearance, and distribution of these organelles within a cell depend on the cell type and its function (see overview figure).

The Cell and Its Membrane

A **cell** or a **plasma membrane** surrounds all cells and forms an important barrier or boundary between the internal and the external environments. Internal to the cell membrane is the **cytoplasm,** a fluid-like medium that contains a variety of **organelles,** microtubules, microfilaments, and membrane-bound secretory granules or ingested material. In most cells, the cytoplasm also surrounds the **nucleus.**

The cell membrane consists of a **bilayer,** or a double layer, of **phospholipid molecules.** Interspersed within and embedded in the phospholipid bilayer of the cell membrane are the **molecules** of **integral** and **peripheral proteins.** Also present in the plasma membrane is **cholesterol,** an important element that stabilizes the membrane and regulates the fluidity of the phospholipid bilayer. On the external surface of the cell membrane is a delicate, fuzzy cell coat called **glycocalyx** that is composed of carbohydrate chains that are attached to the integral proteins of the cell membrane. The lipid bilayer is fluid, and the proteins move freely within the membrane confines. As a result, the composition of the cell membrane is characterized as a **fluid mosaic model.**

The lipid molecules are arranged in two layers with their polar heads arranged on both the inner and outer surfaces of the cell membrane. The nonpolar tails of the lipid layers face each other in the center of the membrane. In electron micrographs, however, the plasma membrane appears as three layers, consisting of the outer and inner dense layers and a less dense, or lighter, middle layer. This discrepancy results from the osmic acid that is used to fix and stain tissues for electron microscopy. Osmic acid binds to the polar heads of the lipids in the cell membrane, and it stains them very densely. The nonpolar tails in the middle of the cell membrane remain light and unstained.

The Cell Organelles

The cell cytoplasm contains numerous organelles, each of which performs a specific function that is essential for cell life. A membrane similar to the cell membrane surrounds most of the cytoplasmic organelles.

Mitochondria

The **mitochondria** are elongated, rod-shaped structures that often vary in size and shape, depending on the cell function. Each mitochondrion (plural, mitochondria) consists of an outer and an inner membrane. The inner membrane exhibits numerous folds in the form of **cristae.** In protein-secreting cells, these cristae project into the interior of the organelle in the form of shelves. In contrast, mitochondria exhibit tubular cristae in steroid-secreting cells of the adrenal cortex or interstitial cells in the testes. Surrounding the mitochondrial cristae is an amorphous **mitochondrial matrix.**

Endoplasmic Reticulum

The **endoplasmic reticulum** in the cytoplasm is an extensive network of sacs, vesicles, and interconnected flat tubules called **cisternae.** There are rough endoplasmic reticulum and smooth endoplasmic reticulum. Their predominance and distribution in a given cell is dependent on cell function.

The **rough endoplasmic reticulum** is characterized by numerous flattened, interconnected cisternae, the cytoplasmic surfaces of which are covered or studded with numerous dark-staining granules called **ribosomes.** This type of reticulum extends throughout the cytoplasm from the nuclear envelope around the nucleus. In contrast, **smooth endoplasmic reticulum** is devoid of ribosomes and consists primarily of anastomosing tubules. In some cells, smooth endoplasmic reticulum is directly continuous with rough endoplasmic reticulum.

Golgi Apparatus

The **Golgi apparatus** is composed of a system of membrane-bound, smooth, flattened, stacked, and slightly curved **cisternae.** These cisternae are not continuous with the endoplasmic reticulum. The concave side of these stacked cisternae faces the nucleus. Numerous small vesicles are located around the terminal ends of the cisternae.

The cisternae on the convex side of the Golgi apparatus are considered to be the *cis*-face, whereas the cisternae at the inner concave side are the *trans*-face. Vesicles from the endoplasmic reticulum move though the cytoplasm to the *cis* side of the Golgi apparatus and bud off from the *trans* side.

Ribosomes

The **ribosomes** are small, dark-staining granules that are found in the cytoplasm of the cell; a membrane does not surround them. A given cell has both free ribosomes and attached ribosomes, as seen on the endoplasmic reticulum.

Lysosomes

The **lysosomes** are membrane-bound organelles formed by the Golgi apparatus. They contain a variety of hydrolyzing or digestive enzymes called **acid hydrolases.** Lysosomes are highly variable in both appearance and size. The main function of lysosomes is digestion of substances taken into the cells or of the cell organelles. Lysosomes digest phagocytosed microorganisms, cell debris, cells, and damaged or excessive cell organelles, such as mitochondria or rough endoplasmic reticulum.

Peroxisomes

The **peroxisomes** are cell organelles that appear similar to lysosomes; however, peroxisomes are smaller. They are found in nearly all cell types. Peroxisomes contain several types of **oxidases,** which are enzymes that oxidize various organic substances and can form hydrogen peroxide, a cytotoxic product. Peroxisomes also contain an enzyme **catalase** that can remove excess hydrogen peroxide by converting it to water and oxygen molecules.

The Cytoskeleton of the Cell

The **cytoskeleton** of a cell consists of a network of tiny protein filaments and tubules that extends throughout the cytoplasm. It serves as an important structural framework for the cells. Three types of filamentous proteins—microfilaments, intermediate filaments, and microtubules—form the cytoskeleton of a cell.

Microfilaments, Intermediate Filaments, and Microtubules

The **microfilaments** are the thinnest structures of the cytoskeleton. They are composed of the protein **actin** and are most prevalent on the peripheral regions of the cell membrane.

The **intermediate filaments** are thicker than the microfilaments and, in terms of size, are between microfilaments and microtubules. These filaments are found in all cell types, and they bind intracellular structures both to each other and to plasma membrane proteins. In many epithelial cells, the intermediate filaments contain the protein **keratin.** In skin cells, these filaments terminate at cell junctions, where they stabilize the shape of the cell and its attachments to adjacent cells.

The **microtubules,** which are also found in almost all cell types, are the largest elements of the cytoskeleton. They are hollow, unbranched tubules that are composed of the protein **tubulin.** These tubules are most visible and are predominant in motile **cilia** and sperm tail or **flagellum,** where they are arranged as nine parallel microtubules around a central pair of microtubules.

Centrosome and Centrioles

The **centrosome** is an area of the cytoplasm near the nucleus. Within the centrosome are two small, cylindrical structures called **centrioles.** The two centrioles are located perpendicular to each other. Each centriole consists of nine evenly spaced clusters of three microtubules arranged in a circle. The microtubules have longitudinal orientation and are parallel to each other.

Cytoplasmic Inclusions

The **cytoplasmic inclusions** are temporary structures in the cytoplasm of certain cells. **Lipids, glycogen, crystals, pigment,** or byproducts of **metabolism** are inclusions and represent the nonliving parts of the cell.

The Nucleus and the Nuclear Envelope

The **nucleus** is the largest organelle of a cell. Most cells have a single nucleus; other cells may exhibit multiple nuclei. The shape of the nucleus usually corresponds to the cell shape. Skeletal muscle cells have numerous nuclei, whereas mature red blood cells in mammals are not nucleated.

A double membrane called the **nuclear envelope** surrounds the nucleus. Both the inner and outer layers of the nuclear envelope contain the lipid bilayer of the cell membrane. In some cells, the outer nuclear membrane exhibits tiny ribosomes and is continuous with the rough endoplasmic reticulum, which it resembles. At intervals around the periphery of the nucleus, the outer and inner membranes of the nuclear envelope fuse to form numerous **nuclear pores.**

The nondividing cells contain regions of dark-staining material called **chromatin** that is located adjacent to the inner nuclear membrane. Inside the nucleus are one or more dark-staining, spherical structures called the **nucleoli** (singular, nucleus).

FIGURE 1.1 ■ Apical Surfaces of Ciliated and Nonciliated Epithelium

A low-magnification electron micrograph shows alternating ciliated and nonciliated cells in the epithelium of the efferent ductules of the testis. The **cilia** (1) in the ciliated cells are attached to the dense **basal bodies** (2) at the cell apices, from which they extend into the **lumen** (7) of the duct. The core of the cilia (1) contains longitudinal microtubules, which are arranged in a consistent pattern of two single central microtubules surrounded by nine double microtubules. In contrast, the **microvilli** (8) in the nonciliated cells are shorter, and their core contains thin actin microfilaments. Note also the dense structures in the apices between the adjacent epithelial cells. These are the **junctional complexes** (3) that hold the cells together. Distinct **cell membranes** (10) separate the individual cells. Located in the cytoplasm of these cells are numerous elongated or rod-shaped **mitochondria** (5), a few stacked **cisternae** of the **rough endoplasmic reticulum** (11), numerous light-staining **vesicles** (4) and some **dense bodies** (6). Each cell also contains **nuclei** (12) of various shapes with dispersed, dense-staining nuclear **chromatin** (13) arranged around the nuclear peripheries.

FIGURE 1.2 ■ Junctional Complex between Epithelial Cells

A high-magnification electron micrograph illustrates a junctional complex between two adjacent epithelial cells. This complex exhibits three distinct parts. In the apical region of the cells, the opposing cells membranes fuse to form a **tight junction** or **zonula occludens** (2a), which extends around the cell peripheries like a belt. Inferior to the zonula occludens (2a) is another junction called the **zonula adherens** (2b). It is characterized by a dense layer of proteins on the inside of the plasma membranes of both cells, that attach to the cytoskeleton filaments of each cell. A small intercellular space with transmembrane adhesion proteins separates the two membranes. This type of junction also extends around the cells like a belt. Below the zonula adherens is a **desmosome** (2c). Desmosomes (2c) do not encircle the cells; rather, they are spot-like plaques that exhibit random distribution in the cells. The cytoplasmic side of each desmosome exhibits dense areas that are composed of attachment proteins. Transmembrane glycoproteins extend into the intercellular space between opposing cell membranes of the desmosome and attach the cells to each other.

Note also the distinct **cell membranes** (3) of each cell, the numerous **mitochondria** (1) in cross section, and the variety of **vesicular structures** (6) in their cytoplasm. Visible on the cell apices are sections of **cilia** (5) with a core of **microtubules** and a few **microvilli** (4) of an adjacent cell.

FUNCTIONAL CORRELATIONS

Junctional Complex

Junctional complexes have a variety of functions, depending on their morphology. In the epithelium that lines the stomach, intestines, and urinary bladder, zonula occludens or tight junctions prevent the passage of corrosive chemicals or waste products between cells and into the bloodstream. Similarly, zonula adherens assists these cells in resisting separation. Desmosomes, however, are most commonly seen in the epithelium of the skin and in cardiac muscle fibers. Here, the cells are subjected to great mechanical stresses. In these organs, desmosomes prevent skin cells from separating and cardiac muscle cells from pulling apart during heart contractions.

Other parts of the junctional complex are hemidesmosomes and gap junctions. Hemidesmosomes are half of the desmosome and are present at the base of epithelial cells. Here, the hemidesmosomes anchor the epithelial cells to the basement membrane and the adjacent connective tissue.

Gap junctions are also spot-like in structure. The plasma membrane at the gap junctions is not fused, however, and tiny fluid channels called connexons connect the adjacent cells. These fluid channels serve an important function by allowing very rapid communication between cells, especially in cardiac muscle cells and nerve cells, where fast impulse transmission through the cells or axons is essential for normal organ function.

1 Cilia

2 Basal bodies

3 Junctional complexes

4 Vesicles

5 Mitochondria

6 Dense bodies

7 Lumen

8 Microvilli

9 Basal bodies

10 Cell membranes

11 Rough endoplasmic reticulum

12 Nuclei

13 Chromatin

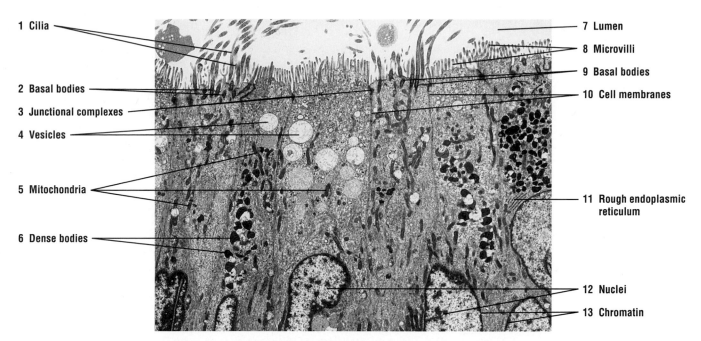

FIGURE 1.1 ▪ Apical surfaces of ciliated and nonciliated epithelium. 10,600×

4 Microvilli

5 Cilia with microtubules

1 Mitochondria

2 Junctinal complex
a. Tight junction
b. Zonula adherens
c. Desmosome

3 Cell membranes

6 Vesicles

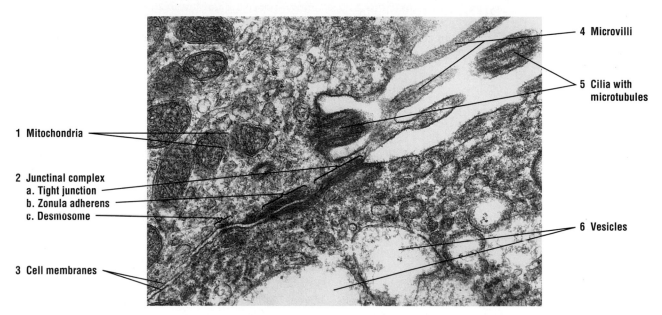

FIGURE 1.2 ▪ Junctional complexes between epithelial cells. 31,200×

FIGURE 1.3 ■ Basal Regions of Epithelial Cells

A medium-magnification electron micrograph illustrates the appearance of the basal region of epithelial cells. Note that the basal regions of the cells are attached to a thin, electron-lucent layer called the **basal lamina (3)**. Deep to the basal lamina (3) is a **connective tissue (2)** layer of fine reticular fibers. The basal lamina (3) itself is seen only with an electron microscope, whereas the basal lamina (3) and the reticular fibers of connective tissue (2) are seen under the light microscope as a basement membrane. Inferior to the epithelial cells is an elongated, spindle-shaped **fibroblast (4)** with its **nucleus (4)** and dispersed **chromatin (5)** surrounded by numerous connective tissue fibers (2) produced by the fibroblasts. In the cytoplasm of one of the epithelial cells also is a **nucleus (8),** dispersed **chromatin (9)**, and a dense, round **nucleolus (7)**. **Cisternae** of **rough endoplasmic reticulum (11)**, elongated **mitochondria (14)**, and various types of **dense bodies (6)** are visible in different cells. Between the individual epithelial cells is a distinct **cell membrane (1)**. Hemidesmosomes (see Fig. 1-4) attach the basal membrane of the cells to the basal lamina (3).

FIGURE 1.4 ■ Basal Region of an Ion-Transporting Cell

A medium-magnification electron micrograph illustrates the basal region of a cell from a distal convoluted tubule of the kidney. In contrast to the basal regions of the epithelial cells, the basal regions of cells in convoluted kidney tubules are characterized by numerous complex **infoldings** of the **basal cell membrane (5)**. These infoldings then form numerous **basal membrane interdigitations (11)** with the similar infoldings of the neighboring cell. Numerous long **mitochondria (4, 10)** with vertical or apical-basal orientations are located between the cell membrane infoldings. Also, numerous dark-staining, spot-like **hemidesmosomes (6, 12)** attach the highly infolded basal cell membrane to the electron-lucent **basal lamina (7, 13)**.

A portion of a large **nucleus (1)** is visible with its dispersed **chromatin (9)**. Surrounding the nucleus is a distinct **nuclear envelope (2)**, which consists of a double membrane. Both the outer and inner membranes of the nuclear envelope (2) fuse at intervals around the periphery of the nucleus to form numerous **nuclear pores (3)**.

FUNCTIONAL CORRELATIONS

Infolded Basal Regions of the Cell

The deep infoldings of the basal and lateral cell membrane are only seen with electron microscopy. These infoldings are found in certain cells of the body; the main function of the infoldings is to transport ions across the cell membrane. The cells in the tubular portions of the kidney (proximal convoluted tubules and distal convoluted tubules) selectively absorb useful or nutritious components from the glomerular filtrate and retain them in the body. At the same time, these cells are eliminating from the body toxic or nonuseful metabolic waste products, such as urea, urine, and others. Because these cells transport numerous ions across their membranes, the infolded basal and lateral cell membranes contain Na^+,K^+-activated ATPase pumps. To perform these vital functions, increased amounts of energy are needed. The numerous mitochondria that are located in these basal infoldings continually supply the cells with the energy source (ATP) that is needed to operate these pumps for membrane transport. Similar basal cell membrane infoldings are seen in the striated ducts of the salivary glands. These glands produce saliva, which is then modified by selective transport of various ions across the cell membrane as it moves through these ducts to the larger excretory ducts.

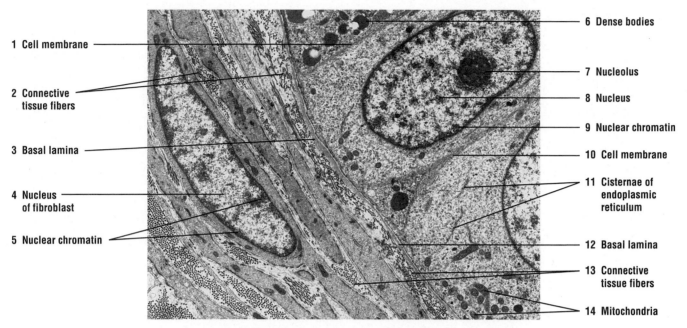

1 Cell membrane

2 Connective tissue fibers

3 Basal lamina

4 Nucleus of fibroblast

5 Nuclear chromatin

6 Dense bodies

7 Nucleolus

8 Nucleus

9 Nuclear chromatin

10 Cell membrane

11 Cisternae of endoplasmic reticulum

12 Basal lamina

13 Connective tissue fibers

14 Mitochondria

FIGURE 1.3 ■ Basal regions of epithelial cells. 9,500×

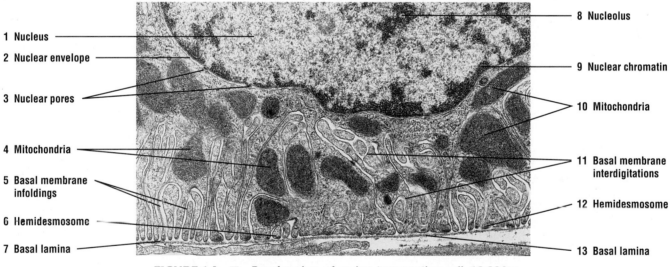

1 Nucleus

2 Nuclear envelope

3 Nuclear pores

4 Mitochondria

5 Basal membrane infoldings

6 Hemidesmosome

7 Basal lamina

8 Nucleolus

9 Nuclear chromatin

10 Mitochondria

11 Basal membrane interdigitations

12 Hemidesmosome

13 Basal lamina

FIGURE 1.4 ■ Basal region of an ion-transporting cell. 16,600×

FIGURE 1.5   ■   Cilia and Microvilli

This high-magnification electron micrograph illustrates the ultrastructural differences between cilia (singular, cilium) and microvilli (singular, microvillus). Both **cilia (1)** and **microvilli (2)** project from the apical surfaces of certain cells in the body. The cilia (1) are long, motile structures with a core of uniformly arranged **microtubules (3)** in a longitudinal orientation. The core of each cilium contains a constant number of nine microtubule doublets that are located peripherally and of two single microtubules in the center. Each cilium is attached to and extends from the **basal body (4)** in the apical region of the cell. Instead of nine microtubule doublets, the basal bodies exhibit nine microtubule triplets and no central microtubules.

In contrast to cilia, microvilli (2) are small, short, closely packed, finger-like extensions that greatly increase the surface area of certain cells. The microvilli (2) are nonmotile and exhibit a core of thin microfilaments called actin. The actin filaments extend from the microvilli (2) into the apical cytoplasm of the cell to form a terminal web, which is a complex network of actin filaments in the cell apices.

FIGURE 1.6   ■   Nuclear Envelope and Nuclear Pores

A high-magnification electron micrograph illustrates in detail part of a **nucleus (8)** and the surrounding membrane, the **nuclear envelope (3)**, which consists of an **inner nuclear membrane (3b)** and an **outer nuclear membrane (3a).** Between the two nuclear membranes (3a, 3b) is a space. The outer nuclear membrane (3b) is in contact with the **cell cytoplasm (4)**, whereas the inner nuclear membrane is associated with the **nuclear chromatin (7).** The nuclear envelope is continuous with the **rough endoplasmic reticulum (1)**, and the outer nuclear membrane (3b) contains ribosomes. At certain intervals around the nucleus, the two membranes of the nuclear envelope (3) fuse and form numerous **nuclear pores (2, 6).**

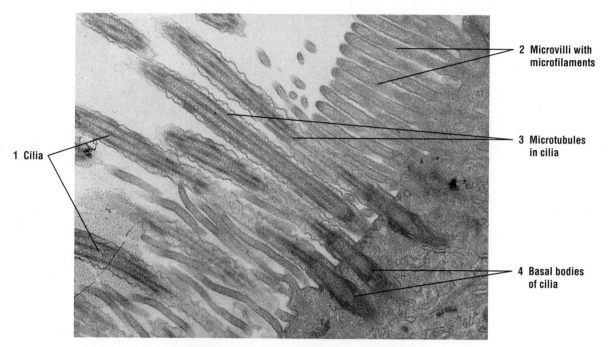

FIGURE 1.5 ■ Cilia and microvilli. 20,000×

- 2 Microvilli with microfilaments
- 3 Microtubules in cilia
- 1 Cilia
- 4 Basal bodies of cilia

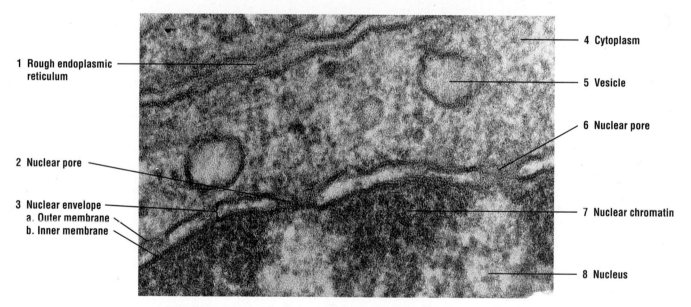

FIGURE 1.6 ■ Nuclear envelope and nuclear pores. 110,000×

- 1 Rough endoplasmic reticulum
- 2 Nuclear pore
- 3 Nuclear envelope
  - a. Outer membrane
  - b. Inner membrane
- 4 Cytoplasm
- 5 Vesicle
- 6 Nuclear pore
- 7 Nuclear chromatin
- 8 Nucleus

FIGURE 1.7 ■ Mitochondria

A high-magnification electron micrograph illustrates the ultrastructure of **mitochondria (1, 4)** in a **longitudinal section (1)** and in **cross section (4)**. Note that the mitochondria (1, 4) also exhibit two membranes. The **outer mitochondrial membrane (5, 9)** is smooth and surrounds the entire organelle. The inner mitochondrial membrane is highly folded, surrounds the matrix of the mitochondria, and projects inward into the organelle to form the numerous, shelf-like **cristae (6)**. Some mitochondrial matrix may contain dense-staining granules. Also visible in the **cytoplasm (8)** of the cell are various sized, light-staining **vacuoles (7)**, a section of **rough endoplasmic reticulum (2)**, and free **ribosomes (3)**. This type of mitochondria with shelf-like cristae (6) is normally found in protein-secreting cells.

FUNCTIONAL CORRELATIONS

Cilia

Cilia are a highly motile surface modification in cells that line the respiratory organs, oviducts or uterine tubes, and efferent ducts in the testes. The major function of cilia is to sweep or move fluids, cells, and/or particulate matter across the cell surfaces. In the lungs, cilia clean the air passages of particulate matter or mucus. In the oviduct, cilia move eggs and sperm along the passageway. In the testes, cilia move mature sperm into the epididymis. The motility exhibited by cilia results from the sliding of adjacent microtubule doublets in the cilia core. Each of the nine doublets in the cilia consists of subfibers A and B. Extending from subfibers A are two arm-like filaments, containing the motor protein dynein, that exhibits ATPase activity. Dynein extensions from one doublet bind to subfiber B of the adjacent doublet, producing a sliding force between these doublets and causing cilia motility.

Microvilli

In contrast to cilia, microvilli are shorter and nonmotile. Also, their core consists of microfilament actin. Microvilli are longest and most developed on epithelia of the small intestine and kidney. Here, the main functions of the microvilli are to absorb nutrients from the digestive tract of the small intestine or the glomerulate filtrate in the kidney.

The Nucleus, Nucleolus, and Nuclear Pores

The nucleus is the control center of each cell; it stores and processes most of the genetic information of the cell. The nucleus directs all the activities of the cells through the process of protein synthesis and, ultimately, controls the structural and functional characteristics of each cell. The cell's genetic material, the DNA, is visible in the cell in the form of chromatin when the cells are not dividing.

The nucleolus is a dense-staining nonmembrane that is bound within the nucleus. One or more may be visible in a given cell. The nucleolus functions in the synthesis, processing, and assembly of ribosomal subunits. Nucleoli are prominent in cells that synthesize large amounts of proteins.

Nuclear pores perform an important role in the cell by controlling protein movements into the nucleus for its function and by transporting RNA from the nucleus into the cytoplasm. The nuclear pores, like other cell membranes, show selective permeability. As a result, some of the larger molecules travel through the pores via an active transport mechanism.

Mitochondria

These organelles produce most of the high-energy ATP of the cells and, therefore, are considered to be the powerhouses of the cells. The numerous cristae in the mitochondria increase the surface area of the inner membrane, which is necessary for the various chemical reactions that eventually produce ATP for cell metabolism. Cells that are highly active metabolically, such as those in the skeletal and cardiac muscles, have an increased number of mitochondria, because they need and use ATP at a very high rate.

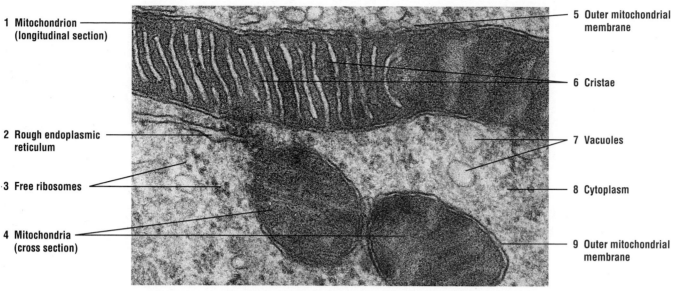

1 **Mitochondrion (longitudinal section)**

2 **Rough endoplasmic reticulum**

3 **Free ribosomes**

4 **Mitochondria (cross section)**

5 **Outer mitochondrial membrane**

6 **Cristae**

7 **Vacuoles**

8 **Cytoplasm**

9 **Outer mitochondrial membrane**

FIGURE 1.7 ■ Mitochondria (longitudinal and cross sections). 49,500×

FIGURE 1.8 ■ Rough Endoplasmic Reticulum

A high-magnification electron micrograph illustrates the components of the **rough endoplasmic reticulum** (3) in the cytoplasm of a cell. It consists of stacked layers of membranous cavities called **cisternae** (3). In the rough endoplasmic reticulum, ribosomes are attached to the outer surface of the membranes. Also present in the cytoplasm are **free ribosomes** (4, 12), some of which attach to other ribosomes and form ribosome groups called **polyribosomes** (4, 13). In addition, visible in the cytoplasm are numerous **mitochondria** (2, 10) in both **longitudinal** (10) and **cross section** (2), **dense secretory granules** (8), and very thin strands of **microfilaments** (5, 11). In the lower right corner of the micrograph are the smooth cisternae and associated vesicles of the **Golgi apparatus** (14). Note the **cell membranes** (1, 9) of adjacent cells, **nuclear envelope** (6), and portions of the **nucleus** (7) and nuclear **chromatin** (12).

FIGURE 1.9 ■ Smooth Endoplasmic Reticulum

This high-magnification electron micrograph illustrates the structure of the **smooth endoplasmic reticulum** (2) in two adjacent cells. Smooth endoplasmic reticulum (2) is devoid of ribosomes, and it consists primarily of smooth, anastomosing tubules. In this micrograph, the tubules of the smooth endoplasmic reticulum (2) are primarily seen in cross section. In other sections, the smooth endoplasmic reticulum (2) can be seen as flattened vesicles. In some cells, smooth endoplasmic reticulum is continuous with **cisternae** of the **rough endoplasmic reticulum** (7), as seen in this micrograph.

Also seen in the micrograph are the **cell membranes** (6, 11) of the two cells, the **cell membrane interdigitations** (10), and the **extracellular matrix** (9) between the two cell membranes. A section of the **nucleus** (4, 5), **nuclear envelope** (8), **nuclear chromatin** (3), and **mitochondrion** (1) in cross section are visible in the two cells as well. The mitochondria (1) in these cells contain tubular cristae, which indicates that the cells synthesize products other than proteins.

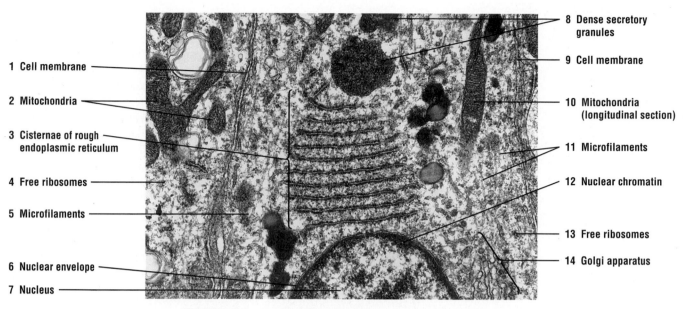

1 Cell membrane

2 Mitochondria

3 Cisternae of rough
endoplasmic reticulum

4 Free ribosomes

5 Microfilaments

6 Nuclear envelope

7 Nucleus

8 Dense secretory
granules

9 Cell membrane

10 Mitochondria
(longitudinal section)

11 Microfilaments

12 Nuclear chromatin

13 Free ribosomes

14 Golgi apparatus

FIGURE 1.8 ■ Rough endoplasmic reticulum. 32,000×

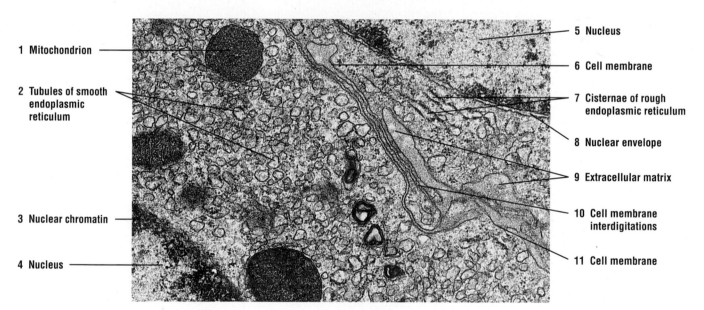

1 Mitochondrion

2 Tubules of smooth
endoplasmic
reticulum

3 Nuclear chromatin

4 Nucleus

5 Nucleus

6 Cell membrane

7 Cisternae of rough
endoplasmic reticulum

8 Nuclear envelope

9 Extracellular matrix

10 Cell membrane
interdigitations

11 Cell membrane

FIGURE 1.9 ■ Smooth endoplasmic reticulum. 11,500×

FIGURE 1.10 ■ Golgi Apparatus

A high-magnification electron micrograph illustrates the components of the **Golgi apparatus** (**2**). This apparatus consists of membrane-bound **Golgi cisternae** (**2**) with numerous membranous **Golgi vesicles** (**1**) near the end of the cisternae. The Golgi apparatus (2) usually exhibits a crescent shape. Its convex side is called the *cis* **face** (**3**), and the opposite, concave side is called the *trans* **face** (**9**), of the Golgi apparatus (2). This micrograph illustrates the Golgi apparatus (2) in the seminiferous tubule of the testis, where a spermatid is undergoing transformation into a sperm. At this stage of the transformation, the Golgi apparatus (2) is packaging and condensing the secretory product into an electron-dense **acrosome granule** (**7**). This acrosome granule (7) is located in the **acrosomal vesicle** (**8**) that adheres to the **nuclear envelope** (**6**) on the anterior end of the spermatid. In the left corner of the micrograph, note a short cisternae of the **rough endoplasmic reticulum** (**4**) and some **free ribosomes** (**5**) in the **cytoplasm** (**11**) of the spermatid. A **cell membrane** (**10**) surrounds the cell.

FUNCTIONAL CORRELATIONS

Rough Endoplasmic Reticulum

Cells that synthesize increased amounts of protein exhibit a highly developed and extensive rough endoplasmic reticulum with numerous stacks of flattened cisternae. Thus, the main function of rough endoplasmic reticulum is the synthesis of all proteins produced by the cell. These proteins can then be transported either to the outside of the cell, to lysosomes, or to the membranes of the cell, endoplasmic reticulum, or Golgi apparatus for further processing.

Smooth Endoplasmic Reticulum

Although the smooth endoplasmic reticulum is continuous with the rough endoplasmic reticulum, the functions of the smooth endoplasmic reticulum are completely different and unrelated to protein synthesis. Smooth endoplasmic reticulum is found in abundance in those cells that synthesize phospholipids, cholesterol, and steroid hormones, such as estrogens, testosterone, and corticosteroids. In liver cells, smooth endoplasmic reticulum performs an important function in the inactivation or detoxification of potentially harmful drugs or chemicals.

Golgi Apparatus

The Golgi apparatus is present in almost all cells. Its size and development varies, depending on the cell function; however, it is most highly developed in secretory cells. Most proteins synthesized by cisternae of the rough endoplasmic reticulum are transported in the cell cytoplasm to the *cis* face of the Golgi apparatus. Here, the proteins are modified, sorted, processed, and packaged, and they exit the Golgi apparatus from the cisternae on its *trans* face. These proteins are then delivered to different locations in the cell, such as to the plasma membrane for export to the outside of the cell, or for incorporation into the cell membrane itself or to other organelles in the cell cytoplasm, such as the lysosomes.

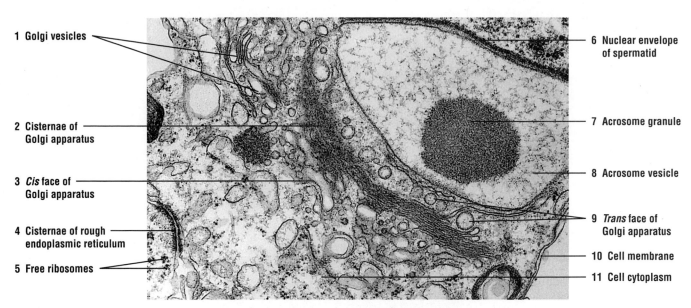

1 Golgi vesicles

2 Cisternae of
Golgi apparatus

3 *Cis* face of
Golgi apparatus

4 Cisternae of rough
endoplasmic reticulum

5 Free ribosomes

6 Nuclear envelope
of spermatid

7 Acrosome granule

8 Acrosome vesicle

9 *Trans* face of
Golgi apparatus

10 Cell membrane

11 Cell cytoplasm

FIGURE 1.10 ■ Golgi apparatus. 23,000×

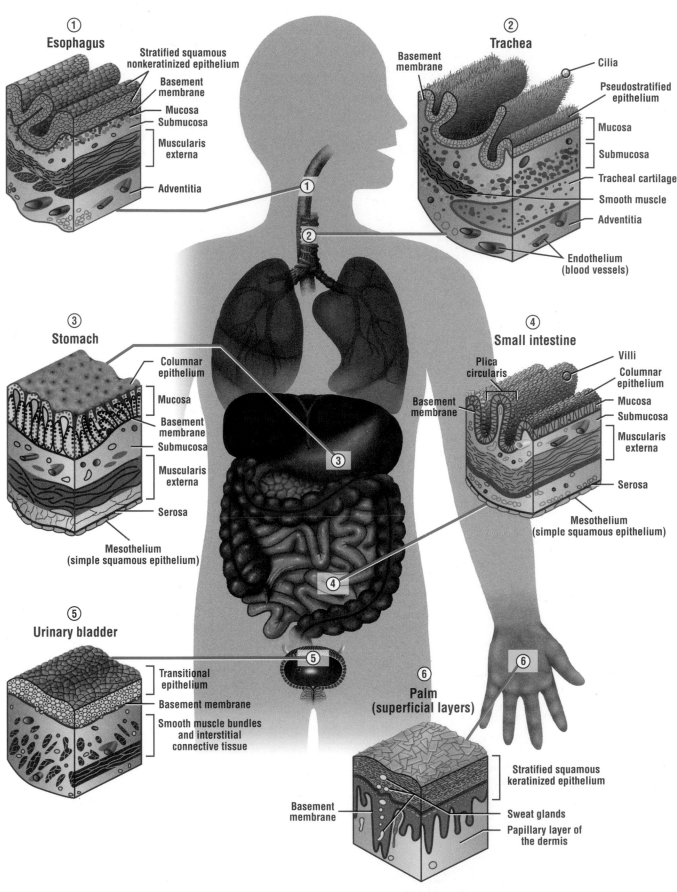

① **Esophagus**

Stratified squamous
nonkeratinized epithelium

Basement
membrane

Mucosa

Submucosa

Muscularis
externa

Adventitia

② **Trachea**

Basement
membrane

Cilia

Pseudostratified
epithelium

Mucosa

Submucosa

Tracheal cartilage

Smooth muscle

Adventitia

Endothelium
(blood vessels)

③ **Stomach**

Columnar
epithelium

Mucosa

Basement
membrane

Submucosa

Muscularis
externa

Serosa

Mesothelium
(simple squamous epithelium)

④ **Small intestine**

Villi

Plica
circularis

Columnar
epithelium

Basement
membrane

Mucosa

Submucosa

Muscularis
externa

Serosa

Mesothelium
(simple squamous epithelium)

⑤ **Urinary bladder**

Transitional
epithelium

Basement membrane

Smooth muscle bundles
and interstitial
connective tissue

⑥ **Palm
(superficial layers)**

Stratified squamous
keratinized epithelium

Basement
membrane

Sweat glands

Papillary layer of
the dermis

OVERVIEW FIGURE ■ Different types of epithelia in selected organs.

CHAPTER 2

Epithelial Tissue

SECTION 1 ■ Classification of Epithelial Tissue

Location of Epithelium

The four basic tissue types in the body are epithelial, connective, muscular, and nervous. These tissues exist and function in close association with one another.

The **epithelial tissue,** or **epithelium,** consists of sheets of cells that cover the **external surfaces** of the body, line the **internal cavities,** form various **organs** and **glands,** and line their **ducts.** Epithelial cells are in contact with each other, either in a single layer or in multiple layers. The structure of the lining epithelium, however, differs from organ to organ, depending on its location and function. For example, epithelium that covers the outer surfaces of the body and that serves as a protective layer differs from epithelium that lines the internal organs.

The overview figure shows different types of epithelia in selected organs.

Classification of Epithelium

Epithelium is classified according to the number of **cell layers** and the **morphology** or structure of the **surface cells.** A **basement membrane** is a thin, noncellular region that separates the epithelium from the underlying **connective tissue.** This membrane is easily seen with a light microscope. An epithelium with a single layer of cells is called **simple,** and that with numerous cell layers is called **stratified.** A **pseudostratified** epithelium consists of a single layer of cells that attach to a basement membrane; however, not all of these cells reach the surface. An epithelium with flat surface cells is called **squamous.** When the surface cells are round, or are as tall as they are wide, the epithelium is called **cuboidal.** When the cells are taller than they are wide, the epithelium is called **columnar.** Epithelium is **nonvascular;** that is, it does not have blood vessels. Oxygen, nutrients, and metabolites **diffuse** from the blood vessels in the underlying connective tissue to the epithelium.

Special Surface Modifications on Epithelial Cells

Epithelial cells in different organs exhibit special cell membrane modifications on their **apical** or upper **surfaces.** These modification are cilia, stereocilia, or microvilli. **Cilia** are motile structures that are found on certain cells in the **uterine tubes, uterus,** and conducting tubes of the **respiratory system. Microvilli** are small, nonmotile projections that cover all absorptive cells in the small intestine and proximal convoluted tubules in the kidney. **Stereocilia** are long, nonmotile, branched microvilli that cover the cells in the **epididymis** and **vas deferens.** The function of microvilli and stereocilia is absorption.

Types of Epithelia

Simple Epithelium

Simple squamous epithelium that covers the external surfaces of the digestive organs, lungs, and heart is called **mesothelium.** Simple squamous epithelium that covers the lumina of the heart chambers, blood vessels, and lymphatic vessels is called **endothelium.**

Simple cuboidal epithelium lines small excretory ducts in different organs. In the proximal convoluted tubules of the kidney, the apical surfaces of the simple cuboidal epithelium are lined with a **brush border** consisting of **microvilli.**

Simple columnar epithelium covers the **digestive organs** (stomach, small and large intestines, and gallbladder). In the small intestine, simple columnar absorptive cells that cover the villi also exhibit **microvilli.** Villi are finger-like structures that project into the lumen of the small intestine.

Pseudostratified Columnar Epithelium

Pseudostratified columnar epithelium lines the **respiratory passages** and lumina of the **epididymis** and **vas deferens.** In the trachea, bronchi, and larger brochioles, the surface cells exhibit motile **cilia;** in the epididymis and vas deferens, the surface cells exhibit nonmotile **stereocilia,** which are branched or modified microvilli.

Stratified Epithelium

Stratified squamous epithelium contains multiple cell layers. The basal cells are cuboidal to columnar; these cells give rise to cells that migrate toward the surface and become squamous. There are two types of stratified squamous epithelia: nonkeratinized and keratinized.

Nonkeratinized epithelium exhibits live surface cells and covers moist cavities, such as the mouth, pharynx, esophagus, vagina, and anal canal. **Keratinized epithelium** is found on exposed surfaces of the body, such as the skin. The surface layers contain nonliving, keratinized cells that are filled with the protein **keratin.** The exposed epithelium that covers the palms and soles exhibits especially thick layers of keratinized cells.

Stratified cuboidal epithelium and **stratified columnar epithelium** have a limited distribution in the body. Both types of epithelia line the larger **excretory ducts** of the pancreas, salivary glands, and sweat glands. In these ducts, the epithelium exhibits two or more layers of cells.

Transitional epithelium lines the minor and major calyxes, pelvis, ureter, and bladder of the **urinary system.** This type of epithelium changes shape and can resemble either stratified squamous or stratified cuboidal epithelia, depending on whether it is stretched or contracted. When transitional epithelium is **contracted,** the surface cells appear **dome-shaped;** when transitional epithelium is **stretched,** the epithelium appears **squamous.**

FIGURE 2.1 ■ Simple Squamous Epithelium: Surface View of Peritoneal Mesothelium

To visualize the surface of the simple squamous epithelium, a small piece of mesentery was fixed and treated with silver nitrate and then counterstained with hematoxylin. The cells of the simple squamous epithelium (**mesothelium**) appear flat, adhere tightly to each other, and form a sheet with the thickness of a single cell layer. The irregular **cell boundaries (1)** of the epithelium stain dark and are highly visible because of silver deposition between the cell boundaries, and they form a characteristic mosaic pattern. The blue-gray **cell nuclei (2)** are centrally located in the yellow- to brown-stained **cytoplasm (3).**

Simple squamous epithelium is common in the body. It covers the surfaces that allow passive transport of gases or fluids, and it lines the pleural (thoracic), pericardial (heart), and peritoneal (abdominal) cavities.

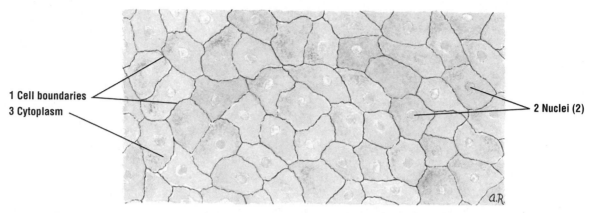

1 Cell boundaries

3 Cytoplasm

2 Nuclei (2)

FIGURE 2.1 ■ Simple squamous epithelium: surface view of peritoneal mesothelium. Stain: silver nitrate with hematoxylin. High magnification.

FIGURE 2.2 ■ Simple Squamous Epithelium: Peritoneal Mesothelium Surrounding Small Intestine (Transverse Section)

The simple squamous epithelium that lines different organs in the pleural and peritoneal cavities is called mesothelium. A transverse section of a wall of the small intestine illustrates **mesothelium (1),** a thin layer of spindle-shaped cells with prominent and oval nuclei. A thin **basement membrane (2)** is located directly under the mesothelium (1). In a surface view, the dispositon of these cells would appear similar to those shown in Figure 2-1.

Mesothelium (1) and the underlying, irregular **connective tissue (5)** form the serosa of the peritoneal cavity. Serosa is attached to a layer of **smooth muscle fibers (6)** called the muscularis externa **serosa** (see the overview figure, 3 and 4). In this illustration, the bundles of smooth muscle fibers (6) are cut in the transverse plane. Also present in the connective tissue are small **blood vessels (4)** that are also lined by a simple squamous epithelium called the **endothelium (4)** and numerous **fat (adipose) cells (3).**

FUNCTIONAL CORRELATIONS

Simple Squamous Epithelium

In the peritoneal cavity, simple squamous epithelium **reduces friction** between visceral organs by producing lubricating fluids, and it also **transports fluid.** In the cadiovascular system, this epithelium or endothelium allows passive **transport** of fluids, nutrients, and metabolites across the thin capillary walls. In the lungs, the simple squamous epithelium provides an efficient means of **gas exchange** or **transport** across the thin-walled capillaries and alveoli.

FIGURE 2.3 ■ Different Epithelial Types in the Kidney Cortex

This high-power photomicrograph of the kidney illustrates the different types of epithelia in the kidney cortex (peripheral region). **Simple squamous epithelium (1)** lines the interior of the **Bowman's capsule (4).** This capsule surrounds the **glomerulus (6)** of the kidney, where blood is filtered through its numerous capillaries. Simple squamous epithelium called **endothelium** (3, 9) lines the capillaries (2) and all other blood vessels (8). **Simple cuboidal epithelium (5)** lines the lumina of the surrounding **convoluted tubules (7).** The blue-staining fibers surrounding the Bowman's capsule (4), convoluted tubules (7), and blood vessels (8) in the kidney cortex are the collagen fibers of the **connective tissue (10).**

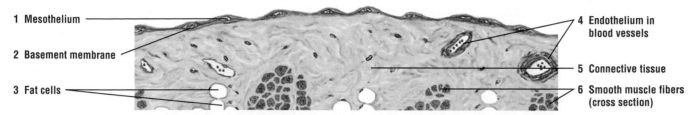

1 Mesothelium

2 Basement membrane

3 Fat cells

4 Endothelium in blood vessels

5 Connective tissue

6 Smooth muscle fibers (cross section)

FIGURE 2.2 ■ Simple squamous epithelium: peritoneal mesothelium surrounding small intestine (transverse section). Stain: hematoxylin and eosin. High magnification.

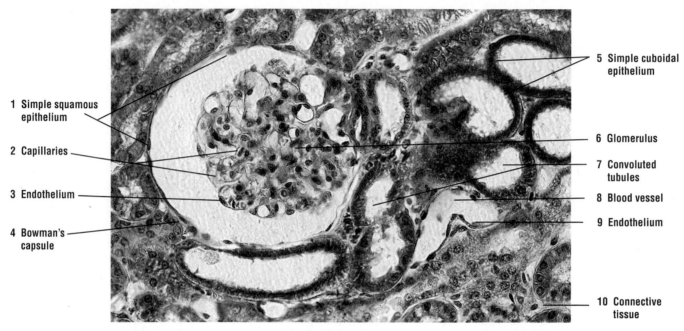

1 Simple squamous epithelium

2 Capillaries

3 Endothelium

4 Bowman's capsule

5 Simple cuboidal epithelium

6 Glomerulus

7 Convoluted tubules

8 Blood vessel

9 Endothelium

10 Connective tissue

FIGURE 2.3 ■ Different epithelial types in the kidney cortex. Stain: Masson's trichrome. 100×

FIGURE 2.4 ■ Simple Columnar Epithelium: Stomach Surface

The surface of the stomach is covered by a tall **simple columnar epithelium (1).** The illustration shows the light-staining **apical cytoplasm (1a)** and the dark-staining **basal nuclei (1b)** of the simple columnar epithelium **(1).** The epithelial cells are in close contact with each other and are arranged in a single row. A thin, connective tissue **basement membrane (2, 9)** separates the surface epithelium (1) from the underlying collagen fibers and cells of the **connective tissue (3, 10),** called the **lamina propria.** Small **blood vessels (5)** lined with endothelium are present in the connective tissue (3, 10).

In some areas, the surface epithelium has been sectioned in the transverse or oblique plane. When a plane of section passes close to the free surface of the epithelium, the sectioned **apices (6)** of the epithelium resemble a layer of stratified, enucleated polygonal cells. When a plane of section passes through **bases (7)** of the epithelial cells, the nuclei resemble a stratified epithelium.

The surface cells of the stomach secrete a protective coat of mucus. The pale appearance of the cytoplasm results from routine histologic preparation of the tissues. The mucigen droplets that filled the apical cytoplasm (1a) were lost during section preparation. The more granular cytoplasm is located basally (1b) and stains more acidophilic.

In an empty stomach, the stomach wall exhibits numerous **temporary folds (8)** that disappear when the stomach is filled with solid or fluid material. Also, the surface epithelium extends downward to form numerous indentations or pits in the surface of the stomach called **gastric pits (11),** which are seen in both logitudinal and transverse section.

FUNCTIONAL CORRELATIONS

Simple Columnar Epithelium of the Stomach

Simple columnar epithelium covers the surface of the stomach. These cells are **secretory** and produce **mucus.** The mucus covers the stomach surface and **protects** its surface lining from the corrosive gastric secretions that are normally found in the stomach during food processing and digestion.

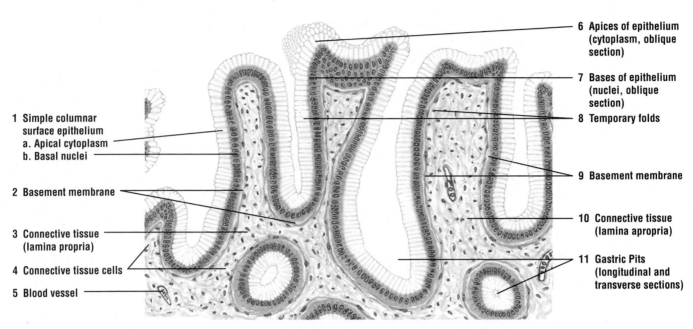

1 **Simple columnar surface epithelium**
   a. Apical cytoplasm
   b. Basal nuclei

2 **Basement membrane**

3 **Connective tissue (lamina propria)**

4 **Connective tissue cells**

5 **Blood vessel**

6 **Apices of epithelium (cytoplasm, oblique section)**

7 **Bases of epithelium (nuclei, oblique section)**

8 **Temporary folds**

9 **Basement membrane**

10 **Connective tissue (lamina apropria)**

11 **Gastric Pits (longitudinal and transverse sections)**

FIGURE 2.4 ■ Simple columnar epithelium: stomach surface. Stain: hematoxylin and eosin. Medium magnification.

FIGURE 2.5 ■ Simple Columnar Epithelium on Villi in Small Intestine: Cells with Striated Borders (Microvilli) and Goblet Cells

The intestinal **villi (1),** illustrated in transverse section (t.s.) and longitudinal section (l.s.), are covered by simple columnar epithelium. In the small intestine, the epithelium consists of two cell types: columnar cells with **striated borders (5, 7)** and oval-shaped **goblet cells (6, 13).** The striated border (5, 7) is seen as a reddish outer cell layer with faint vertical striations; these striations represent microvilli on the apices of columnar cells.

Pale-staining goblet cells (6, 13) are interspersed among the columnar cells. During routine histologic preparation, the mucus is lost; hence, the goblet cell cytoplasm appears clear or only lightly stained (6, 13). Normally, the mucigen droplets occupy **cell apices (4)** and the nucleus cell **bases (4).** When the epithelium at the tip of a villus is sectioned in an oblique plane, the cell apices (4) of the columnar cells appear as a mosaic of enucleated cells, whereas the cell bases appear as stratified epithelium (4).

A thin connective tissue **basement membrane (8)** is visible directly under the epithelium. The connective tissue **lamina propria (12)** contains an empty lymphatic vessel with a very thin endothelium called the **central lacteal (2, 9).** Also present in the lamina propria (12) are numerous **blood vessels (10)** and a **capillary (14)** lined with endothelium. **Smooth muscle fibers (3, 11)** extend into the villi. In this illustration, smooth muscle fibers (3, 11) are cut in transverse section (3) and longitudinal section (11).

The lamina propria also contains numerous other connective tissue cells, such as plasma cells, lymphocytes, macrophages, and fibroblasts. These cells are normally seen with higher magnification.

FUNCTIONAL CORRELATIONS

Epithelium with Striated Borders (Small Intestine) and Brush Borders (Kidney)

The main function of the epithelium in the small intestine is **absorption.** This function is enhanced by the presence of finger-like **villi,** which increase the absorptive surface area and which are covered by simple columnar epithelium with **striated borders** or **microvilli.** These microvilli absorb nutrients and fluids from the intestinal contents. The intestinal epithelium also contains numerous **goblet cells.** These cells secrete **mucus,** which **protects** the surface lining from corrosive secretions that enter the small intestine from the stomach during digestion.

Production of urine by the kidney involves filtration, absorption, and exretion. The apical surfaces of the simple cuboidal epithelium in the proximal convoluted tubules of the kidney are also covered with **brush borders** or **microvilli.** The main function of these microvilli is to **absorb** the nutrient material and fluid from the filtrate that passes through the tubules.

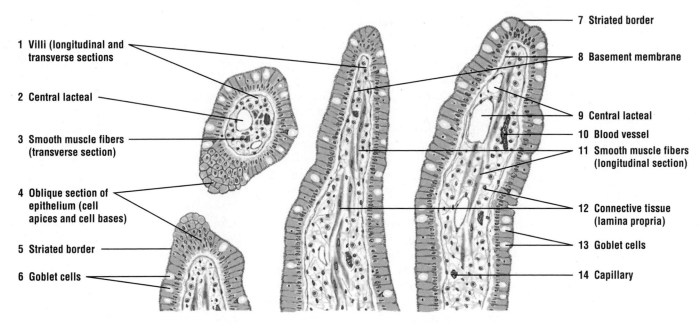

1 Villi (longitudinal and transverse sections

2 Central lacteal

3 Smooth muscle fibers (transverse section)

4 Oblique section of epithelium (cell apices and cell bases)

5 Striated border

6 Goblet cells

7 Striated border

8 Basement membrane

9 Central lacteal

10 Blood vessel

11 Smooth muscle fibers (longitudinal section)

12 Connective tissue (lamina propria)

13 Goblet cells

14 Capillary

FIGURE 2.5 ■ Simple columnar epithelium on villi in small intestine: cells with striated borders (microvilli) and goblet cells. Stain: hematoxylin and eosin. Medium magnification.

FIGURE 2.6 ■ Pseudostratified Columnar Ciliated Epithelium: Respiratory Passages (Trachea)

Pseudostratified columnar ciliated epithelium lines the upper respiratory passages, such as the trachea and bronchi. In this type of epithelium, the cells appear to form several layers. Serial sections show that all cells reach **the basement membrane (4, 13);** however, because the epithelial cells are of different shapes and heights, not all of them reach the surface. For this reason, this type of epithelium is called pseudostratified rather than stratified.

Numerous motile and closely spaced **cilia (1, 8)** (singular, cilium) cover all cell apices of the ciliated cells except those of the light-staining, oval **goblet cells (3, 11)** that are interspersed among the ciliated cells. Each cilium arises from a **basal body (9),** the internal morphology of which is identical to the centriole. The basal bodies (9) are located directly beneath the apical cell membrane and are adjacent to each other; they often give the appearance of a continuous, dark, apical membrane (9).

In pseudostratified epithelium, the deeper nuclei belong to the intermediate and short **basal cells (12).** The more superficial, oval nuclei belong to the columnar ciliated cells (1, 8). The small, round, heavily stained nuclei without any visible surrounding cytoplasm are those of **lymphocytes (2, 10).** These cells migrate from the underlying connective tissue (5) through the epithelium.

A clearly visible **basement membrane (4, 13)** separates the pseudostratified epithelium from the underlying **connective tissue (5).** Visible in the connective tissue (5) are **fibrocytes (5a),** dense **collagen fibers (5b),** scattered lymphocytes, and small **blood vessels (14).** Deeper in the connective tissue are glands with **mucous acini (6)** and **serous acini (7, 15).** These provide secretions that moisten the respiratory passages.

FUNCTIONAL CORRELATIONS

Epithelium with Cilia or Stereocilia

In most **respiratory passages** (trachea and bronchi), **psedostratified epithelium** contains both **goblet cells** and **ciliated cells.** Ciliated cells cleanse the inspired air and transport **mucus** and **particulate material** across the cell surfaces to the oral cavity for expulsion.

Simple columnar ciliated cells in the **uterine tubes** facilitate the conduction of oocyte and sperm across their surfaces. In the **efferent ductules** of the **testes,** ciliated cells assist in **transporting** sperm out of the testis and into the ducts of the epididymis.

The **epididymis** and **vas deferens** are lined by pseudostratified epithelium with **stereocilia.** The major function of the stereocilia in these organs is to absorb fluid that is produced by cells in the testes.

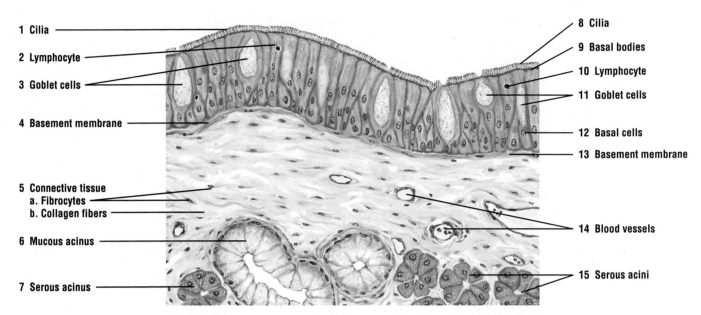

1 Cilia

2 Lymphocyte

3 Goblet cells

4 Basement membrane

5 Connective tissue
   a. Fibrocytes
   b. Collagen fibers

6 Mucous acinus

7 Serous acinus

8 Cilia

9 Basal bodies

10 Lymphocyte

11 Goblet cells

12 Basal cells

13 Basement membrane

14 Blood vessels

15 Serous acini

FIGURE 2.6 ■ Pseudostratified columnar ciliated epithelium: respiratory passages (trachea). Stain: hematoxylin and eosin. High magnification.

FIGURE 2.7 ■ Transitional Epithelium: Bladder (Contracted)

Transitional epithelium (2) is found exclusively in the excretory passages of the urinary system. It covers the lumina of renal calyces, pelvis, ureters, and bladder. This stratified epithelium is composed of several layers of similar cells. The epithelium changes its shape in response to stretching, resulting from fluid accumulation, or contraction while voiding of urine.

In a relaxed, unstretched condition, the **surface cells (8)** are usually cuboidal and bulge outward. Frequently, **binucleate (two-nuclei) cells (1, 7)** are visible in the superficial layers or **surface cells (8)** of the bladder. When the bladder fills and the transitional epithelium (2) is distended or stretched, the number of cell layers is reduced. The cells in the outer layers appear to be more elongated or flattened, but not to the degree that is seen in the squamous epithelium. In the stretched condition, the transitional epithelium may resemble the stratified squamous epithelium found in other regions of the body. (Compare transitional epithelium with the stratified squamous epithelium of the esophagus; see Fig. 2-8.)

Transitional epithelium (2) rests on a **connective tissue (4, 10)** layer that is composed primarily of **fibroblasts (10a)** and **collagen fibers (10b).** Between the connective tissue (4, 10) and the transitional epithelium (2) is a thin **basement membrane (3, 9).** The base of the epithelium is not indented by connective tissue papillae, and it exhibits an even contour.

Small **blood vessels (venules) (5)** and **arterioles (11)** of various sizes are present in the connective tissue (4, 10). Deeper in the connective tissue are strands of **smooth muscle fibers (6, 12),** which are sectioned in both the cross and longitudinal planes in this illustration. The muscle layers in the bladder are located deep to the connective tissue (4, 10).

FUNCTIONAL CORRELATIONS

Transitional Epithelium

Transitional epithelium allows **distention** of the urinary organs (calyces, pelvis, ureters, and bladder) during urine accumulation and **contraction** of these organs during the emptying process without breaking the cell contacts in the epithelium. In addition, transitional epithelium forms a **protective osmotic barrier** between urine in the bladder and the underlying tissue fluids.

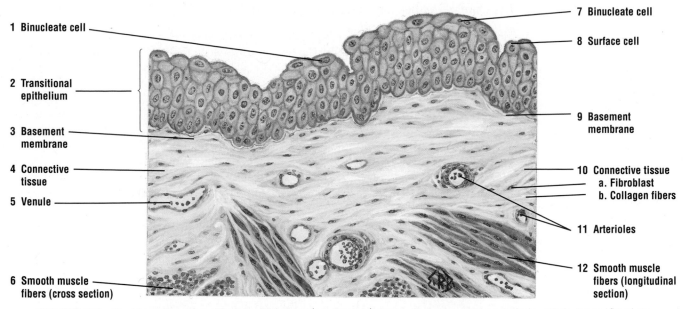

1 Binucleate cell

2 Transitional epithelium

3 Basement membrane

4 Connective tissue

5 Venule

6 Smooth muscle fibers (cross section)

7 Binucleate cell

8 Surface cell

9 Basement membrane

10 Connective tissue
 a. Fibroblast
 b. Collagen fibers

11 Arterioles

12 Smooth muscle fibers (longitudinal section)

FIGURE 2.7 ■ Transitional epithelium: bladder (contracted). Stain: hematoxylin and eosin. High magnification.

FIGURE 2.8 ■ Stratified Squamous Nonkeratinized Epithelium: Esophagus

Stratified squamous epithelium is characterized by numerous cell layers, with the outermost layer consisting of flat or squamous cells. The thickness of the epithelium varies among different regions of the body; as a result, the composition of the epithelium also varies. This illustration provides an example of a moist, **nonkeratinized stratified squamous epithelium (1)** that lines the oral cavity, esophagus, vagina, and anal canal.

Cuboidal or low columnar **basal cells (5)** are located at the base of the stratified epithelium. The cytoplasm is finely granular, and the oval, chromatin-rich nucleus occupies most of the cell. Cells in the intermediate layers of the epithelium are **polyhedral (4)**, with round or oval nuclei and more visible cell cytoplasm and membranes. **Mitoses (6)** are frequently observed in the deeper cell layers and in the basal cells (5). Cells and their nuclei become progressively flatter as the cells migrate toward the free surface of the epithelium. Above the polyhedral cells (4) are several rows of flattened or **squamous cells (3).**

A fine **basement membrane (7)** separates the epithelium (1) from the underlying **connective tissue,** the **lamina propria (2). Papillae (10),** or extensions, of connective tissue indent the lower surface of the epithelium (1), giving it a characteristic wavy appearance. The connective tissue (2) contains **collagen fibers (11), fibrocytes (9), capillaries (12),** and **arterioles (8).**

In areas where stratified squamous epithelium is exposed to increased wear and tear, the outermost layer, or the stratum corneum, becomes thick and keratinized. An example of one such area is found in the epidermis of the palm (see Fig. 2-9).

An example of thin, stratified squamous epithelium without connective tissue papillae indentation is found in the cornea of the eye; here, the surface underlying the epithelium is smooth. This type of epithelium is only a few cell layers thick, but it has the characteristic arrangement of basal columnar, polyhedral, and superficial squamous cells.

FIGURE 2.9 ■ Stratified Squamous Keratinized Epithelium: Palm of the Hand

This medium-power photomicrograph illustrates the **stratified squamous keratinized epithelium (1)** of the palm and the cell layers **stratum granulosum (6), stratum spinosum (7)** and the basal cell layer, **stratum basale (8).** The outermost layer of the skin contains dead cells and is called the **stratum corneum (5).** In the palms and soles, the stratum corneum (5) is thick, whereas in the rest of the body, it is thinner. Inferior to the stratum corneum (5) are the different cell layers that give rise to it.

The epithelium is attached to the underlying **connective tissue (3)** layer composed of dense collagen fibers and fibroblasts. The underlying surface of the epithelium (1) is indented by the connective tissue (3) extensions called the **papillae (2)** that form the characteristic wavy boundary between the epithelium (1) and the connective tissue (3). Passing through the connective tissue (3) and the epithelium (1) are **excretory ducts of the sweat glands (4)** that are located deep to the epithelium.

FUNCTIONAL CORRELATIONS

Stratified Epithelium

Stratified squamous epithelium is well suited to withstand the increased wear and tear that occur in the moist cavities of the esophagus, vagina, and mouth. Its multilayered cellular composition protects the surfaces of these organs. In the larger excretory ducts of the kidney, salivary glands, and pancreas, another cell layer is added to form either stratified cuboidal or stratified columnar epithelium for even more protection (see Fig. 2-10).

Formation of dead **keratin layers,** or keratinization, on the skin surface provides additional protection from abrasion, desiccation, and bacterial invasion.

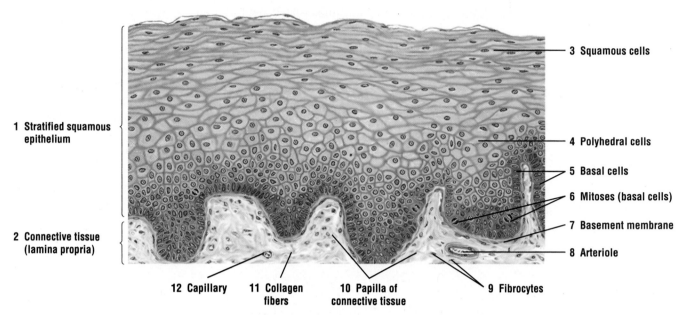

FIGURE 2.8 ■ Stratified squamous nonkeratinized epithelium: esophagus. Stain: hematoxylin and eosin. Medium magnification.

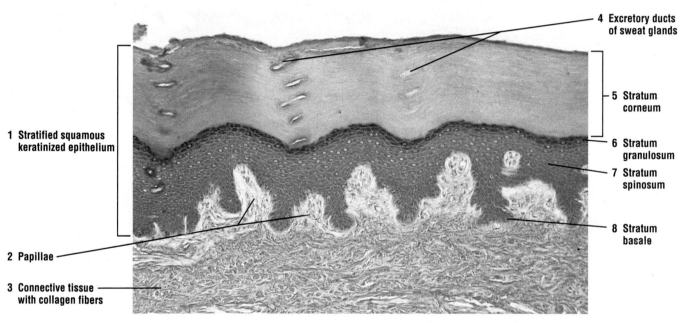

FIGURE 2.9 ■ Stratified squamous keratinized epithelium: palm of the hand. Stain: hematoxylin and eosin. 40×

FIGURE 2.10 ■ Stratified Cuboidal Epithelium: Excretory Duct in Salivary Gland

Stratified cuboidal epithelium has a limited distribution and is seen in only a few organs. The larger excretory ducts in the salivary glands and in the pancreas are lined the stratified cuboidal epithelium. This figure illustrates a high-power photomicrograph of a large excretory duct of a salivary gland. The luminal lining consists of two layers of cuboidal cells, forming the **stratified cuboidal epithelium (1).** Surrounding the excretory duct are collagen fibers of the **connective tissue (2,7)** and **blood vessels (3, 5)** that are lined by simple squamous epithelium called **endothelium (4,6).**

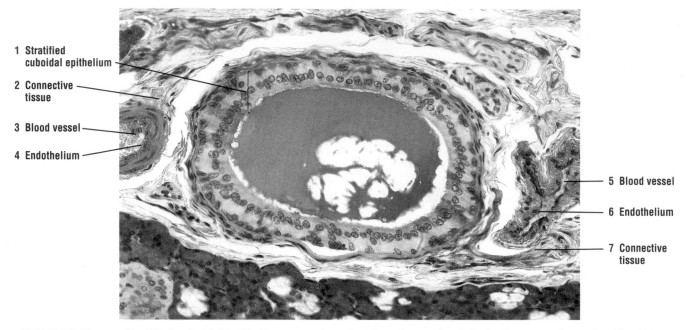

1 Stratified
  cuboidal epithelium

2 Connective
  tissue

3 Blood vessel

4 Endothelium

5 Blood vessel

6 Endothelium

7 Connective
  tissue

FIGURE 2.10 ■ Stratified cuboidal epithelium: excretory duct in salivary gland. Stain: hematoxylin and eosin. 100×

The body contains a variety of glands, which are classified as either **exocrine glands** or **endocrine glands.** The cells or parenchyma of these glands develop from epithelial tissue. Exocrine glands secrete their products into **ducts,** whereas endocrine glands deliver their secretory products into the **circulatory system.**

Exocrine Glands

Exocrine glands are either **unicellular** or **multicellular.** Unicellular glands consist of single cells. The mucus-secreting **goblet cells** in the epithelia of the small and large intestines and in the respiratory passages are the best examples of unicellular glands.

Multicellular glands are characterized by a **secretory portion,** an end piece in which the epithelial cells secrete a product, and an epithelium-lined **ductal portion,** through which the secretion from the secretory regions is delivered to the exterior of the gland. Larger ducts are usually lined by stratified epithelium.

Simple and Compound Exocrine Glands

Multicellular exocrine glands are divided into two major categories, depending on the structure of their ductal portion. A **simple exocrine gland** exhibits an unbranched duct, which may be straight or coiled. Also, if the terminal secretory portion of the gland is shaped in a form of a tube, the gland is called a **tubular gland.**

An exocrine gland that shows a repeated, branching pattern of the ducts that drain the secretory portions is called a **compound exocrine gland.** Furthermore, if the secretory portions are shaped like a flask or a tube, the glands are called **acinar (alveolar) glands** or **tubular glands,** respectively. Certain exocrine glands exhibit a mixture of both tubular and acinar secretory portions; such glands are called **tubuloacinar glands.**

Exocrine glands may also be classified based on the secretory products of their cells. Glands containing cells that produce a viscous secretion that lubricates and/or protects the inner lining of organs are called **mucous glands.** Glands with cells that produce watery secretions, which are often rich in enzymes, are called **serous glands.** Certain glands in the body contain a mixture of both mucous and serous secretory cells; these are called **mixed glands.**

Merocrine and Holocrine Glands

Exocrine glands may also be classified according to the method by which their secretory product is discharged. **Merocrine glands,** such as the pancreas, release their secretion by exocytosis without any loss of cellular components. Most exocrine glands in the body secrete their product in this manner. In **holocrine glands,** such as the sebaceous glands of the skin, the cells themselves become the secretory product. Gland cells accumulate lipids, die, and degenerate to become **sebum,** the secretory product. Another type of gland, the apocrine glands (mammary glands), discharge part of the secretory cell as the secretory product. However, almost all glands that were once classified as apocrine are now regarded as merocrine glands.

Endocrine Glands

Endocrine glands differ from exocrine glands in that they do not have ducts for their secretory products. Instead, endocrine glands are highly vascularized, and their secretory cells are surrounded by rich **capillary networks.** The close proximity of the secretory cells to the capillaries allows efficient release of the secretory products into the **bloodstream** and their distribution to different organs via the systemic circulation.

The endocrine glands can be either **individual cells** (unicellular glands), **endocrine tissue** in mixed glands (both endocrine and exocrine), or separate and distinct **endocrine organs.** Individual endocrine cells, or enteroendocrine cells, are found in the digestive organs. Endocrine tissues are seen in such mixed glands as the pancreas and the reproductive organs of both sexes.

FIGURE 2.11 ■ Unbranched Simple Tubular Exocrine Glands: Intestinal Glands

Unbranched simple tubular glands without excretory ducts are best represented by the **intestinal glands** (crypts of Lieberkühn) in the **large intestine** and **rectum.** The **surface epithelium** and the **secretory cells** of the glands in the intestines are lined with numerous goblet cells; these are unicellular exocrine glands. Similar, but shorter, intestinal glands with goblet cells are also found in the small intestine.

FIGURE 2.12 ■ Simple Branched Tubular Exocrine Glands: Gastric Glands

Simple or slightly branched tubular glands without excretory ducts are found in the stomach. These are the **gastric glands.** In the fundus and body of the stomach, they are lined with modified columnar cells that are highly specialized for secreting hydrochloric acid and the precursor for the proteolytic enzyme pepsin.

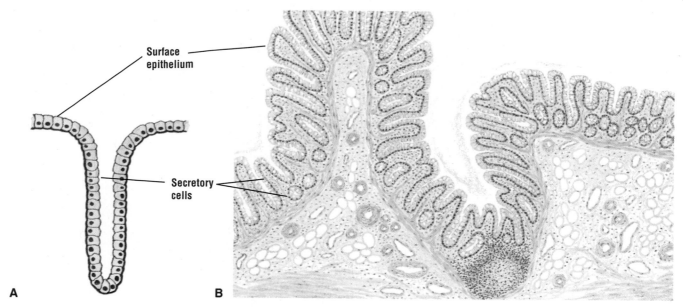

FIGURE 2.11 ■ Unbranched simple tubular exocrine glands: intestinal glands. **(A)** Diagram of gland. **(B)** Transverse section. Stain: hematoxylin and eosin. Medium magnification.

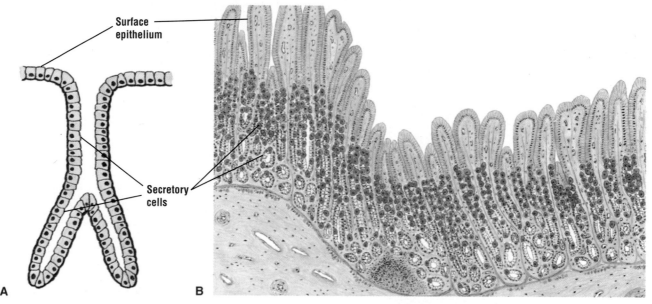

FIGURE 2.12 ■ Simple branched tubular exocrine gland: gastric glands. **(A)** Diagram of gland. **(B)** Transverse section. Stain: hematoxylin and eosin. Low magnification.

FIGURE 2.13 ▪ Coiled Tubular Exocrine Glands: Sweat Glands

Sebaceous glands in the skin are coiled tubular glands with long, unbranched ducts. Note the **secretory cells** of the gland and the **excretory ducts,** lined by stratified cuboidal epithelium, which deliver the secretory product to the surface.

FIGURE 2.14 ▪ Compound Acinar (Exocrine) Gland: Mammary Gland

The mammary gland is an example of a **compound acinar (alveolar) gland.** The lactating mammary gland contains enlarged **secretory acini (alveoli)** with large lumina that are filled with milk. Draining these acini (alveoli) are **excretory ducts,** some of which contain secretory material and are lined by stratified epithelium.

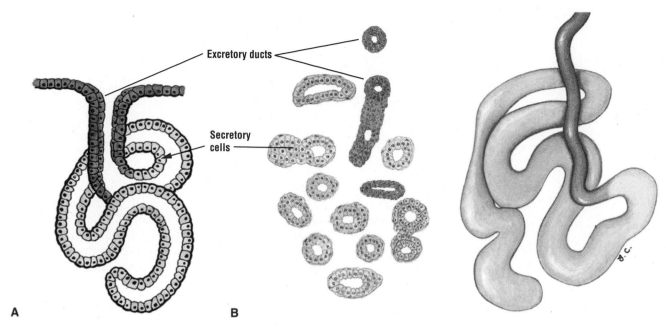

FIGURE 2.13 ■ Coiled tubular exocrine glands: sweat glands. **(A)** Diagram of gland. **(B)** Cross section. Stain: hematoxylin and eosin. Medium magnification.

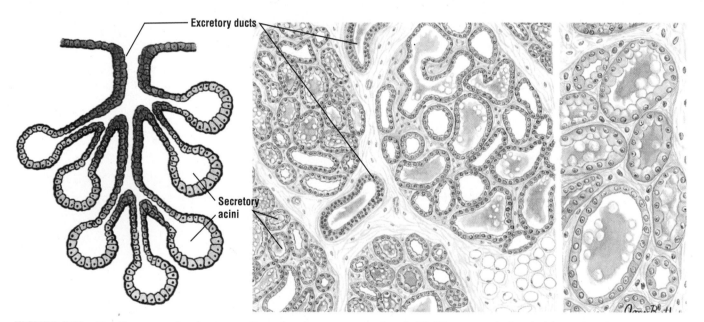

FIGURE 2.14 ■ Compound acinar exocrine gland: mammary gland. **(A)** Diagram of gland. **(B)** During lactation. Stain: hematoxylin and eosin. (A) Low magnification. (B) Medium magnification.

FIGURE 2.15 ■ Compound Tubuloacinar (Exocrine) Gland: Salivary Gland

The salivary glands (parotid, submandibular, and sublingual) best illustrate **compound tubuloacinar glands.** The glands contain **secretory acinar elements** and **secretory tubular elements.** In addition, the submandibular and sublingual salivary glands contain both serous and mucous acini. Details and comparisons of these acini are described in Chapter 11. The **excretory ducts** are lined with cuboidal, columnar, or stratified epithelium and are named according to their location in the gland.

FIGURE 2.16 ■ Compound Tubuloacinar (Exocrine) Gland: Submaxillary Salivary Gland

A photomicrograph of a submaxillary salivary gland shows the secretory units of a compound tubuloacinar gland. The grape-like **secretory acinar elements** (1) are circular in transverse section and are distinguished from the longer **secretory tubular elements** (7) of the gland. Empty lumina can be seen in some sections of both types of secretory elements. This salivary gland is a mixed gland and contains both the **mucous cells** (4), which stain light, and the **serous cells** (5), which stain dark. Draining the secretory elements of the gland are **excretory ducts** (3, 6, 8). The small excretory ducts are lined by simple cuboidal epithelium and are surrounded by **connective tissue** (2), which also surrounds all the secretory elements.

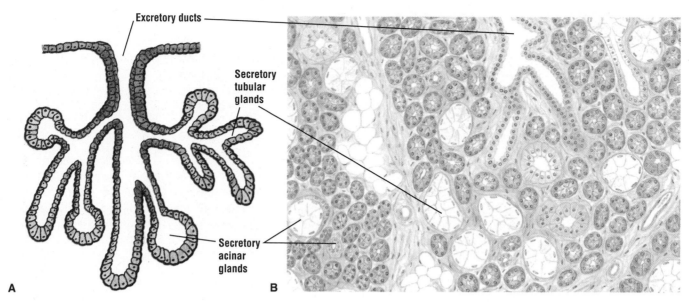

FIGURE 2.15 ■ Compound tubuloacinar (exocrine) gland: salivary gland. **(A)** Diagram of gland. **(B)** Submandibular salivary gland. Stain: hematoxylin and eosin. Low magnification.

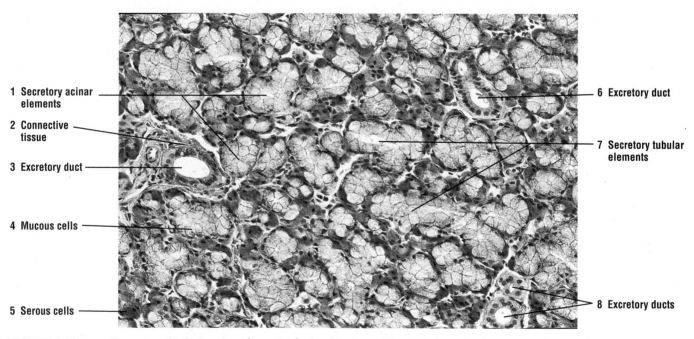

1 Secretory acinar elements

2 Connective tissue

3 Excretory duct

4 Mucous cells

5 Serous cells

6 Excretory duct

7 Secretory tubular elements

8 Excretory ducts

FIGURE 2.16 ■ Compound tubuloacinar (exocrine) gland: submaxillary salivary gland. Stain: hematoxylin and eosin. 64×

FIGURE 2.17 ◼ Endocrine Gland: Pancreatic Islet

An example of an endocrine gland is illustrated as a pancreatic islet from the pancreas. The pancreas is a mixed gland, containing both an **exocrine portion** and **endocrine portion.** In the pancreas, the exocrine acini surround the endocrine pancreatic islets.

The structure and function of other endocrine organs (glands) are presented in greater detail in Chapter 17.

FIGURE 2.18 ◼ Pancreas

A photomicrograph of the pancreas shows a mixed gland. The endocrine portion of the pancreas, the **pancreatic islet (4),** is separated from the secretory acini of the **exocrine pancreas (1)** by a thin connective tissue. The pancreatic islet does not contain excretory ducts. Instead, it is highly vascularized, and all its secretory products leave the islet via numerous **blood vessels (capillaries) (3).** In contrast, the secretory elements of the exocrine pancreas deliver their secretory product directly into an **excretory duct (2).**

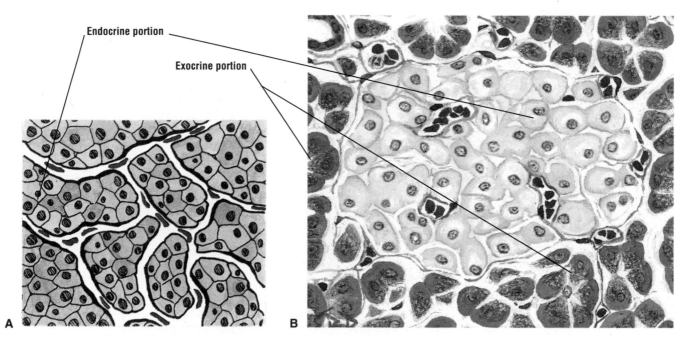

FIGURE 2.17   ■   Endocrine gland: pancreatic islet. **(A)** Diagram of gland. **(B)** High magnification. Stain: hematoxylin and eosin.

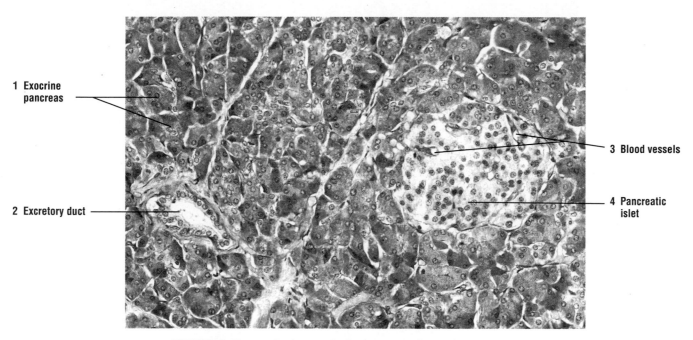

FIGURE 2.18   ■   Pancreas. Stain: hematoxylin and eosin. 80×

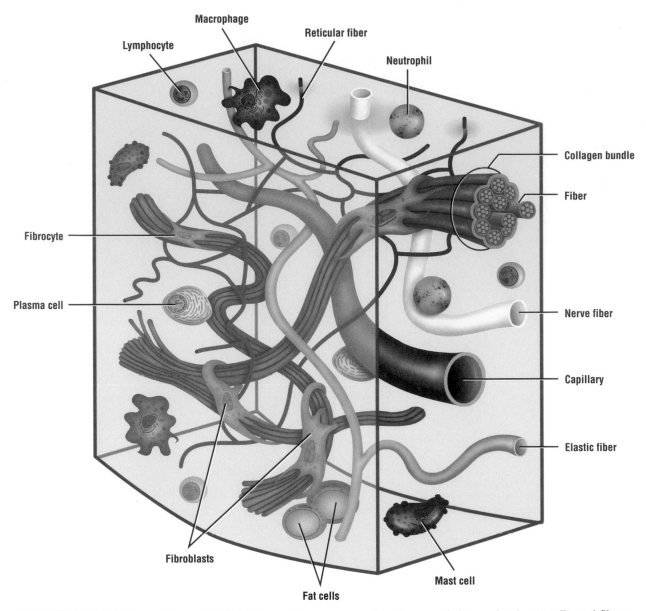

Lymphocyte

Macrophage

Reticular fiber

Neutrophil

Collagen bundle

Fiber

Fibrocyte

Nerve fiber

Plasma cell

Capillary

Elastic fiber

Fibroblasts

Mast cell

Fat cells

OVERVIEW FIGURE ■ Composite Illustration of loose connective tissue with its predominant cells and fibers.

CHAPTER 3

Connective Tissue

Classification of Connective Tissue

Connective tissue develops from **mesenchyme,** an embryonic type of tissue. With the exceptions of blood and lymph, **connective tissue** consists of **cells** and **extracellular material** called **matrix.** The matrix consists of connective tissue **fibers, ground substance,** and **tissue fluid.** The connective tissue binds, anchors, and supports various cells, tissues, and organs in the body. This tissue is classified into loose connective tissue and dense connective tissue, depending on the amount, type, arrangement, and abundance of cells, fibers, and ground substance.

Loose Connective Tissue

Loose connective tissue is more prevalent than dense connective tissue. It is characterized by a loose, irregular arrangement of connective tissue fibers and abundant ground substance. Numerous connective tissue cells are found in its matrix. **Collagen fibers, fibroblasts, adipose cells, mast cells,** and **macrophages** predominate in loose connective tissue, with fibroblasts being the most common cell type. The overview figure shows the various types of cells and fibers that are present in loose connective tissue.

Dense Connective Tissue

In contrast to loose connective tissue, **dense connective tissue** contains thicker and more densely packed collagen fibers, with fewer cell types and less ground substance. The collagen fibers in **dense irregular connective tissue** exhibit a random and irregular orientation. Dense irregular connective tissue is present in the dermis of skin, in capsules of different organs, and in areas that need strong support. **Dense regular connective tissue** contains densely packed collagen fibers that exhibit a regular and parallel arrangement. This type of dense connective tissue is found in the **tendons** and **ligaments.** In both dense irregular and dense regular connective tissue types, **fibroblasts** are the most abundant cells and are located between the dense collagen bundles.

Cells of the Connective Tissue

The two most common connective tissue cells are the fibrocytes and fibroblasts. Fusiform-shaped **fibroblasts** synthesize connective tissue fibers and the surrounding ground substance. **Fibrocytes** are inactive or resting fibroblasts. **Adipose (fat) cells** in the connective tissue store fat and may occur either singly or in groups. When adipose cells predominate, the connective tissue is called an **adipose tissue.**

    Macrophages or **histiocytes** are phagocytic and are most numerous in the loose connective tissue. They are difficult to distinguish from fibroblasts, unless they are performing phagocytic activity.

    Mast cells, which usually are closely associated with blood vessels, are widely distributed in the connective tissue of the skin and in digestive and respiratory organs. Mast cells are spherical cells that are filled with fine, regular, dark-staining granules.

    Plasma cells arise from lymphocytes that migrate into the connective tissue. These cells are found in great abundance in loose connective tissue and lymphatic tissue of the respiratory and digestive tracts.

White blood cells, or **leukocytes,** neutrophils, and eosinophils, migrate into the connective tissue from the blood vessels. Their main function is to defend the organism against bacterial invasion or foriegn matter.

Fibroblasts and adipose cells are permanent connective tissue cells. Neutrophils, eosinophils, plasma cells, mast cells, and macrophages migrate from the blood into the connective tissue of different regions of the body.

Fibers of the Connective Tissue

Connective tissue fibers are classified as collagen, elastic, and reticular. The amount and arrangement of these types of fibers depend on the function of the tissues or the organs in which they are found.

Collagen Fibers

Collagen fibers are tough, fibrous proteins that are thick and do not branch. They are the most abundant fibers, and they are found in almost all connective tissue of all organs.

Elastic Fibers

Elastic fibers are thin, small, branching fibers and have less tensile strength than collagen fibers. When stretched, elastic fibers return to their original size (recoil) without deformation. Elastic fibers are abundant in the lungs, bladder, and skin. In the walls of the aorta and pulmonary trunk, elastic fibers allow stretching of these vessels during powerful blood ejection from the heart ventricles without breakage or distortion, which is essential for their function.

Reticular Fibers

Reticular fibers are thin and form a delicate, net-like framework in the liver, lymph nodes, spleen, hemopoietic organs, and other organs where they filter blood and lymph. Reticular fibers also support capillaries, nerves, and muscle cells. These fibers are visible when stained with silver.

FIGURE 3.1 ■ Loose Connective Tissue

This illustration presents a composite image of a mesentery that has been stained to show different fibers and cells. A **mesentery** is a thin sheet that is composed of loose connective tissue.

The pink **collagen fibers (3)** are the thickest, largest, and most numerous fibers. In this connective tissue preparation, the collagen fibers (3) course in all directions. The **elastic fibers (5, 10)** are thin, fine, single fibers that are usually straight; however, after tissue preparation, the fibers may become wavy because of the release of tension. Elastic fibers (5, 10) form branching and anastomosing networks. Fine reticular fibers are also present in loose connective tissue but are not included in this illustration.

Fibroblasts (2) are the fixed, permanent cells of the connective tissues. Fibroblasts are flattened cells with an oval nucleus, sparse chromatin, and one or two nucleoli. Fixed **macrophages,** or **histiocytes (12),** are always present in connective tissue. Inactive macrophages appear similar to fibroblasts, although their processes may be more irregular and their nuclei smaller. Phagocytic inclusions are present in the cytoplasm of the macrophages. In this illustration, the cytoplasm of different macrophages (12) is filled with dense-staining particles that were ingested by these cells (12).

Mast cells (1, 9) are also present in loose connective tissue and appear as single or grouped cells along small blood vessels **(capillary, 7).** Mast cells are usually ovoid, with a small, centrally placed nucleus and a cytoplasm filled with fine, closely packed granules that stain dense or deep red with neutral red stain.

Numerous blood cells are also seen in the loose connective tissue. **Small lymphocytes (6)** exhibit a dense-staining nucleus that occupies most of the cell cytoplasm. **Large lymphocytes (8)** also exhibit a dense nucleus but have more cytoplasm than small lymphocytes do. Loose connective tissue contains blood cells, such as eosinophils and neutrophils, as well as adipose cells. These cells are illustrated in greater detail in Figures 3-2, 3-4, and 3-11.

The faint background around the fibers and cells is ground substance.

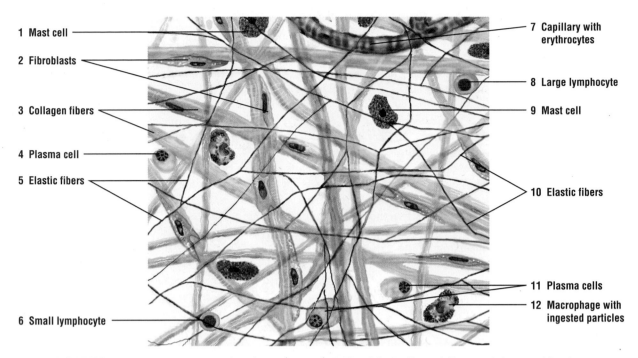

1 Mast cell

2 Fibroblasts

3 Collagen fibers

4 Plasma cell

5 Elastic fibers

6 Small lymphocyte

7 Capillary with erythrocytes

8 Large lymphocyte

9 Mast cell

10 Elastic fibers

11 Plasma cells

12 Macrophage with ingested particles

FIGURE 3.1 ■ Loose connective tissue (spread). Stained for cells and fibers. High magnification.

FIGURE 3.2 ■ Individual Cells of Connective Tissue

The main cells of connective tissue are fibroblasts and fibrocytes. The **fibroblast (1)** is an elongated cell with cytoplasmic projections, an ovoid nucleus with sparse chromatin, and one or two nucleoli. The **fibrocyte (6)** is a more mature, smaller, spindle-shaped cell without cytoplasmic projections. The nucleus in the fibrocyte is similar to, but smaller than, the nucleus in the fibroblast.

The **plasma cell (2)** has a smaller, eccentrically placed nucleus with condensed, coarse chromatin clumps that are distributed peripherally in a characteristic radial (cartwheel) pattern around one central mass. A prominent, clear area in the cytoplasm is adjacent to the nucleus.

The large **adipose cell (3)** exhibits a narrow rim of cytoplasm and a flattened, eccentric nucleus. In histologic sections, the large fat globules of adipose cells are dissolved by different chemicals, leaving a large, highly characteristic empty space.

The **large lymphocyte (4)** and **small lymphocyte (10)** are spherical cells that differ primarily in their amount of cytoplasm. The dense-staining nuclei of all lymphocytes have condensed chromatin but no nucleoli.

The free **macrophage (5)** usually appears round, with irregular cell outlines, but it can exhibit a variable appearance. In this illustration, the macrophage exhibits a small nucleus that is rich in chromatin and a cytoplasm that is filled with dense, ingested particles.

The **eosinophil (7)** is a large, white blood cell with a bilobed nucleus and large, eosinophilic cytoplasmic granules that fill the cytoplasm.

The **neutrophil (8)** is also a large, white blood cell and is characterized by a multilobed nucleus and a lack of stained granules in the cytoplasm.

Cells with **pigment granules (9)** may also be seen in connective tissue, especially in the epithelial cells of the skin. Here, the basal epithelial cells contain brown-staining pigment or melanin granules.

The **mast cell (11)** is usually ovoid, with a small, centrally placed nucleus. Its cytoplasm is normally filled with fine, closely packed, and dense-staining granules.

FUNCTIONAL CORRELATIONS

Individual Cells in Connective Tissue

Macrophages or histiocytes are **phagocytes** that ingest bacteria, dead cells, cell debris, and other foreign matter. They **present antigens** to immune cells called lymphocytes, and they perform an important function in the immune response.

Fibroblasts are the dominant cells in the connective tissue. These highly active cells, with irregularly branched cytoplasm, synthesize **collagen, reticular,** and **elastic fibers** as well as the carbohydrates of the **extracellular matrix.**

The spindle-shaped *fibrocytes* are smaller than fibroblasts. They are the mature and less active cells of the fibroblast line.

Lymphocytes are the most numerous cells in the loose connective tissue of the respiratory and gastrointestinal tracts. They mediate immune responses to antigens by producing antibodies, and they kill virus-infected cells by inducing cell death or apoptosis.

Plasma cells are derived from lymphocytes that have been exposed to antigens. They synthesize and secrete **antibodies** that destroy specific antigens and defend the body against infections.

Adipose cells **store fat** (lipid) and provide protective packing material both in and around numerous organs.

Neutrophils are active phagocytes. They engulf and destroy bacteria at sites of infections.

Eosinophils increase in number following parasitic infections or allergic reactions. They phagocytize antigen-antibody complexes that are formed during allergic reactions.

Mast cells synthesize and release **heparin** and **histamine.** Heparin is a weak anticoagulant. Histamine is a potent mediator of inflammation that dilates blood vessels, increases their permeability to fluid, and induces signs and symptoms of immediate hypersensitive (allergic) reactions.

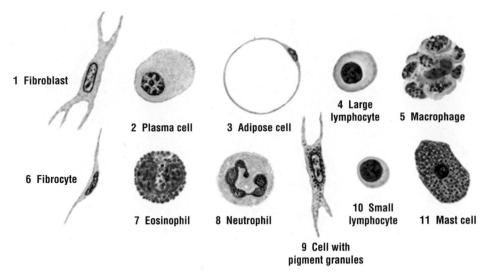

1 Fibroblast

2 Plasma cell

3 Adipose cell

4 Large lymphocyte

5 Macrophage

6 Fibrocyte

7 Eosinophil

8 Neutrophil

9 Cell with pigment granules

10 Small lymphocyte

11 Mast cell

FIGURE 3.2 ■ Cells of the connective tissue. Stain: hematoxylin and eosin. High magnification and/or oil immersion.

FIGURE 3.3 ■ Embryonic Connective Tissue

Embryonic connective tissue resembles mesenchyme or mucous connective tissue in that it is considered to be loose irregular connective tissue. Its ground substance, however, is semifluid, not jelly-like. This feature is not apparent in these sections.

Fibroblasts (4) are numerous, and fine collagen fibers (1) are found between them. Some of the collagen figures come in close contact with the fibroblasts. Embryonic connective tissue is vascular. Capillaries (3) lined with endothelium and filled with red blood cells (2) are visible in the ground substance.

At higher magnification, primitive fibroblasts (5) are seen as large, branching cells with prominent cytoplasmic processes, an ovoid nucleus with fine chromatin, and one or more nucleoli. The widely separated collagen fibers (6) are more apparent at this magnification.

FIGURE 3.4 ■ Loose Connective Tissue

Collagen fibers (9) predominate in loose connective tissue, course in different directions, and form a loose fiber meshwork. In this illustration, collagen fibers (9) are sectioned in various planes, and transverse ends may be seen. The fibers are acidophilic and stain pink with eosin. Thin elastic fibers are also present in loose connective tissue but are difficult to distinguish with this stain and at this magnification.

Fibroblasts (2) are the most numerous cells in loose connective tissue. They may be sectioned in various planes, so only parts of the cells may be seen. Also, during section preparation, the cytoplasm of these cells may shrink. A typical fibroblast (2) has an oval nucleus with sparse chromatin and lightly acidophilic cytoplasm with few short processes.

Loose connective tissue also contains various white blood cells, such as neutrophils (6) with lobulated nuclei, eosinophils (3) with red-staining granules, and small lymphocytes (7) with dense-staining nuclei and sparse cytoplasm. Fat or adipose cells (5) characteristically appear empty, with a thin rim of cytoplasm and peripherally displaced flat nuclei (4).

The connective tissue is highly vascular; capillaries (8) sectioned in different planes are visible. Larger blood vessels, such as an arteriole (1) with red blood cells, are also seen.

FIGURE 3.5 ■ Dense Irregular and Loose Irregular Connective Tissue (Elastin Stain)

This illustration shows a transition zone between loose irregular connective tissue in the upper region and a more dense irregular connective tissue in the lower region. In addition, this tissue section has been especially prepared to show the presence and distribution of elastic fibers in the connective tissue.

Elastic fibers (1, 7) have been selectively stained a deep blue using Verhoeff's method. With Van Gieson's as a counterstain, acid fuchsin stains collagen fibers red (2, 6). Cellular details of fibroblasts are not obvious, but the fibroblast nuclei (3, 5) stain deep blue.

The characteristic features of dense irregular and loose connective tissues become apparent with this staining technique. In dense irregular connective tissue, the collagen fibers (2) are larger, more numerous, and more concentrated. Elastic fibers are also larger and more numerous (1). In contrast, both fiber types in the loose connective tissue are smaller (6, 7) and more loosely arranged. Fine elastic networks are seen in both types of connective tissue.

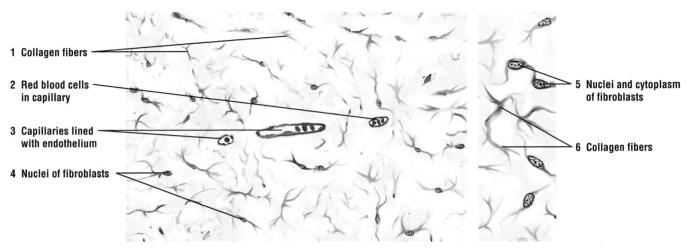

1 Collagen fibers

2 Red blood cells
   in capillary

3 Capillaries lined
   with endothelium

4 Nuclei of fibroblasts

5 Nuclei and cytoplasm
   of fibroblasts

6 Collagen fibers

FIGURE 3.3 ■ Embryonic connective tissue. Stain: hematoxylin and eosin. Left, low magnification; right, high magnification.

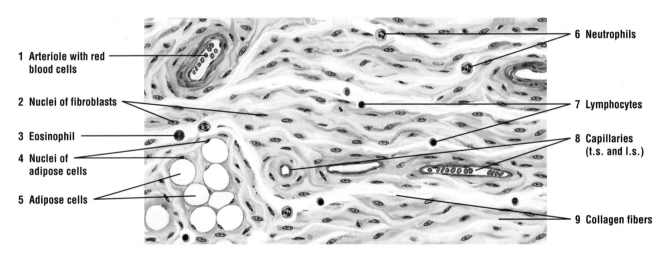

1 Arteriole with red
   blood cells

2 Nuclei of fibroblasts

3 Eosinophil

4 Nuclei of
   adipose cells

5 Adipose cells

6 Neutrophils

7 Lymphocytes

8 Capillaries
   (t.s. and l.s.)

9 Collagen fibers

FIGURE 3.4 ■ Loose connective tissue with blood vessels and adipose cells. Stain: hematoxylin and eosin. High magnification.

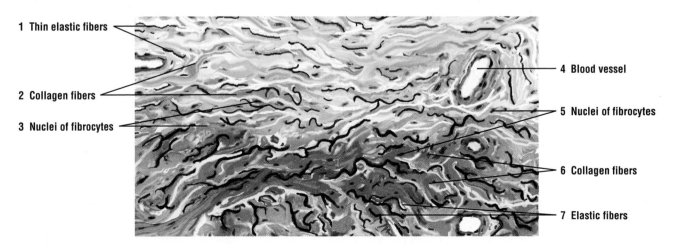

1 Thin elastic fibers

2 Collagen fibers

3 Nuclei of fibrocytes

4 Blood vessel

5 Nuclei of fibrocytes

6 Collagen fibers

7 Elastic fibers

FIGURE 3.5 ■ Dense irregular and loose irregular connective tissue. Stain: Verhoeff's elastin stain and Van Gieson's. Medium magnification.

FIGURE 3.6 ■ Loose Irregular and Dense Irregular Connective Tissue

This illustration shows a gradual transition from **loose irregular connective tissue (5)** to **dense irregular connective tissue (1)**. Where firmer support and strength are required, dense irregular connective tissue replaces the loose type.

Collagen fibers **(2, 9)** in both types of tisse are large, typically are found in bundles, and are sectioned in several planes (because they course in various directions). Also present are thin, wavy elastic fibers that form fine networks. However, these fibers are not obvious in routine histological preparations.

In dense connective tissue (1), **fibroblasts (3, 10)** are often found compressed among the collagen fibers (2). In loose irregular connective tissue (5), collagen fibers (9) are less compressed, and fibroblasts (10) are more visible. Also illustrated in the connective tissue are **capillaries (4); a small venule (11);** an **eosinophil (6)** with a lobulated nucleus; **lymphocytes (7)** with large, round nuclei without visible cytoplasm; a **plasma cell (8);** and numerous **adipose cells (12)**.

FIGURE 3.7 ■ Dense Irregular Connective Tissue and Adipose Tissue

This photomicrograph illustrates a deep section of the skin called the dermis. This region contains **dense irregular connective tissue (1)** and the collagen-producing cells, **fibroblasts (3)**. In this type of connective tissue, **collagen fibers (2)** show a random and irregular orientation. Adjacent to the dense irregular connective tissue (1) is a region of **adipose tissue (4)** with numerous adipose cells. Because of the tissue preparation with different chemicals, individual adipose cells appear empty, and only their flattened, dense-staining nuclei are visible. Numerous sweat glands are also found in the dermis. The light-staining regions are the **secretory cells of the sweat gland (7)**. The dark-staining cells form a **stratified cuboidal epithelium of the excretory duct of the sweat gland (6, 8)**. The excretory duct (6, 8) continues through the connective tissue and the stratified squamous epithelium of the skin and finally exits on the surface of the skin (see Fig. 2-9).

FUNCTIONAL CORRELATIONS

Ground Substance and Connective Tissue

The **ground substance** in connective tissue consists primarily of amorphous, transparent, and colorless **extracellular matrix,** which has the properties of a semifluid gel and a high water content. It supports and surrounds the connective tissue and all its cells and fiber types. The ground substance contains different types of mixed, unbranched polysacchride chains of **glycosaminoglycans** and **adhesive glycoproteins. Hyaluronic acid** constitutes the principal glycosaminoglycan of connective tissue. Except for hyaluronic acid, the various glycosaminoglycans are bound to a core protein to form much larger molecules called **proteoglycan aggregates.** These proteoglycans attract water, which forms the hydrated gel of the ground substance.

The semifluid consistency of ground substance in the connective tissue facilitates **diffusion** of oxygen, electrolytes, nutrients, fluids, metabolites, and other water-soluble molecules between the cells and the blood vessels. Similarly, waste products from the cells diffuse through the ground substance back into the blood vessels. Because of its viscosity, the ground substance also serves as an efficient **barrier,** preventing the movement of large molecules and the spread of pathogens from the connective tissue into the bloodstream. However, certain bacteria can produce hyaluronidase, an enzyme that hydrolyzes the hyaluronic acid and reduces the viscosity of the gel-like ground substance, thereby allowing pathogens to invade the surrounding tissues.

The density of ground substance depends on the amount of extracellular tissue fluid or water that it contains. Mineralization, caused by increased calcium deposition or mineralization, changes the density, rigidity, and permeability of ground substance, as seen in normally developing cartilage models and bones.

In addition to proteoglycans, connective tissue also contains several cell **adhesive glycoproteins,** which bind cells to the fibers. One glycoprotein, **fibronectin,** binds cells, collagen fibers, and proteoglycans, thereby interconnecting all three components of the connective tissue. Integral proteins of the plasma membrane, called **integrins,** bind to extracellular collagen fibers. **Laminin** is a large glycoprotein and a major component of the cell basement membrane; this protein binds epithelial cells to the basal lamina.

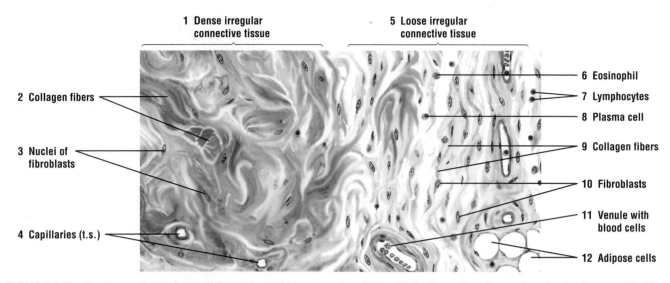

1 Dense irregular connective tissue

5 Loose irregular connective tissue

2 Collagen fibers

3 Nuclei of fibroblasts

4 Capillaries (t.s.)

6 Eosinophil

7 Lymphocytes

8 Plasma cell

9 Collagen fibers

10 Fibroblasts

11 Venule with blood cells

12 Adipose cells

FIGURE 3.6 ■ Dense irregular and loose irregular connective tissue. Stain: hematoxylin and eosin. High magnification.

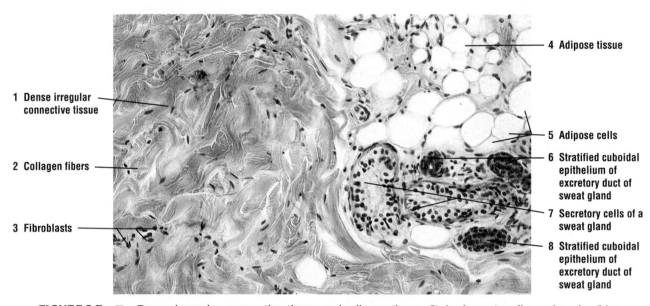

1 Dense irregular connective tissue

2 Collagen fibers

3 Fibroblasts

4 Adipose tissue

5 Adipose cells

6 Stratified cuboidal epithelium of excretory duct of sweat gland

7 Secretory cells of a sweat gland

8 Stratified cuboidal epithelium of excretory duct of sweat gland

FIGURE 3.7 ■ Dense irregular connective tissue and adipose tissue. Stain: hematoxylin and eosin. 64×

FIGURE 3.8 ■ Dense Regular Connective Tissue: Tendon (Longitudinal Section)

Dense regular connective tissue is present in ligaments and tendons. This illustration shows a section of a tendon in the longitudinal plane in which some of the collagen fibers are stretched and some are relaxed.

Collagen fibers (2, 5, 8) are arranged in compact, parallel bundles. Between the collagen bundles (2, 5, 8) are thin partitions of looser connective tissue that contain parallel rows of **fibroblasts (1, 3).** The fibroblasts (1, 3) have short processes (not visible here) and nuclei that appear ovoid when seen in the **surface view (3)** or flat and rod-like in the **lateral view (1).** When the tendon is stretched, the bundles of collagen fibers (2) are straight. When the tendon is relaxed, the bundles of collagen fibers (8) become wavy.

Dense irregular connective tissue with less regular fiber arrangement than in the tendon also surrounds and partitions the collagen bundles as the **interfascicular connective tissue (4).** Fibroblasts (6) and numerous blood vessels, such as **arterioles (7),** that supply the connective tissue cells are found here.

FIGURE 3.9 ■ Dense Regular Connective Tissue: Tendon (Longitudinal Section)

A photomicrograph of the dense regular connective tissue of a tendon shows a compact, regular, and parallel arrangement of **collagen fibers (1).** Between the densely packed collagen fibers are the flattened nuclei of **fibroblasts (2).** A small **blood vessel (3)** containing red blood cells courses between the dense bundles of collagen fibers to supply the connective tissue cells of the tendon.

FUNCTIONAL CORRELATIONS

Dense Irregular Connective Tissue

Dense irregular connective tissue consists primarily of **collagen fibers** with minimal amounts of surrounding ground substance. Except for the **fibroblasts,** cells in this type of connective tissue are sparse. Collagen fibers exhibit great **tensile strength,** and their main function is **support.** Collagen fibers also exhibit **random orientation** and are most highly concentrated where strong support is needed to resist pulling forces from different directions.

Dense Regular Connective Tissue

Dense regular connective tissue is present where **great tensile strength** is required, such as in **ligaments** and **tendons.** The parallel and dense arrangements of collagen fibers offer strong resistance to forces pulling along a **single axis or direction.**

Tendons and ligaments are attached to bones and are constantly subjected to strong pulling forces. Because of the dense arrangement of collagen fibers, little ground substance is present, and the predominant cell types are the **fibroblasts,** which are located between rows of collagen fibers.

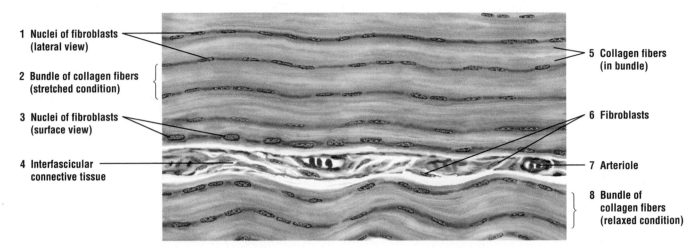

1 **Nuclei of fibroblasts (lateral view)**

2 **Bundle of collagen fibers (stretched condition)**

3 **Nuclei of fibroblasts (surface view)**

4 **Interfascicular connective tissue**

5 **Collagen fibers (in bundle)**

6 **Fibroblasts**

7 **Arteriole**

8 **Bundle of collagen fibers (relaxed condition)**

FIGURE 3.8 ■ Dense regular connective tissue: tendon (longitudinal section). Stain: hematoxylin and eosin. Medium magnification.

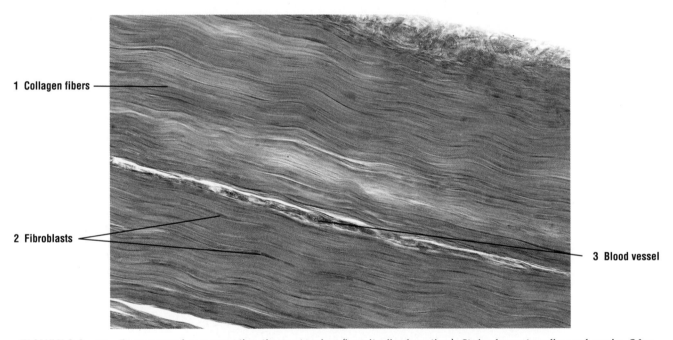

1 **Collagen fibers**

2 **Fibroblasts**

3 **Blood vessel**

FIGURE 3.9 ■ Dense regular connective tissue: tendon (longitudinal section). Stain: hematoxylin and eosin. 64×

FIGURE 3.10 ■ Dense Regular Connective Tissue: Tendon (Transverse Section)

A transverse section of a tendon is illustrated at low magnification (left side) and high magnification (right side).

Between the large collagen bundles are **interfascicular connective tissue (5)** partitions. These partitions contain blood vessels, including an **arteriole** and **venules (1),** nerves, and occasionally, the sensitive pressure-receptors, **Pacinian corpuscles (7).**

Also illustrated in the upper left is a transverse section of several **skeletal muscle fibers (2, 3).** These are adjacent to the tendon but are separated from it by a connective tissue partition. Note that the **nuclei (2)** of skeletal muscles fibers (3) are located on the periphery of the fibers, whereas the nuclei of fibroblasts (6, 8) are located between bundles of collagen fibers (4, 9).

FIGURE 3.11 ■ Adipose Tissue in the Intestine

A small section of a mesentery of an intestine, in which large accumulations of **adipose (fat) cells (4, 8)** are organized into an adipose tissue, is illustrated. The **connective tissue (9)** that surrounds the adipose tissue is covered by a simple squamous epithelium called **mesothelium (10).**

Adipose cells (4, 8) are closely packed and separated by thin strips of connective tissue septa (3), in which are found compressed **fibroblasts (7); blood vessels,** including an **arteriole (1), venules (2, 6),** and **capillaries (5);** and nerves.

Individual adipose cells appear as empty cells (4), because the fat was dissolved by the chemicals used during routine histologic preparation of the tissue. The nuclei of **adipose cells (8)** are compressed to the peripheral rim of the cytoplasm, and in certain sections, it is difficult to distinguish fibroblast nuclei (7) from adipose cell nuclei (8).

FUNCTIONAL CORRELATIONS

Adipose Tissue

The two distinct types of adipose tissue in the body are **white adipose tissue** and **brown adipose tissue.** These two types of adipose tissue represent the main sites of **lipid storage** and **metabolism** in the body. Cells of the white adipose tissue are large and store lipids as a single, large droplet; cells of brown adipose tissue are smaller and store lipids as multiple, small droplets.

White adipose tissue is more widely distributed compared to brown adipose tissue. White adipose tissue is distributed throughout the body, with the distribution pattern showing variations that are dependent on the sex and age of the individual. In addition to serving as an energy source, white adipose tissue provides **insulation** under the skin and forms cushioning **fat pads** around organs. Adipose tissue is also highly vascularized because of its high metabolic activity. In addition, white adipose tissue cells secrete a hormone called **leptin,** which increases carbohydrate and lipid metabolism in cells while inhibiting or suppressing appetite and food intake.

Brown adipose tissue is found in all mammals, but it is best developed in animals that **hibernate.** The main function of brown adipose tissue is to supply the body with **heat.** Newborn humans and animals with fur that emerge from hibernation use brown adipose tissue to generate and increase body heat during these critical periods. The amount of brown adipose tissue gradually decreases in older individuals, and it is mainly found around the adrenal glands and great vessels as well as in the neck region.

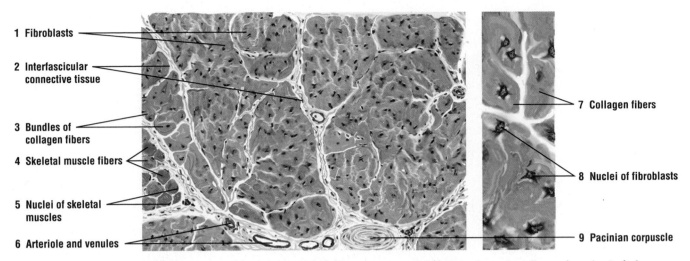

1 Fibroblasts

2 Interfascicular connective tissue

3 Bundles of collagen fibers

4 Skeletal muscle fibers

5 Nuclei of skeletal muscles

6 Arteriole and venules

7 Collagen fibers

8 Nuclei of fibroblasts

9 Pacinian corpuscle

FIGURE 3.10 ■ Dense regular connective tissue: tendon (transverse section). Stain: hematoxylin and eosin. Left, low magnification; right: high magnification.

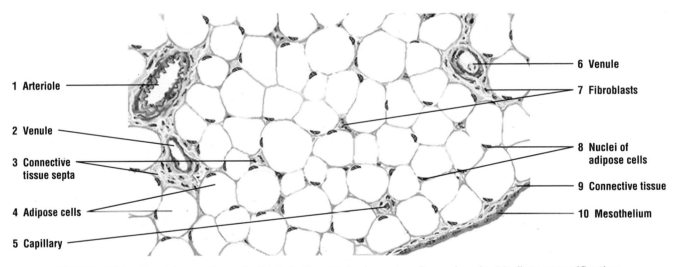

1 Arteriole

2 Venule

3 Connective tissue septa

4 Adipose cells

5 Capillary

6 Venule

7 Fibroblasts

8 Nuclei of adipose cells

9 Connective tissue

10 Mesothelium

FIGURE 3.11 ■ Adipose tissue in the intestine. Stain: hematoxylin and eosin. Medium magnification.

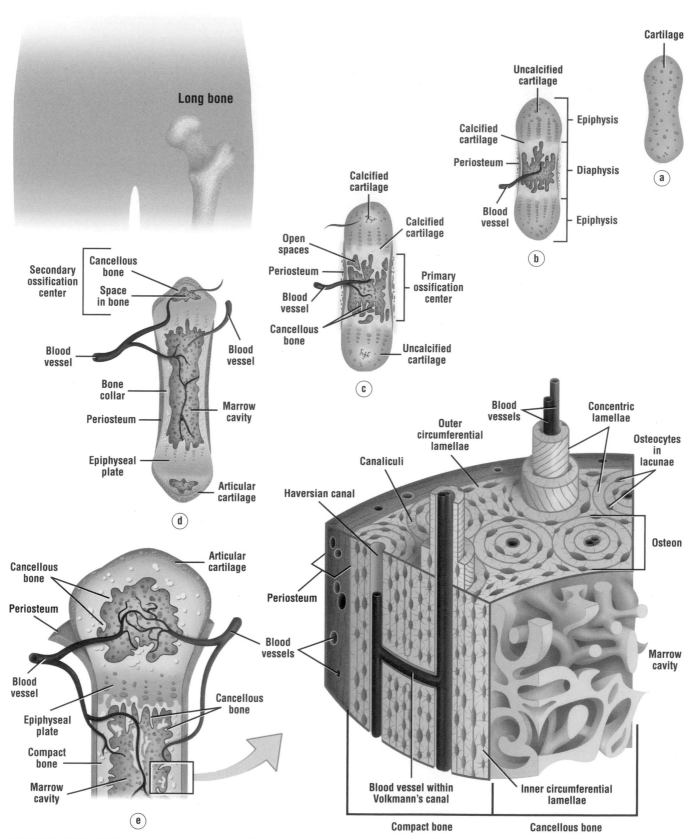

OVERVIEW FIGURE ■ Endochondral ossification, illustrating the progressive stages of bone formation (from cartilage model to bone) and including the histology of a section of formed bone.

CHAPTER 4

Cartilage and Bone

SECTION 1 ■ Cartilage

Types of Cartilage

Cartilage is a special form of connective tissue. It exhibits tensile strength, provides firm structural support for soft tissues, allows flexibility without distortion, and is resilient to compression. Cartilage consists mainly of cells called **chondrocytes** and **chondroblasts** that synthesize the extensive **extracellular matrix** (connective tissue fibers and ground substance). Three main types of cartilage are found in the body: hyaline, elastic, and fibrocartilage. Cartilage is classified based on the amount and types of fibers that are present in the extracellular matrix.

Hyaline Cartilage

Hyaline cartilage is the most common type. In embryos, hyaline cartilage serves as a skeletal model for most bones. As the individual grows, the cartilage bone model is gradually replaced with bone through a process called **endochondral ossification.** In adults, most of the hyaline cartilage has been replaced with bone, except on the articular surfaces of bones, ends of ribs (costal cartilage), nose, larynx, and trachea as well as in bronchi. Here, hyaline cartilage persists throughout life and does not calcify.

Elastic Cartilage

Elastic cartilage is similar in appearance to hyaline cartilage, except for the presence of numerous branching elastic fibers in its matrix. Elastic cartilage is highly flexible and is found in the external ear, walls of the auditory tube, epiglottis, and larynx.

Fibrocartilage

Fibrocartilage is characterized by large amounts of irregular and dense bundles of collagen fibers in its matrix. In contrast to hyaline and elastic cartilage, fibrocartilage consists of alternating layers of cartilage matrix and thick, dense layers of collagen fibers. The collagen fibers normally orient themselves toward the direction of functional stress. Fibrocartilage has a limited distribution and is found in the intervertebral disks, symphysis pubis, and certain joints.

Perichondrium

Most of the hyaline and elastic cartilage in the body is surrounded by a peripheral layer of vascularized, dense irregular connective tissue called the **perichondrium.** The inner layer of perichondrium is **chondrogenic:** It gives rise to new chondroblasts that secrete cartilage matrix. An exception to this arrangement, however, is the hyaline cartilage on the articulating surfaces of bones, which is devoid of perichondrium. Also, because fibrocartilage is always associated with dense connective tissue, it does not exhibit an identifiable perichondrium.

Cartilage Matrix

Cartilage matrix is produced and maintained by chondrocytes and chondroblasts. The collagen or elastic fibers give cartilage matrix its firmness and resilience. Similar to that of loose connective tissue, the extracellular **ground substance** of cartilage contains sulfated glycosaminoglycans and hyaluronic acid that are closely associated with elastic and collagen fibers. Also, cartilage matrix is highly hydrated because of its high water content. Cartilage is a semirigid tissue. Embedded within its matrix are varying proportions of collagen and elastic fibers. The presence of these fibers characterizes cartilage as hyaline cartilage, elastic cartilage, or fibrocartilage.

Hyaline cartilage matrix consists of fine **type II collagen fibrils** embedded in a firm, amorphous, hydrated matrix rich in proteoglycans and structural glycoproteins. Most proteoglycans in cartilage matrix exist as large proteoglycan aggregates, which contain sulfated glycosaminoglycans linked to core proteins and molecules of nonsulfated glycosaminoglycan hyaluronic acid. The proteoglycan aggregates bind to the thin fibrils of the collagen matrix.

In addition to type II collagen fibrils and proteoglycans, cartilage also contains an adhesive glycoprotein called **chondronectin.** These macromolecules bind to glycosaminoglycans and collagen fibers, thereby providing adherence of chondroblasts and chondrocytes to collagen fibers of the surrounding matrix.

FIGURE 4.1 ▪ Fetal Hyaline Cartilage

This illustration shows hyaline cartilage during an early stage of development. Superficial **mesenchyme (1)** with **blood vessels (5)** surrounds the nonvascular fetal cartilage. At this stage, lacunae around the **fetal chondroblasts (4, 7)** are not visible, and the chondroblasts (4, 7) resemble superficial mesenchymal cells (1). Fetal chondroblasts (4, 7) are randomly distributed, without forming isogenous groups, and secrete the **intercellular cartilage matrix (8).**

During development, mesenchyme cells (1) concentrate on the periphery of the cartilage, and their nuclei become elongated. This region develops into **perichondrium (2, 6),** which is a sheath of dense irregular connective tissue with fibroblasts (2, 6) that surrounds hyaline and elastic cartilage. The inner layer of the perichondrium (2, 6) becomes the **chondrogenic layer (3),** which gives rise to chondroblasts (4, 7).

FIGURE 4.2 ▪ Hyaline Cartilage and Surrounding Structures: Trachea

This illustration depicts a section of a hyaline cartilage plate from the trachea. **Perichondrium (5)** with **fibroblasts (7)** surrounds the cartilage. The inner **chondrogenic layer (4)** produces **chondroblasts (8)** that differentiate into chondrocytes. **Chondrocytes** in lacunae appear either singly or in **isogenous groups (3).** Lacunae and chondrocytes (3) in the middle of the cartilage plate are large and spherical, but they become progressively flatter toward the periphery, where these cells are differentiating chondroblasts (8). The **interterritorial** (intercellular) **matrix (1)** stains lighter, whereas the **territorial matrix (2)** around the lacunae stains darker.

Vascular (9) and **connective tissue (10)** as well as tracheal glands with grape-like secretory units called acini are visible near the cartilage. **Serous acini (11)** produce watery secretions, whereas **mucous acini (12)** secrete a lubricating mucus. An **excretory duct (6)** delivers these secretions into the tracheal lumen.

FUNCTIONAL CORRELATIONS

Cartilage Cells

Cartilage develops from primitive **mesenchyme cells** that differentiate into **chondroblasts.** These cells divide mitotically and synthesize the cartilage **matrix** and **extracellular material.** As the cartilage model grows, the individual chondroblasts are surrounded by extracellular matrix and become trapped in compartments called **lacunae** (singular, lacuna). In the lacunae are mature cartilage cells called **chondrocytes.** The main function of chondrocytes is to maintain the cartilage matrix. Some lacunae may contain more than one chondrocyte; these groups of chondrocytes are called **isogenous groups.**

Mesenchyme cells can also differentiate into fibroblasts that form the **perichondrium,** a dense irregular connective tissue layer that invests the cartilage. The inner layer of perichondrium contains chondrogenic cells, which can differentiate into chondroblasts, secrete cartilage matrix, and become trapped in lacunae as chondrocytes.

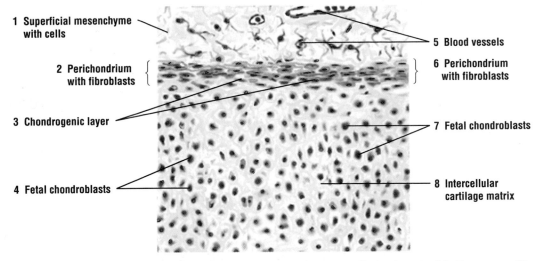

1 Superficial mesenchyme with cells

2 Perichondrium with fibroblasts

3 Chondrogenic layer

4 Fetal chondroblasts

5 Blood vessels

6 Perichondrium with fibroblasts

7 Fetal chondroblasts

8 Intercellular cartilage matrix

FIGURE 4.1 ■ Developing fetal hyaline cartilage. Stain: hematoxylin and eosin. Medium magnification.

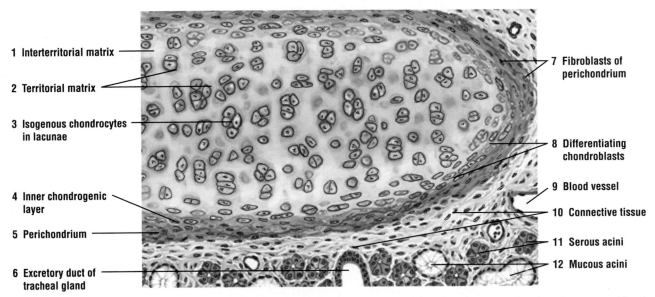

1 Interterritorial matrix

2 Territorial matrix

3 Isogenous chondrocytes in lacunae

4 Inner chondrogenic layer

5 Perichondrium

6 Excretory duct of tracheal gland

7 Fibroblasts of perichondrium

8 Differentiating chondroblasts

9 Blood vessel

10 Connective tissue

11 Serous acini

12 Mucous acini

FIGURE 4.2 ■ Hyaline cartilage and surrounding structures: trachea. Stain: hematoxylin and eosin. Medium magnification.

FIGURE 4.3 ◼ Cells and Matrix of Mature Hyaline Cartilage

Higher magnification illustrates an interior or central region of mature hyaline cartilage. Distributed throughout the homogeneous ground substance, the **matrix (4, 5),** are ovoid spaces called **lacunae (3),** which contain mature cartilage cells, the **chondrocytes (1, 2).** In intact cartilage, chondrocytes fill the lacunae. Each chondrocyte has a granular cytoplasm and a **nucleus (1).** During histologic preparations, chondrocytes (1, 2) shrink, and the lacunae (3) appear as clear spaces. Cartilage cells in the matrix are seen either singly or in isogenous groups.

Hyaline cartilage matrix (4, 5) appears homogeneous and, usually, basophilic. The lighter-staining matrix between chondrocytes (2) is called the **interterritorial matrix (5).** The more basophilic or darker-staining matrix adjacent to the chondrocytes is called the **territorial matrix (4).**

FIGURE 4.4 ◼ Hyaline Cartilage: Developing Bone

A photomicrograph of a section through a developing bone shows a portion of the hyaline cartilage and its characteristic homogeneous **matrix (1).** Located within the matrix (1) are the mature hyaline cartilage cells, or **chondrocytes (3),** in their **lacunae (2).** Surrounding the hyaline cartilage is the dense irregular connective tissue **perichondrium (5).** On the inner surface of the perichondrium (5) is the **chondrogenic layer (4).**

FUNCTIONAL CORRELATIONS

Cartilage (Hyaline, Elastic, and Fibrocartilage)

Cartilage is nonvascular, but it is surrounded by the vascular connective tissue **perichondrium.** All nutrients enter and metabolites leave the cartilage by diffusing through the matrix. Because cartilage matrix is soft, pliable, and not as hard as bone, cartilage can simultaneously grow by two different means: interstitial and appositional.

Interstitial growth involves mitosis of chondrocytes within the matrix and deposition of new matrix between and around the cells. This growth process increases cartilage size from within. **Appositional growth** occurs on the periphery of the cartilage. In this type of growth, chondroblasts differentiate from the inner connective tissue perichondrium and deposit a layer of cartilage matrix that is apposed to the existing cartilage layer. This growth process increases cartilage width.

Hyaline cartilage provides firm structural and flexible support. Elastic cartilage, because of the numerous branching elastic fibers in its matrix, confers structural support as well as increased flexibility. In contrast to the matrix of hyaline cartilage, which can calcify with aging, that of elastic cartilage does not calcify. The main function of fibrocartilage is to provide tensile strength, to bear weight, and to resist stretch or compression.

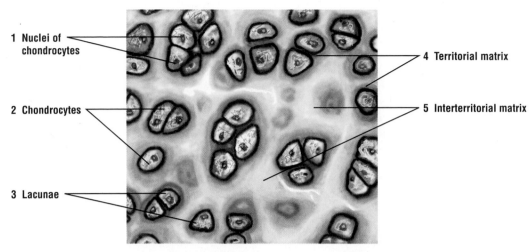

1 Nuclei of chondrocytes

2 Chondrocytes

3 Lacunae

4 Territorial matrix

5 Interterritorial matrix

FIGURE 4.3 ■ Cells and matrix of mature hyaline cartilage. Stain: hematoxylin and eosin. High magnification.

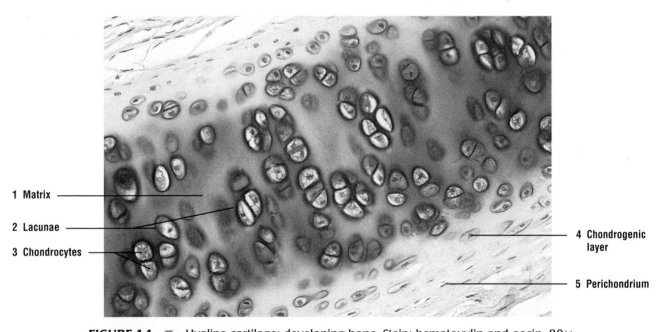

1 Matrix

2 Lacunae

3 Chondrocytes

4 Chondrogenic layer

5 Perichondrium

FIGURE 4.4 ■ Hyaline cartilage: developing bone. Stain: hematoxylin and eosin. 80×

FIGURE 4.5 ▪ Elastic Cartilage: Epiglottis

Elastic cartilage differs from hyaline cartilage principally by the presence of numerous **elastic fibers (4)** in its **matrix (7).** Staining the cartilage of the epiglottis with silver reveals the thin elastic fibers **(4).** Elastic fibers **(4, 7)** enter the cartilage matrix from the surrounding connective tissue **perichondrium (1)** and become distributed as branching and anastomosing fibers of various sizes. The density of the fibers varies among elastic cartilages as well as among different areas of the same cartilage.

As in hyaline cartilage, larger **chondrocytes** in **lacunae (3, 8)** are more prevalent in the interior of the plate. The smaller and flatter chondrocytes are located peripherally in the inner **chondrogenic layer** of the **perichondrium (2),** from which chondroblasts develop to synthesize the cartilage matrix. Also visible in the perichondrium **(1)** are the connective tissue cells, or **fibrocytes (5),** and a **venule (6).**

FIGURE 4.6 ▪ Elastic Cartilage: Epiglottis

A photomicrograph of a section of an epiglottis shows that this type of structure is characterized by a cartilage with fine, branching **elastic fibers (2)** in its **matrix (5)** in addition to distinct **chondrocytes (3)** and **lacunae (4).** The presence of elastic fibers **(2)** gives this cartilage flexibility as well as support. Surrounding the elastic cartilage is a layer of dense irregular connective tissue **perichondrium (1).**

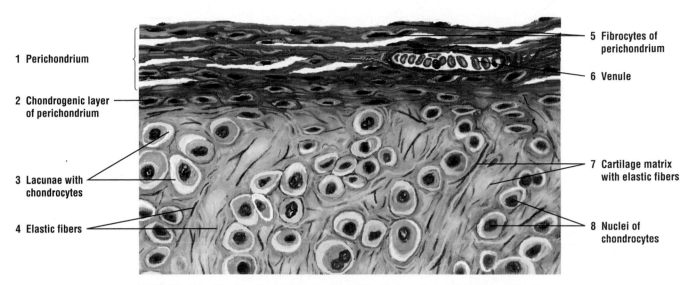

1 Perichondrium

2 Chondrogenic layer
   of perichondrium

3 Lacunae with
   chondrocytes

4 Elastic fibers

5 Fibrocytes of
   perichondrium

6 Venule

7 Cartilage matrix
   with elastic fibers

8 Nuclei of
   chondrocytes

FIGURE 4.5 ■ Elastic cartilage: epiglottis. Stain: silver. High magnification.

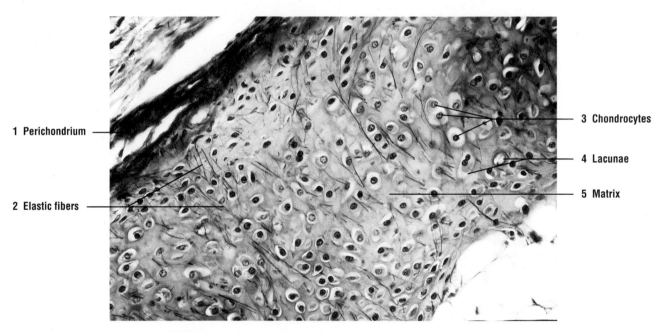

1 Perichondrium

2 Elastic fibers

3 Chondrocytes

4 Lacunae

5 Matrix

FIGURE 4.6 ■ Elastic cartilage: epiglottis. Stain: silver. 80×

FIGURE 4.7 ■ Fibrous Cartilage: Intervertebral Disk

In fibrous cartilage, the **matrix (5)** is filled with dense **collagen fibers (2, 6),** which frequently exhibit parallel arrangement, as seen in tendons. Small **chondrocytes (1, 4)** in **lacunae (3)** are usually distributed in **rows (4)** within the fibrous cartilage matrix (5) rather than at random or in isogenous groups, as seen in hyaline or elastic cartilage. All chondrocytes and lacunae (1, 3, 4) are of similar size; no gradation is observed from larger central chondrocytes to smaller and flatter peripheral cells.

A perichondrium, which normally is present around hyaline cartilage and elastic cartilage, is absent, because fibrous cartilage usually forms a transitional area between hyaline cartilage and tendon or ligament.

The proportion of collagen fibers (2, 6) to cartilage matrix (5), the number of chondrocytes, and the arrangement of chondrocytes in the matrix (5) may vary. Collagen fibers (2, 6) may be so dense that the matrix (5) is invisible. In such cases, chondrocytes and lacunae appear flattened. Collagen fibers within a bundle are normally parallel, but collagen bundles may course in different directions.

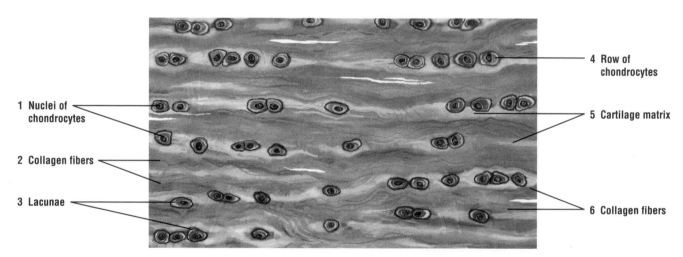

FIGURE 4.7   ■   Fibrous cartilage: intervertebral disk. Stain: hematoxylin and eosin. High magnification.

SECTION 2 ■ Bone

Similar to cartilage, **bone** is also a special form of connective tissue and consists of **cells, fibers, and extracellular matrix.** Because of mineral deposition in the matrix, bones become calcified. As a result, they can bear more weight than cartilage, serve as a rigid skeleton for the body, and provide attachment sites for muscles and organs.

Bones also protect the brain in the skull, the heart and lungs in the thorax, and the urinary and reproductive organs between the pelvic bones. In addition, bones function in **hemopoiesis** (blood cell formation), and they serve as crucial **reservoirs** for calcium, phosphate, and other minerals. Almost all (99%) of the calcium in the body is stored in bones, from which the body receives its daily calcium supply.

The Process of Bone Formation (Ossification)

Bone development begins in the embryo by two distinct processes: endochondral ossification and intramembranous ossification (see the overview figure). Although bones are produced by two different methods, they exhibit the same histologic structures.

Endochondral Ossification

Most bones in the body develop by the process of **endochondral ossification,** in which a temporary hyaline cartilage model precedes bone formation. This cartilage model continues to grow by both interstitial and appositional means. The chondrocytes then divide, hypertrophy (enlarge), and mature, and the hyaline cartilage model begins to calcify. As the calcification of the cartilage model continues, diffusion of nutrients and gases through the calcified matrix decreases. Consequently, chondrocytes die, and the fragmented, calcified matrix serves as a structural framework for the deposition of bony material.

As soon as a layer of bony material has been deposited around the calcifying cartilage, the external surrounding connective tissue is called the **periosteum. Osteoprogenitor cells** from the inner layer of periosteum and blood vessels from the connective tissue invade the calcified and degenerating cartilage model. Osteoprogenitor cells proliferate and differentiate into **osteoblasts** that secrete the bony matrix. Osteoprogenitor cells also arise from the inner surface of bone called the **endosteum.** Endosteum lines all internal cavities in the bone, and it consists of a single layer of osteoprogenitor cells.

Mesenchyme tissue, osteoblasts, and blood vessels form an **ossification center** in the developing bone. In developing long bones, the primary **ossification center** first appears in the **diaphysis,** followed by a secondary ossification center in the **epiphysis. Osteoid matrix** is initially produced by osteoblasts, after which it is mineralized into bone. In all developing long bones, cartilage in the diaphysis and epiphysis is replaced by bone, except in the epiphyseal plate region, where growth continues and is responsible for lengthening the bone until bone growth stops. Expansion of the two ossification centers eventually replaces all cartilage, including the epiphyseal plate, with bone. The only exceptions are the free ends of the long bones, where a layer of permanent hyaline cartilage covers the bone and is called the **articular cartilage.**

Intramembranous Ossification

In **intramembranous ossification,** bone develops not from a cartilage model but from the connective tissue **mesenchyme.** Some mesenchyme cells differentiate directly into osteoblasts and produce the surrounding osteoid matrix, which quickly calcifies. The osteoblasts then become surrounded by bone in the cave-like lacunae and are called **osteocytes.** Osteocytes establish complex cell-to-cell connections through a system of tiny canals called **canaliculi.**

The **mandible, maxilla, clavicles,** and most of the **flat bones of the skull** are formed by the intramembranous method. In the developing skull, the centers of bone development grow radially, replace the connective tissue, and then fuse. In newborns, the fontanelles in the skull represent the soft membranous regions where intramembranous ossification of skull bones has not been completed.

Types of Bone

Examination of bone in cross section shows two types: **compact bone** and **cancellous (spongy) bone** (see the overview figure). In long bones, the outer, cylindrical part is the dense compact bone. The inner surface of compact bone adjacent to the marrow cavity is the cancellous bone. Cancellous bone contains numerous interconnecting areas and is not dense; however, both types of bone have the same microscopic appearance. In newborns, the marrow cavity is red and produces blood cells. In adults, the marrow cavity normally is yellow and filled with adipose (fat) cells.

In compact bone, the collagen fibers are arranged in thin layers of bone called **lamellae** that are parallel to each other in the periphery of the bone or are concentrically arranged around a blood vessel. In a long bone, the **outer circumferential lamellae** are deep to the periosteum. The **inner circumferential lamellae** surround the bone marrow cavity. **Concentric lamellae** that surround a canal with blood vessels, nerves, and loose connective tissue are called **osteons** (Haversian systems). The space in the osteon that contains blood vessels and nerves is the **central (Haversian) canal.** Most of the compact bone consists of osteons. Lacunae that have osteocytes and are connected via canaliculi are found between the lamellae in each osteon (see the overview figure).

Bone Matrix

The bone matrix consists of living cells and extracellular material. Because bone matrix is calcified or mineralized, it is harder than cartilage. Diffusion is not possible through the calcified matrix; therefore, bone matrix is highly vascularized. Bone matrix contains both organic and inorganic components. The organic components enable bones to resist tension, whereas the mineral components enable bones to resist compression.

The major organic components of bone matrix are the coarse **type I collagen fibers.** The other organic components are sulfated glycosaminoglycans and hyaluronic acid that form larger proteoglycan aggregates. The glycoproteins osteocalcin and osteopontin bind tightly to calcium crystals during mineralization of bone. Another matrix protein, sialoprotein, binds osteoblasts to the extracellular matrix through the integrins of the plasma membrane proteins.

The inorganic component of bone matrix consists of the minerals calcium and phosphate in the form of hydroxyapatite crystals. The association of coarse collagen fibers with hydroxyapatite crystals provides the bone with its hardness, durability, and strength. In addition, the stored calcium and phosphate deposits in the matrix can be quickly mobilized by hormones to maintain proper mineral content in the blood.

FIGURE 4.8 ■ Endochondral Ossification: Development of a Long Bone (Panoramic View, Longitudinal Section)

During endochondral ossification, the bone is first formed as a model of embryonic hyaline cartilage. As bone development progresses, the cartilage model is replaced by bone. The process of endochondral ossification can be followed by examining the upper part of the illustration and then proceeding downward.

In the upper part, the hyaline cartilage is surrounded by connective tissue **perichondrium (13).** The **zone of reserve cartilage (1)** shows chondrocytes in their lacunae distributed either singly or in small groups. Below this region is the **zone of proliferating chondrocytes (2),** where the chondrocytes divide and become arranged in vertical columns. **Chondrocytes in lacunae (14)** increase in size in the **zone of chondrocyte hypertrophy (3)** because of swelling of the nucleus and cytoplasm. The hypertrophied chondrocytes degenerate, forming thin **plates of calcified cartilage matrix (15).** Below this region is the **zone of ossification (4),** where a bony material is deposited on the plates of calcified cartilage matrix (15).

Blood sinusoids (20) or capillaries invade the calcifying cartilage. Lacunar walls and the calcified cartilage (15) are eroded, and the **red bone marrow cavity (16)** is formed. The connective tissue around the newly formed bone is called **periosteum (5, 6, 17),** and this region is now the **zone of ossification (4).** In this illustration, bone is stained dark red. Osteoprogenitor cells from the **inner periosteum (6)** continue to differentiate into osteoblasts, to deposit **osteoid** and **bone**

(**8**) around the remaining plates of calcified cartilage (15), and to form the **periosteal bone collar (7).**

Formation of new periosteal bone (7) keeps pace with the formation of new endochondral bone. The bone collar (7) increases in thickness and compactness as development of bone proceeds. The thickest portion of the bone collar (7) is seen in the central part of the developing bone called the diaphysis. The primary center of ossification is located in the diaphysis, where the initial periosteal bone collar (7) is formed.

Red bone marrow (16) fills the cavity of newly formed bone with hemopoietic (blood-forming) cells. Fine reticular connective tissue fibers in the bone marrow (16) are obscured by masses of developing erythrocytes, granulocytes, **megakaryocytes (12), bony spicules (22),** numerous **blood sinusoids (20),** capillaries, and blood vessels.

Surrounding the shaft of the developing bone are the soft tissues. The **epidermis (18)** of skin is lined by stratified squamous epithelium. Below the epidermis (18) is the subcutaneous **connective tissue** of the **dermis (19),** in which **hair follicles (9), blood vessels (10), adipose cells (21),** and **sweat glands (23)** are seen.

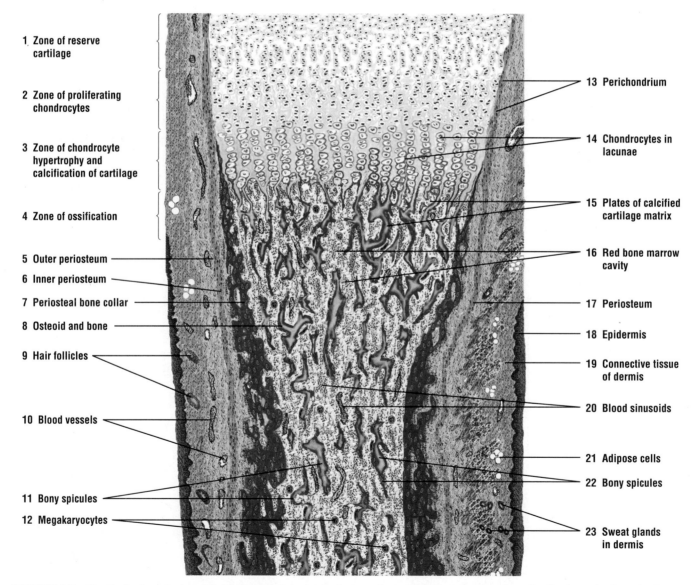

1 Zone of reserve cartilage

2 Zone of proliferating chondrocytes

3 Zone of chondrocyte hypertrophy and calcification of cartilage

4 Zone of ossification

5 Outer periosteum

6 Inner periosteum

7 Periosteal bone collar

8 Osteoid and bone

9 Hair follicles

10 Blood vessels

11 Bony spicules

12 Megakaryocytes

13 Perichondrium

14 Chondrocytes in lacunae

15 Plates of calcified cartilage matrix

16 Red bone marrow cavity

17 Periosteum

18 Epidermis

19 Connective tissue of dermis

20 Blood sinusoids

21 Adipose cells

22 Bony spicules

23 Sweat glands in dermis

FIGURE 4.8 ■ Endochondral ossification: development of a long bone (panoramic view, longitudinal section). Stain: hematoxylin and eosin. Low magnification.

FIGURE 4.9   ■   Endochondral Ossification: Zone of Ossification

This illustration shows endochondral ossification at higher magnification and in greater detail and corresponds to the upper region of Figure 4-8.

Proliferating **chondrocytes (1, 14)** are arranged in distinct vertical columns, below which is the zone of **hypertrophied chondrocytes (2, 15)**. Chondrocytes and lacunae undergo hypertrophy because of increased glycogen and lipid accumulations in their cytoplasm and nuclear swelling. The cytoplasm of hypertrophied chondrocytes (2, 15) becomes **vacuolized (16)**, the nuclei become pyknotic, and the thin cartilage plates become surrounded by **calcified matrix (5, 17)**.

Osteoblasts (6, 20) line up along remaining plates of calcified cartilage (5, 17), and lay down a layer of **osteoid (19)** and bone. Osteoblasts that are trapped in the osteoid or bone become **osteocytes (9, 21)**. **Capillaries (8, 18)** from the **marrow cavity (10)** invade the newly ossified area.

The developing marrow cavity (10) contains numerous **megakaryocytes (13, 24)** and pluripotential stem cells that give rise to erythrocytic and granulocytic **blood cells (23)**. Multinucleated **osteoclasts (11, 22)** lie in shallow depressions called the **Howship's lacunae (11, 22)** and adjacent to bone that is being resorbed.

On the left side is an area of **periosteal bone (7)** with osteocytes (9) in their lacunae. The new bone is added peripherally by osteoblasts (6), which develop from osteoprogenitor cells of the **inner periosteum (12)**. The outer layer of periosteum continues as the connective tissue **perichondrium (3)**.

FIGURE 4.10   ■   Endochondral Ossification: Zone of Ossification

This photomicrograph illustrates the transformation of hyaline cartilage into bone through the process of endochondral ossification. The **hyaline cartilage matrix (6)** contains **proliferating chondrocytes (7)** and **hypertrophied chondrocytes (1)** with **vacuolated cytoplasm (2)**. Below these cells are plates or **spicules of calcified cartilage (3)** that are surrounded by **osteoblasts (4)**. As the cartilage calcifies, a **marrow cavity (5)** is formed with blood vessels, **hematopoietic tissue (10)**, osteoprogenitor cells, and osteoblasts (4). The hyaline cartilage is surrounded by the connective tissue **perichondrium (8)**. The marrow cavity in the new bone is surrounded by the connective tissue **periosteum (9)**.

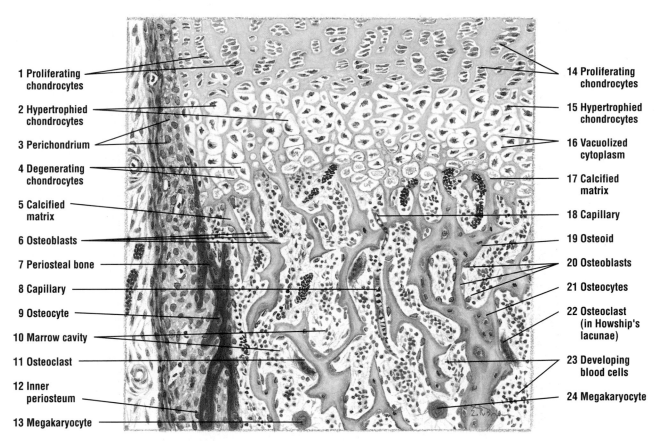

1 Proliferating chondrocytes
2 Hypertrophied chondrocytes
3 Perichondrium
4 Degenerating chondrocytes
5 Calcified matrix
6 Osteoblasts
7 Periosteal bone
8 Capillary
9 Osteocyte
10 Marrow cavity
11 Osteoclast
12 Inner periosteum
13 Megakaryocyte

14 Proliferating chondrocytes
15 Hypertrophied chondrocytes
16 Vacuolized cytoplasm
17 Calcified matrix
18 Capillary
19 Osteoid
20 Osteoblasts
21 Osteocytes
22 Osteoclast (in Howship's lacunae)
23 Developing blood cells
24 Megakaryocyte

FIGURE 4.9 ■ Endochondral ossification: zone of ossification. Stain: hematoxylin and eosin. Medium magnification.

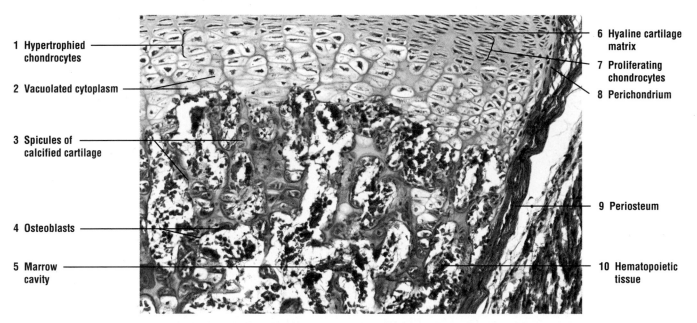

1 Hypertrophied chondrocytes
2 Vacuolated cytoplasm
3 Spicules of calcified cartilage
4 Osteoblasts
5 Marrow cavity

6 Hyaline cartilage matrix
7 Proliferating chondrocytes
8 Perichondrium
9 Periosteum
10 Hematopoietic tissue

FIGURE 4.10 ■ Endochondral ossification: zone of ossification. Stain: hematoxylin and eosin. 50×

FIGURE 4.11 ▪ Endochondral Ossification: Formation of Secondary (Epiphyseal) Centers of Ossification and Epiphyseal Plate in Long Bones (Decalcified Bone, Longitudinal Section)

The hyaline cartilage in the epiphyseal ends of two developing bones is illustrated. Both bones exhibit **secondary centers of ossification (5, 11).** Although cartilage is nonvascular, numerous **blood vessels (1, 6),** sectioned in different planes, pass through the cartilage matrix to supply the osteoblasts and osteocytes in the secondary centers of ossification (5, 11). **Articular cartilage (4, 12)** covers both articulating ends of the future bone. A **synovial** or **joint cavity (3)** separates the two cartilage models. The inner synovial membrane of squamous cells lines the synovial cavity (3), except over the articular cartilage (4, 12). A synovial membrane, together with the connective tissue, may extend into the joint cavity as **synovial folds (2, 13).** The synovial cavity (3) is covered by a connective tissue capsule.

In the lower bone, an active **epiphyseal plate (16)** is seen between the secondary ossification center (5) and the developing shaft of the bone. A **zone of proliferating chondrocytes (7)** and a **zone of chondrocyte hypertrophy and calcification of cartilage (8)** are clearly visible in the epiphyseal plate (16). Small **spicules of calcified cartilage (9, 15),** surrounded by red-stained bony material and **primitive bone marrow cavities with hemopoiesis (14, 17),** are seen in the shaft of the bone and secondary center of ossification (5). A **megakaryocyte (18)** is also visible in the lower bone marrow cavity (17). A connective tissue **periosteum (19)** surrounds the compact **bone (10).**

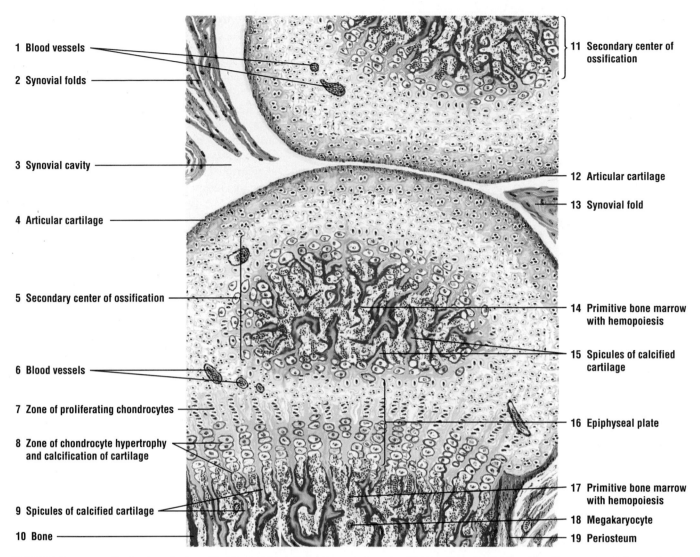

1 Blood vessels

2 Synovial folds

3 Synovial cavity

4 Articular cartilage

5 Secondary center of ossification

6 Blood vessels

7 Zone of proliferating chondrocytes

8 Zone of chondrocyte hypertrophy and calcification of cartilage

9 Spicules of calcified cartilage

10 Bone

11 Secondary center of ossification

12 Articular cartilage

13 Synovial fold

14 Primitive bone marrow with hemopoiesis

15 Spicules of calcified cartilage

16 Epiphyseal plate

17 Primitive bone marrow with hemopoiesis

18 Megakaryocyte

19 Periosteum

FIGURE 4.11 ■ Endochondral ossification. Formation of secondary (epiphyseal) centers of ossification and epiphyseal plate in long bone (decalcified bone, longitudinal section). Stain: hematoxylin and eosin. Low magnification.

FIGURE 4.12 ■ Bone Formation: Development of Osteons (Haversian Systems) (Decalcified Bone, Transverse Section)

This illustration shows the development of osteons in a compact bone. Vascular tufts of connective tissue from the periosteum or endosteum invade and erode the bone and form primitive osteons. Bone reconstruction or remodeling will continue as the initial osteons, and then later ones, are broken down or eroded, followed by the formation of new osteons.

Bone matrix (12) of an immature compact bone is stained deep red with eosin. Numerous primitive osteons are visible in transverse section, with large **central (Haversian) canals (2, 9, 11)** surrounded by a few concentric **lamellae (8)** of bone and **osteocytes** in **lacunae (10)**. The central (Haversian) canals (2, 9, 11) contain primitive connective tissue and **blood vessels (2, 9, 11)**. Bone deposition is continuing in some of the primitive osteons (11), as indicated by the presence of **osteoblasts (1, 15)** along the central (Haversian) canal (2, 9, 11) and the margin of the innermost bone lamella. In some osteons, the multinucleated **osteoclasts (6)** have formed and eroded shallow depressions called **Howship's lacunae (5)** in the bone. Osteoclasts (6) resorb and remodel the bone.

Osteogenic connective tissue (14) passes through the bone, from which arise tufts of vascular connective tissue that, in turn, give rise to new central (Haversian) canals (2, 9). Osteoblasts (1, 15) are located along the periphery of the developing central canals.

In the lower left corner is a **primitive bone marrow cavity (7),** in which hemopoiesis (blood cell formation) is in progress; this is the red marrow. Also present in the bone marrow cavity (7) are developing erythrocytes and granulocytes, **megakaryocytes (4, 16), blood sinusoids (vessels) (3),** and osteoclasts (6) in the eroded Howship's lacunae (5).

FUNCTIONAL CORRELATIONS

Bone Cells

Developing and adult bones contain four different cell types: osteoprogenitor cells, osteoblasts, osteocytes, and osteoclasts.

Osteoprogenitor cells are undifferentiated, pleuropotential stem cells that are derived from the connective tissue mesenchyme. These cells are located on the inner layer of connective tissue periosteum and in the single layer of internal endosteum that lines the marrow cavities, osteons (Haversian system), and perforating canals in the bone (see overview figure). The main functions of periosteum and endosteum are nutrition of bone and to provide a continuous supply of new osteoblasts for growth, remodeling, and repair of bones. During bone development, osteoprogenitor cells proliferate by mitosis and differentiate into osteoblasts, which then secrete collagen fibers and the bony matrix.

Osteoblasts are present on the surfaces of bone. Osteoblasts synthesize, secrete, and deposit osteoid, the organic components of new bone matrix. Osteoid is uncalcified and does not contain any minerals; however, shortly after its deposition, it is rapidly mineralized and becomes bone.

Osteocytes are the mature form of osteoblasts and are the principal cells of the bone; they are also smaller then osteoblasts. Like the chondrocytes in cartilage, osteocytes are trapped by the surrounding bone matrix that was produced by the osteoblasts. Osteocytes lie in the cavelike lacunae and are very close to a blood vessel. In contrast to cartilage, only one osteocyte is found in each lacuna. Also, because mineralized bone matrix is much harder than cartilage, nutrients and metabolites cannot freely diffuse through it to the osteocytes. Consequently, bone is highly vascular and possesses a unique system of channels or tiny canals called canaliculi.

Osteocytes are branched cells. Their cytoplasmic extensions enter the canaliculi, radiate in all directions from each lacuna, and make contact with neighboring cells through gap junctions. These connections allow the passage of ions and small molecules from cell to cell. The canaliculi contain extracellular fluid, and the gap junctions in the cytoplasmic extensions allow individual osteocytes to communicate with adjacent osteocytes and with materials in the nearby blood vessels. In this manner, the canaliculi form complex connections around the blood vessels and constitute an efficient exchange mechanism: Nutrients are brought to the osteocytes, gaseous exchange occurs between the blood and cells, and metabolic wastes are removed from the osteocytes. The canaliculi keep the osteocytes alive, and the osteocytes maintain the structural integrity of the surrounding bone matrix. When an osteocyte dies, the surrounding bone matrix is reabsorbed by osteoclasts.

Osteoclasts are large, multinucleated cells that are found along bone surfaces where resorption (removal), remodeling, and repair of bone take place. They do not belong to the osteoprogenitor cell line. The main function of osteoclasts is to resorb bone during remodeling (renewal or restructuring). Osteoclasts are often located on resorbed surfaces or in shallow depressions of the bone matrix called Howship's lacunae. Lysosomal enzymes released by osteoclasts erode these depressions. The multinucleated osteoclasts originate from the fusion of blood or hemopoietic progenitor cells that belong to the mononuclear phagocytic system.

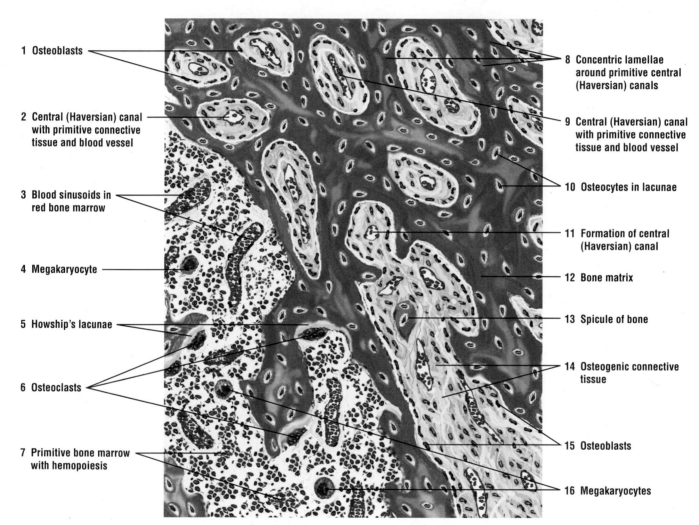

1 Osteoblasts

2 Central (Haversian) canal with primitive connective tissue and blood vessel

3 Blood sinusoids in red bone marrow

4 Megakaryocyte

5 Howship's lacunae

6 Osteoclasts

7 Primitive bone marrow with hemopoiesis

8 Concentric lamellae around primitive central (Haversian) canals

9 Central (Haversian) canal with primitive connective tissue and blood vessel

10 Osteocytes in lacunae

11 Formation of central (Haversian) canal

12 Bone matrix

13 Spicule of bone

14 Osteogenic connective tissue

15 Osteoblasts

16 Megakaryocytes

FIGURE 4.12 ■ Bone formation: development of osteons (Haversian systems) (decalcified bone, transverse section). Stain: hematoxylin and eosin. Medium magnification.

FIGURE 4.13 ■ Intramembranous Ossification: Developing Mandible (Decalcified Bone, Transverse Section)

This illustration depicts a section of mandible in the process of intramembranous ossification. External to the developing bone is the stratified squamous keratinized epithelium of the **skin (1)**. Inferior to the skin (1), the embryonic mesenchyme has differentiated into the highly vascular primitive **connective tissue (2),** with **nerves** and **blood vessels (9),** and a denser connective tissue **periosteum (3, 10).**

Below the periosteum (3, 10) is the developing bone. The cells in the periosteum (3, 10) have differentiated into **osteoblasts (6, 10)** and formed numerous anastomosing **trabeculae of bone (7, 11)** that surround the primitive **marrow cavities (8, 15).** In the marrow cavities (8, 15) are embryonic connective tissue cells and fibers, **blood vessels (4),** and nerves. Peripherally, collagen fibers of the periosteum (3, 10) are in continuity with fibers of the embryonic connective tissue of adjacent marrow cavities (3) and with collagen fibers within the **trabeculae of bone (7, 11).**

Osteoblasts (6, 10) actively deposit the bony matrix and are seen in a linear arrangement along the developing trabeculae of bone (7, 11). **Osteoid (14),** the newly synthesized bony matrix, is seen on the margins of certain bone trabeculae. The **osteocytes (5)** are located in lacunae of the trabeculae (7, 11). **Osteoclasts (13)** are large, multinucleated cells that are associated with bone resorption and remodeling during bone formation.

Although collagen fibers embedded in the bony matrix are obscured, the continuity with embryonic connective tissue fibers in the marrow cavities may be seen at the margins of numerous trabeculae (3).

Formation of new bone is not a continuous process. Inactive areas appear where ossification has temporarily ceased. Osteoid and osteoblasts are not present in these areas. In some primitive marrow cavities, fibroblasts differentiate into **osteoblasts (6, 10).**

FIGURE 4.14 ■ Intramembranous Ossification: Developing Skull Bone

A higher-power photomicrograph illustrates the development of skull bone by the process of intramembranous ossification. The connective tissue **periosteum (5)** surrounds the developing bone and gives rise the **osteoblasts (6)** that form the **bone (7).** Osteoblasts (6) are located along the developing **bony trabeculae (3).** Trapped within the formed bone (7) and the bony trabeculae (3) are the **osteocytes (2)** in their lacunae. Also associated with the bony trabeculae (3) are the multinuclear cells, **osteoclasts (8),** that remodel the developing bone. A primitive **marrow cavity (4)** with **blood vessels (9), blood cells (9),** and hematopoietic tissue is located between the formed bony trabeculae (3).

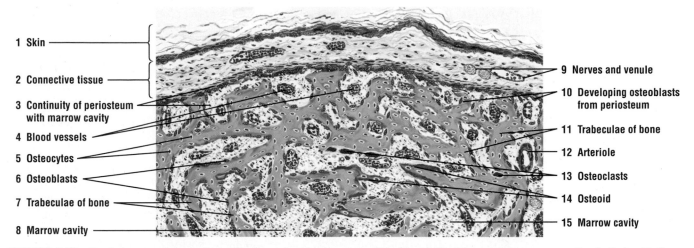

1 Skin
2 Connective tissue
3 Continuity of periosteum with marrow cavity
4 Blood vessels
5 Osteocytes
6 Osteoblasts
7 Trabeculae of bone
8 Marrow cavity

9 Nerves and venule
10 Developing osteoblasts from periosteum
11 Trabeculae of bone
12 Arteriole
13 Osteoclasts
14 Osteoid
15 Marrow cavity

FIGURE 4.13 ■ Intramembranous ossification: developing mandible (decalcified bone, transverse section). Stain: Mallory-Azan. Low magnification.

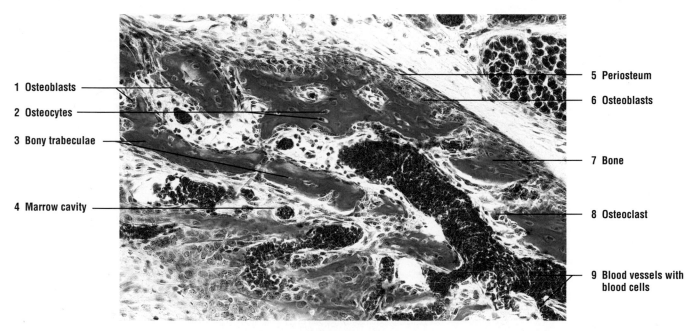

1 Osteoblasts
2 Osteocytes
3 Bony trabeculae
4 Marrow cavity

5 Periosteum
6 Osteoblasts
7 Bone
8 Osteoclast
9 Blood vessels with blood cells

FIGURE 4.14 ■ Intramembranous ossification: developing skull bone. Stain: Mallory-Azan. 64×

FIGURE 4.15 ■ Cancellous Bone with Trabeculae and Marrow Cavities: Sternum (Decalcified Bone, Transverse Section)

Cancellous bone consists primarily of slender bone **trabeculae (5)** that ramify, anastomose, and enclose irregular **marrow cavities** with **blood vessels (4)**. The **periosteum (2, 7)** that surrounds the trabeculae (5) of cancellous bone merges with adjacent dense irregular **connective tissue** with **blood vessels (1)**. Inferior to the periosteum (2, 7), the bone trabeculae (5) merge with a thin layer of **compact bone (9)** that contains a forming or **primitive osteon (6)** and a mature **osteon (Haversian system) (8)** with concentric lamellae.

Except for concentric lamellae in the primitive osteon (6) and mature osteon (8), the bone inferior to the periosteum (2, 7) and the bone trabeculae (5) exhibit parallel lamellae. **Osteocytes (3)** in lacunae are visible in trabeculae (5) and compact bone (9).

Between bone trabeculae (5) are the **marrow cavities** with **blood vessels (4)** and **hemopoeitic tissue (11)** that gives rise to new blood cells. Because of the low magnification, individual red and white blood cells are not recognizable. Lining the bone trabeculae (5) in the marrow cavities (4) is a thin, inner layer of cells called the **endosteum (10)**. Cells in the periosteum (2, 7) and in the endosteum (10) give rise to bone-forming osteoblasts.

FIGURE 4.16 ■ Cancellous Bone: Sternum (Decalcified Bone, Transverse Section)

This photomicrograph shows a section of cancellous bone from the sternum. Cancellous bone is composed of numerous **bony trabeculae (1)** that are separated by the **marrow cavity (5)**, in which are found **blood vessels (7)** and different types of **blood cells (8)**. Bony trabeculae (1) are lined by a thin, inner layer of cells called the **endosteum (4, 6)**. Osteoprogenitor cells in the endosteum (4, 6) give rise to osteoblasts. Formed bone matrix contains numerous **osteocytes in lacunae (2)**. Eroding or remodeling the formed bone matrix are the large, multinuclear cells called **osteoclasts (3)**. Osteoclasts (3) erode part of the bone and become housed in the eroded depressions called the Howship's lacunae.

FUNCTIONAL CORRELATIONS

Bone

Bones are dynamic structures. They are continually renewed or remodeled in response to mineral needs of the body, mechanical stress, bone thinning caused by age or disease, and fracture healing. Calcium and phosphate either are stored in the bone matrix or are released into the blood to maintain proper levels. Maintenance of a normal blood calcium level is critical to life, because calcium is essential for muscle contraction, blood coagulation, cell membrane permeability, transmission of nerve impulses, and other functions.

Hormones regulate the release of calcium into the blood and its deposition in bones. When the calcium level falls below normal, parathyroid hormone, which is released from the parathyroid glands, stimulates osteoclasts to resorb the bone matrix. This action releases more calcium into the blood. When the calcium level is above normal, a hormone called calcitonin, which is released by parafollicular cells in the thyroid gland, inhibits osteoclast activity and decreases bone resorption. These glands and hormones are discussed in more detail in Chapter 17.

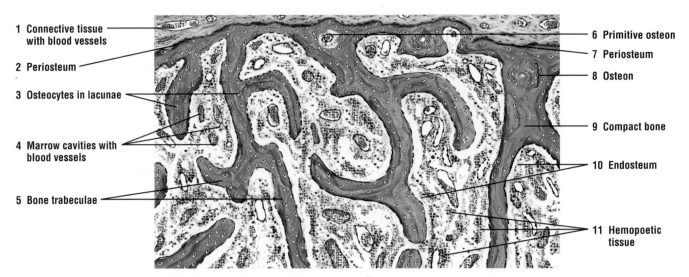

1 Connective tissue with blood vessels
2 Periosteum
3 Osteocytes in lacunae
4 Marrow cavities with blood vessels
5 Bone trabeculae
6 Primitive osteon
7 Periosteum
8 Osteon
9 Compact bone
10 Endosteum
11 Hemopoetic tissue

FIGURE 4.15 ■ Cancellous bone with trabeculae and marrow cavities: sternum (decalcified bone, transverse section). Stain: hematoxylin and eosin. Low magnification.

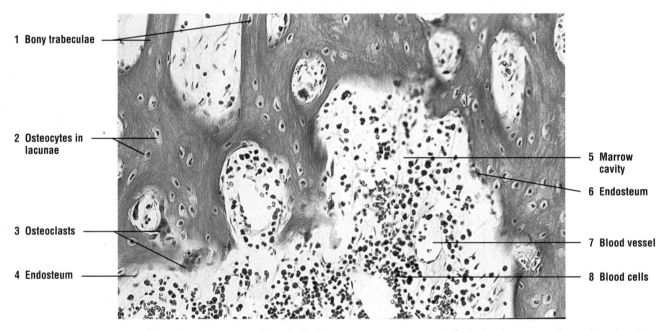

1 Bony trabeculae
2 Osteocytes in lacunae
3 Osteoclasts
4 Endosteum
5 Marrow cavity
6 Endosteum
7 Blood vessel
8 Blood cells

FIGURE 4.16 ■ Cancellous bone: sternum (decalcified bone, transverse section). Stain: hematoxylin and eosin. 64×

FIGURE 4.17 ▪ Compact Bone, Dried (Transverse Section)

This illustration depicts a transverse section of a dried compact bone. The bone was ground to a thin section to show empty canals for blood vessels, lacunae for osteocytes, and the connecting canaliculi.

The structural units of a compact bone matrix are the **osteons (Haversian systems) (3, 10)**. Each osteon (3, 10) consists of layers of concentric **lamellae (3b)** that are arranged around a **central (Haversian) canal (3a)**. Central canals are shown in cross section (3a) and in oblique section (10, middle leader). Lamellae are thin plates of bone that contain osteocytes in almond-shaped spaces called **lacunae (3c, 9)**. Radiating from each lacunae in all directions are tiny canals, the **canaliculi (2)**. Canaliculi (2) penetrate the lamellae (3b, 8), anastomose with canaliculi (2) from other lacunae (3c, 9), and form a network of communicating channels with other osteocytes. Some of the canaliculi (2) open directly into central (Haversian) canals (3a) of the osteon (3) and the marrow cavities of the bone. The small, irregular areas of bone between osteons (3, 10) are the **interstitial lamellae (5, 12)**, which represent the remnants of eroded or remodeled osteons.

External circumferential lamellae (7) form the external wall of a compact bone (beneath the connective tissue periosteum) and run parallel both to each other and to the long axis of the bone. The internal wall of the bone (the endosteum along the marrow cavity) is lined by **internal circumferential lamellae (1)**. Osteons (3, 10) are located between the internal circumferential lamellae (1) and external circumferential lamellae (7).

In living bone, the lacunae of each osteon (3c, 9) house osteocytes. The central canals (3a) contain reticular connective tissue, blood vessels, and nerves. The boundary between each osteon (3, 10) is outlined by a refractile line of modified bone matrix called the **cement line (4, 11)**. Anastomoses between central canals (3a) are called **perforating (Volkmann's) canals (6)**.

FIGURE 4.18 ▪ Compact Bone, Dried (Longitudinal Section)

This figure represents a small area of a dried compact bone that has been ground in a longitudinal plane. Because **central canals (1, 9)** course longitudinally, each central canal is seen as a vertical tube that shows branching. Central canals (1, 9) are surrounded by **lamellae (2)** with **lacunae (4)** and radiating **canaliculi (5)**. The lamellae (2), lacunae (4), and the osteon boundaries, or the **cement lines (3, 8)**, course parallel to the central canals (1, 9).

Other canals that extend in either a transverse or an oblique direction are called **perforating (Volkmann's) canals (7)**. Perforating canals (7) join the central canals (1, 9) of osteons and with the marrow cavity. The perforating canals (7) do not have concentric lamellae; instead, they penetrate directly through the lamellae (2).

1 Internal circumferential lamellae

6 Perforating (Volkmann's) canal

7 External circumferential lamellae

2 Canaliculi

3 Osteon (Haversian system)
  a. central (Haversian) canal
  b. lamellae
  c. lacunae

4 Cement line

5 Interstitial lamellae

8 Lamellae

9 Lacunae

10 Osteons (Haversian systems)

11 Cement line

12 Interstitial lamellae

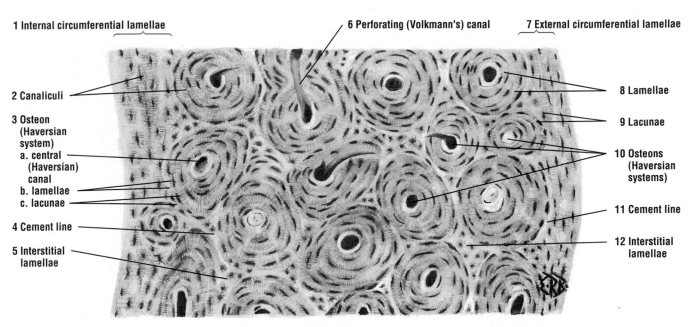

FIGURE 4.17 ■ Compact bone, dried (transverse section). Low magnification.

1 Central (Haversian) canals

2 Lamellae

3 Cement line

4 Lacunae

5 Canaliculi

6 Lamellae

7 Perforating (Volkmann's) canal

8 Cement lines

9 Central (Haversian) canal

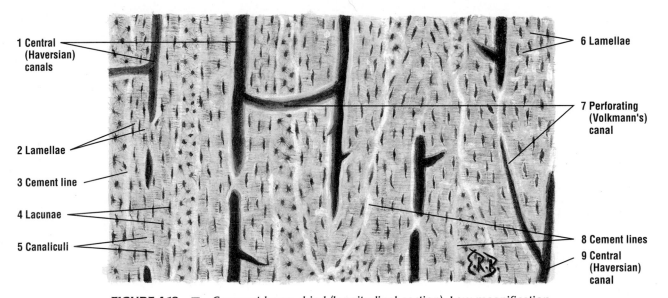

FIGURE 4.18 ■ Compact bone, dried (longitudinal section). Low magnification.

FIGURE 4.19 ■ Compact Bone, Dried: An Osteon (Transverse Section)

A higher-magnification view illustrates the details of one osteon and portions of adjacent osteons. Located in the center of the osteon is the dark-staining **central (Haversian) canal (3)**, which is surronded by the concentric **lamellae (4)**. Between adjacent osteons are the interstitial **lamellae (5).** The dark, almond-shaped structures between the lamellae (4) are the **lacunae (1, 7),** which house osteocytes in living bone.

Tiny **canaliculi (2)** radiate from individual lacunae (1, 7) to adjacent lacunae and form a system of communicating canaliculi (2) throughout the bony matrix and within the central canal (3). The canaliculi (2) contain tiny cytoplasmic extensions of the osteocytes. In this manner, osteocytes around the osteon communicate with each other and with the blood vessels in the central canals. The outer boundary of the osteon is separated by a **cement line (6).**

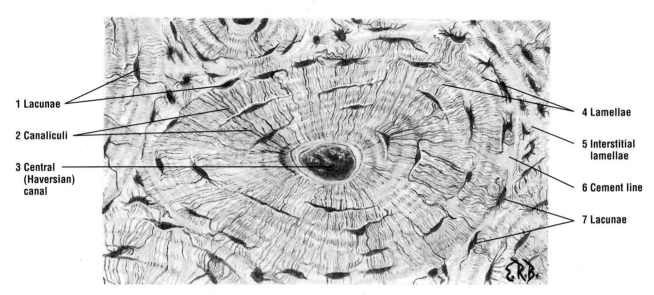

1 Lacunae

2 Canaliculi

3 Central (Haversian) canal

4 Lamellae

5 Interstitial lamellae

6 Cement line

7 Lacunae

FIGURE 4.19 ■ Compact bone, dried: An osteon (transverse section). High magnification.

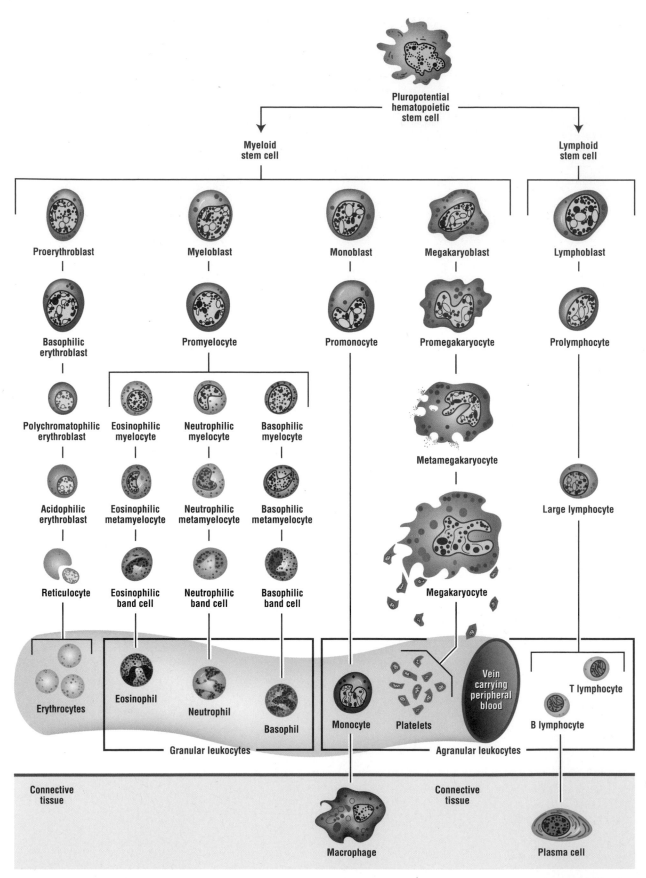

OVERVIEW FIGURE ■ Differentiation of a pluripotential hemopoietic stem cell into the myeloid stem cell line and lymphoid stem cell line during hemopoiesis.

CHAPTER 5

Blood

Blood is a unique form of **connective tissue** that consists of three major cell types: erythrocytes (red blood cells), leukocytes (white blood cells), and platelets (thrombocytes). These cells, which are also called the **formed elements** of blood, are suspended in a liquid medium called **plasma.** Blood cells transport gases, nutrients, waste products, hormones, antibodies, various chemicals, ions, and other substances in the plasma both to and from different cells in the body.

Hemopoieses

Blood cells have a limited life span, and as a result, they are continuosly replaced in the body by a process called **hemopoiesis.** In this process, all blood cells are derived from a single type of stem cell in **red bone marrow.** Because the stem cell is capable of producing all blood cell types, it is called the **pluripotential hemopoietic stem cell.** Pluritpotential stem cells produce two descendants that form pluripotential myeloid stem cells and pluripotential lymphoid stem cells. Before a mature blood cell is produced, the stem cells from each line undergo numerous divisions and exhibit several intermediate stages of differentiation (see the overview figure).

    Myeloid stem cells develop in red bone marrow and give rise to **erythrocytes, eosinophils, neutrophils, basophils, monocytes,** and **megakaryocytes. Lymphoid stem cells** also develop in red bone marrow. Some lymphoid cells remain in the bone marrow, proliferate, and become **B lymphocytes,** whereas others leave the bone marrow and migrate via the bloodstream to **lymph nodes** and the **spleen.** Here, they proliferate and differentiate into B lymphocytes.

    Early in their development, some undifferentiated lymphoid cells migrate to the **thymus gland,** where they proliferate and differentiate into immunocompetent **T lymphocytes.** Afterward, T lymphocytes enter the bloodstream and migrate to specific regions of peripheral lymphoid organs. Both B and T lymphocytes reside in numerous peripheral lymphoid tissues, lymph nodes, and the spleen. Here, they initiate immune responses when exposed to antigens.

    Because all blood cells have a limited life span, hemopoietic stem cells continually divide and differentiate to produce new progeny. When the blood cells wear out and die, they are destroyed in different lymphoid organs, such as the spleen (see Chapter 9).

Sites of Hemopoiesis

Hemopoiesis occurs in different organs of the body, depending on the stage of development of the individual. In the **embryo,** hemopoiesis initially occurs in the **yolk sac.** Later in development, it occurs in the liver, spleen, and lymph nodes. After birth, hemopoiesis continues almost exclusively in the red marrow of different bones. (In the newborn, all bone marrow is red).

    The active red bone marrow is highly cellular, and it consists of hemopoietic stem cells and precursors of different blood cells. Red marrow also contains a loose arrangement of fine reticular fibers. In adults, red marrow is found primarily in the flat bones of the skull, sternum and ribs, vertebrae, and pelvic bones. The remaining bones (normally the long bones) gradually accumulate fat. The marrow of these bones becomes yellow and loses its hemopoietic functions.

Major Blood Cell Types

Microscopic examination of a stained blood smear reveals the major blood cell types. **Erythrocytes,** or red blood cells, are nonnucleated cells, whereas **platelets** are cytoplasmic remnants of larger bone marrow cells called **megakaryocytes.** Erythrocytes and platelets both perform their major functions within the blood vessels.

In contrast, **leukocytes,** or white blood cells, perform their major functions outside the blood vessels. Leukocytes migrate out of the blood vessels through capillary walls and enter connective tissue, lymphatic tissue, and bone marrow. Leukocytes are **nucleated cells,** and they are subdivided into **granulocytes** and **agranulocytes,** depending on the presence or absence, respectively, of granules in their cytoplasm.

The primary function of leukocytes is to defend the body against bacterial invasion or the presence of foreign material. Consequently, most leukocytes are concentrated in the connective tissue.

Platelets

Platelets, or **thrombocytes,** are the smallest formed elements in the blood. They are present in the blood of all mammals and are the nonnucleated, cytoplasmic fragments of megakaryocytes, which are the largest cells in the bone marrow. Platelets are produced when small, uneven portions of the cytoplasm separate or fragment from the peripheries of the megakaryocytes.

The main function of platelets is to continually monitor the vascular system and detect any damage to the endothelial lining of the vessels. If a break is detected in the endothelial lining of a blood vessel, the platelets adhere to the damaged site and initiate a complex process that results in formation of a blood clot.

FIGURE 5.1 ■ Human Blood Smear

A smear of human blood examined at lower magnification illustrates the formed elements. **Erythrocytes** or **red blood cells (1)** are the most abundant elements and are the easiest to identify. Erythrocytes are enucleated (are without a nucleus) and stain pink with eosin. They are uniform in size and measure approximately 7.5 μm in diameter. Erythrocytes can be used as a size reference for other cell types.

Several leukocytes or white blood cells are also visible in the blood smear. Leukocytes are subdivided into categories according to the shape of their nuclei, the absence or presence of cytoplasmic granules, and the staining affinities of the granules. Two **neutrophils (2, 4),** one **eosinophil (7),** and one small **lymphocyte (5)** are visible. Scattered among the blood cells are small, blue-staining fragments called **platelets (3, 6).**

FIGURE 5.2 ■ Human Blood Smear: Red Blood Cells, Neutrophils, Large Lymphocyte, and Platelets

A photomicrograph of a human blood smear shows different blood cell types. The most numerous blood cells are the **erythrocytes** or **red blood cells (1).** Also visible are two **neutrophils (2, 4),** a **large lymphocyte (5),** and numerous **platelets (3).**

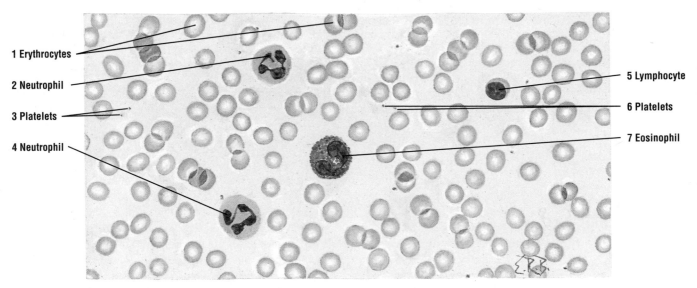

1 Erythrocytes
2 Neutrophil
3 Platelets
4 Neutrophil
5 Lymphocyte
6 Platelets
7 Eosinophil

FIGURE 5.1 ■ Human blood smear. Stain: Wright's stain. High magnification.

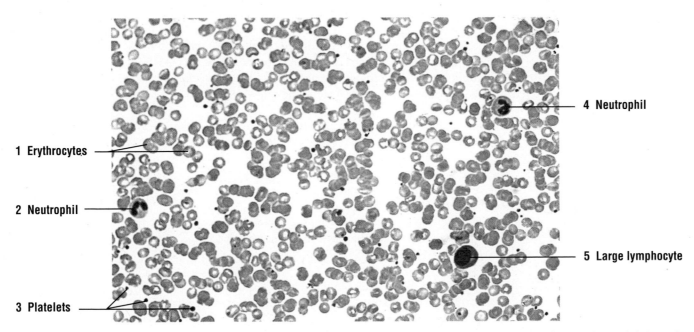

1 Erythrocytes
2 Neutrophil
3 Platelets
4 Neutrophil
5 Large lymphocyte

FIGURE 5.2 ■ Human blood smear: red blood cells, neutrophils, large lymphocytes, and platelets. Stain: Wright's stain. 205×

FIGURE 5.3 ■ Erythrocytes and Platelets

This illustration shows numerous **erythrocytes (1)** and the tiny **platelets (2)** that usually are seen in a blood smear. Blood platelets (2) are the smallest of the formed elements and are nonnucleated, cytoplasmic remnants of large-cell megakaryocytes, which are found in red bone marrow. Platelets (2) appear as irregular masses of basophilic (blue) cytoplasm, and they tend to form clumps in blood smears. Each platelet exhibits a light-blue peripheral zone and a dense central zone containing purple granules.

FIGURE 5.4 ■ Neutrophils

The leukocytes with granules and lobulated nuclei are the polymorphonuclear granulocytes, of which the **neutrophils (1)** are the most abundant. The neutrophil cytoplasm (1) contains fine violet or pink granules that are difficult to see with a light microscope. As a result, the cytoplasm (1) appears clear. The nucleus (1) consists of several lobes that are connected by narrow chromatin strands. Immature neutrophils (1) contain fewer nuclear lobes.

The neutrophils (1) constitute approximately 60% to 70% of the blood leukocytes.

FUNCTIONAL CORRELATIONS

Erythrocytes

Mature erythrocytes are specialized to transport **oxygen** and **carbon dioxide.** This specialization depends on the presence of the protein **hemoglobin** in the erythrocytes. Iron molecules in hemoglobin bind with oxygen molecules. As a result, most oxygen in the blood is carried in the form of **oxyhemoglobin,** which is responsible for the bright red color of arterial blood. Carbon dioxide diffuses from the cells and tissues into the blood and then is carried to the lungs partly dissolved in the blood and partly in combination with hemoglobin as **carbaminohemoglobin,** which gives venous blood its bluish color.

During differentiation and maturation, erythrocytes synthesize large amounts of hemoglobin. Before an erythrocyte is released into the systemic circulation, the nucleus is extruded from the cytoplasm, and the mature erythrocyte assumes a biconcave shape. This shape provides more surface area for carrying respiratory gases. Thus, mature mammalian erythrocytes in the circulation are **nonnucleated,** biconcave disks that are surrounded by a membrane and filled with hemoglobin and some enzymes.

The life span of erythrocytes is approximately 120 days, after which the worn-out cells are removed from the blood and phagocytosed by macrophages in the spleen, liver, and bone marrow.

Platelets

The main function of platelets is to promote **blood clotting.** When the wall of the blood vessel is broken or damaged, the platelets **adhere** to the damaged region of the wall, become activated, and release chemicals that initiate the very complex process of blood clotting. After a blood clot has formed and the bleeding ceased, the aggregated platelets contribute to **clot retraction.**

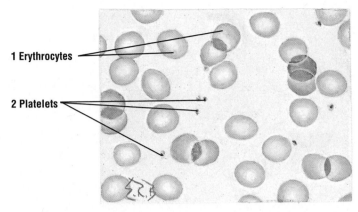

FIGURE 5.3 ■ Erythrocytes and platelets. Stain: Wright's stain. Oil immersion.

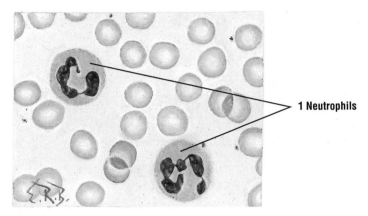

FIGURE 5.4 ■ Neutrophils. Stain: Wright's stain. Oil immersion.

FIGURE 5.5 ■ Eosinophils

Eosinophils (1) are identified in a blood smear by their cytoplasm, which is filled with distinct, large, eosinophilic (bright-pink) granules. The nucleus in eosinophils (1) typically is bilobed, but a small, third lobe may be present.

Eosinophils (1) constitute approximately 2% to 4% of the blood leukocytes.

FIGURE 5.6 ■ Lymphocytes

Agranular leukocytes have few or no cytoplasmic granules and exhibit round to horseshoe-shaped nuclei. **Lymphocytes (1, 2)** vary in size from cells that are smaller than erythrocytes to cells that are almost twice as large. For size comparison among lymphocytes and erythrocytes, this illustration of a human blood smear depicts a **large lymphocyte (1)** and a **small lymphocyte (2)** surrounded by the red-staining erythrocytes. In small lymphocytes (2), the densely stained nucleus occupies most of the cytoplasm, which appears as a thin, basophilic rim around the nucleus. The cytoplasm in lymphocytes is usually agranular, but it sometimes may contain a few granules. In large lymphocytes (1), basophilic cytoplasm is more abundant, and the larger and paler nucleus may contain one or two nucleoli.

Lymphocytes (1, 2) constitute approximately 20% to 30% of the blood leukocytes.

FIGURE 5.7 ■ Monocytes

Monocytes (1) are the largest agranular leukocytes. The nucleus (1) varies from round or oval to indented or horseshoe-shaped, and it stains lighter than the lymphocyte nucleus. The nuclear chromatin is finely dispersed in monocytes (1), and the abundant cytoplasm is lightly basophilic, with few fine granules.

Monocytes (1) constitute approximately 3% to 8% of the blood leukocytes.

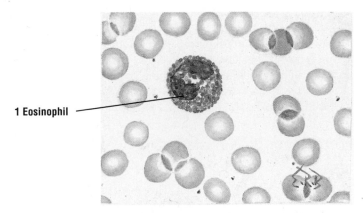

FIGURE 5.5 ■ Eosinophil. Stain: Wright's stain. Oil immersion.

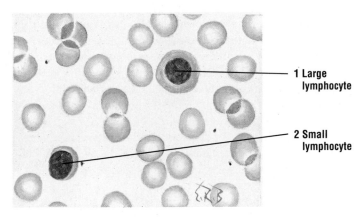

FIGURE 5.6 ■ Lymphocytes. Stain: Wright's stain. Oil immersion.

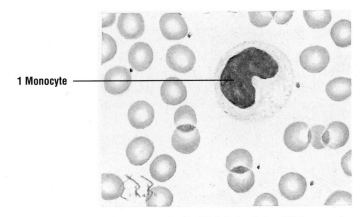

FIGURE 5.7 ■ Monocyte. Stain: Wright's stain. Oil immersion.

FIGURE 5.8 ■ Basophils

The granules in **basophils (1)** are not as numerous as in eosinophils (see Fig. 5–5); however, they are more variable in size, are less densely packed, and stain dark blue or brown. The nucleus is not lobulated and stains pale basophilic, but it is usually obscured by the density of the granules.

The basophils (1) constitute less than 1% of the blood leukocytes; therefore, they are the most difficult to find and identify.

FUNCTIONAL CORRELATIONS

Leukocytes

Neutrophils have a short life span. They circulate in the blood for approximately 10 hours and then enter the connective tissue, where they survive for another 2 or 3 days. Neutrophils are active **phagocytes.** They are attracted by **chemotactic factors** to microorganisms, especially bacterial, which they ingest and quickly destroy with their lysosomal enzymes.

Eosinophils also have a short life span. They remain in the blood for as long as 10 hours and then migrate into the connective tissue, where they remain for up to 10 days. Eosinophils are also **phagocytic** cells, with a particular affinity for **antigen-antibody complexes** that are formed during allergic conditions. The cells also increase in number during **parasitic infestation** and play an important role in the immune response to parasites.

Lymphocytes have a variable life span, ranging from days to months, and have a central role in the **immunological defense** of the body. Some lymphocytes (B lymphocytes), when stimulated by specific antigens, differentiate into **plasma cells** and produce **antibodies** to counteract or destroy the invading organisms.

Monocytes can live in the blood for 2 to 3 days, after which they move into the connective tissue, where they may remain for a few months or longer. Blood monocytes are precursors of the mononuclear phagocyte system. In the connective tissue, monocytes become powerful **phagocytes.** At the site of infection, monocytes differentiate into **tissue macrophages** and then destroy bacteria, foreign matter, and cellular debris.

Basophils have a short life span, and their function is similar to that of mast cells. Their granules contain **histamine** and **heparin.** Release of histamine is associated with severe allergic reactions. These reactions cause vascular changes that lead to increased fluid leakage from blood vessels and may result in hypersensitivity responses and anaphylaxis.

FIGURE 5.9 ■ Human Blood Smear: Basophil, Neutrophil, Red Blood Cells, and Platelets

A high-magnification photomicrograph of a human blood smear shows **erythrocytes (3),** a **basophil (1),** a **neutrophil (5),** and **platelets (4).** The basophil cytoplasm (1) is filled with dense **basophilic granules (2)** that obscure the nucleus. In contrast, the neutrophil cytoplasm (5) does not show granules, and its **nucleus** is **multilobed (6).**

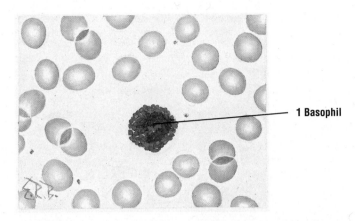

FIGURE 5.8 ■ Basophil. Stain. Wright's stain. Oil immersion.

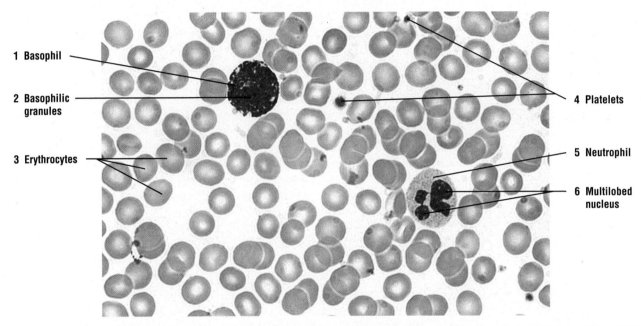

FIGURE 5.9 ■ Human blood smear: basophil, neutrophil, red blood cells, and platelets. Stain: Wright's stain. 320×

FIGURE 5.10 ■ Human Blood Smear: Monocyte, Red Blood Cells, and Platelets

A high-magnification photomicrograph shows numerous **erythrocytes (1)**, **platelets (2)**, and a large **monocyte (3)** with a characteristic, kidney-shaped nucleus and a nongranular cytoplasm.

FIGURE 5.11 ■ Hemopoiesis in Bone Marrow (Decalcified Section)

In a section of red bone marrow, all types of developing blood cells are difficult to distinguish. The cells are densely packed, and different cell types are intermixed. During the maturation process, hemopoeitic cells become smaller and their nuclear chromatin more condensed. As the blood cells pass through a series of developmental stages, they exhibit morphological changes and become identifiable microscopically.

This section of bone marrow is stained with hematoxylin and eosin. At this magnification, little differentiation of cytoplasm is visible. In the erythrocytic line, early **basophilic erythroblasts (7, 21)** are recognized by a large, but not very dense, nuclei and basophilic cytoplasm. These cells give rise to the smaller **polychromatophilic erythroblasts (8, 22)**, with a more condesed chromatin and a more variable color to the cytoplasm. The most recognizable cells of the erythrocytic line are **normoblasts (1, 23)**, which are characterized by small, dark-staining nuclei and a reddish or eosinophilic cytoplasm. Normoblasts (1, 23) exhibit **mitotic activity (6)** in the bone marrow. As normoblasts (1, 23) mature, they extrude their nuclei and become **erythrocytes (2)**. Erythrocytes (2) are abundant in bone marrow and can be seen here in a **sinusoid (4)**, **venule (13)**, and **arteriole (15)**. Cells of the erythrocytic lineage do not display any granules in their cytoplasm.

The early granulocytes initially exhibit numerous primary or azurophilic granules in their cytoplasm. As a result, the immature forms of neutrophils, eosinophils, and basophils are morphologically indistinguishable and become recognizable only at the myelocyte stage, when specific granules appear in quantity in their cytoplasm. In neutrophilic cells, the specific granules are only faintly stained, and the cytoplasm appears clear. In the eosinophilic line, the specific granules stain deep red or eosinophilic. Basophilic granulocytes are rarely observed in the bone marrow because of their small numbers. The cytoplasm of mature basophils exhibits a bilobed nucleus and dense blue or basophilic granules.

The granulocytic **myelocytes (12, 19)** exhibit a large, spherical nucleus and a cytoplasm with many azurophilic granules. The myelocytes (12) give rise to **metamyelocytes (3, 11, 20)**, the nuclei of which are bean- or horseshoe-shaped. The **neutrophilic metamyelocytes (17)** exhibit a deeply indented nuclei and cytoplasm with azurophilic granules and faintly stained, specific granules. In contrast, a cell with bright-staining red or eosinophilic granules in the cytoplasm is the **eosinophilic myelocyte (18)**.

The stroma of the reticular connective tissue in the bone marrow is almost obscured by hemopoietic cells. In less dense areas, the **reticular connective tissue (14)** and the elongated **reticular cells (9, 16)** are recognized. Different types of **blood vessels (4, 13, 15)** containing erythrocytes and leukocytes are seen in the bone marrow. Also conspicuous are large **adipose cells (5)**, each exhibiting a large vacuole (because of fat removal during section preparation) and a small, peripheral cytoplasm that surrounds the **nucleus (5)**. Other identifiable cells in the bone marrow are the large **megakaryocytes (10)** with varied nuclear lobulation.

Selected blood cells from the bone marrow are illustrated at the bottom at a higher magnification.

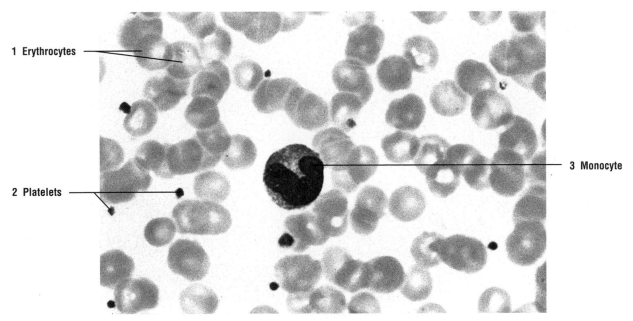

FIGURE 5.10 ▪ Human blood smear: monocyte, red blood cells, and platelets. Stain: Wright's stain. 320×

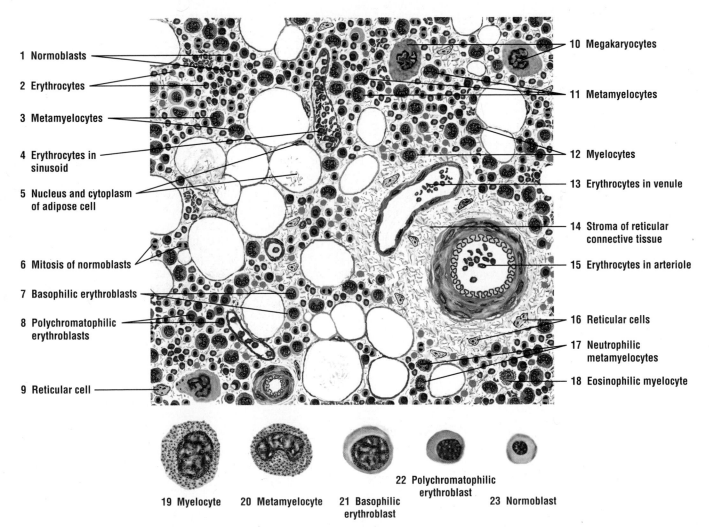

1 Normoblasts

2 Erythrocytes

3 Metamyelocytes

4 Erythrocytes in sinusoid

5 Nucleus and cytoplasm of adipose cell

6 Mitosis of normoblasts

7 Basophilic erythroblasts

8 Polychromatophilic erythroblasts

9 Reticular cell

10 Megakaryocytes

11 Metamyelocytes

12 Myelocytes

13 Erythrocytes in venule

14 Stroma of reticular connective tissue

15 Erythrocytes in arteriole

16 Reticular cells

17 Neutrophilic metamyelocytes

18 Eosinophilic myelocyte

19 Myelocyte   20 Metamyelocyte   21 Basophilic erythroblast   22 Polychromatophilic erythroblast   23 Normoblast

FIGURE 5.11 ▪ Hemopoiesis in bone marrow (decalcified section). Stain: hematoxylin and eosin. Upper image, high magnification; lower image, oil immersion.

FIGURE 5.12 ■ Bone Marrow Smear: Development of Different Cell Types

A bone marrow smear shows a few typical blood cells in different stages of development. In the erythrocytic series, the precursor cell, or **proerythroblast (3),** exhibits a thin rim of basophilic cytoplasm and a large, oval nucleus that occupies most of the cell. The chromatin is dispersed uniformly, and two or more nuclei may be present. Azurophilic granules are absent from the cytoplasm in all cells of the erythrocytic series. The proerythroblasts (3) divide to form the smaller, **basophilic erythroblasts (8, 16).**

Basophilic erythroblasts (8, 16) are characterized by a rim of basophilic cytoplasm and a decreased cell and nuclear size. The nuclear chromatin is coarse and exhibits the characteristic "checkerboard" pattern. Nucleoli are either inconspicuous or absent. Basophilic erythroblasts (8, 16) give rise to the **polychromatophilic erythroblasts (12),** which are similar in size than the basophilic erythroblasts (8, 16). The cytoplasm of the polychromatophilic erythroblast (12) becomes progressively less basophilic and more acidophilic because of increased accumulation of hemoglobin. The nuclei of polychromatophilic erythroblasts (12) are smaller and exhibit a coarse, "checkerboard" pattern.

When the polychromatophilic cells (12) acquire a more acidophilic (pink) cytoplasm because of increased hemoglobin accumulation, their size decreases, and they become **orthochromatophilic erythroblasts (normoblasts) (1).** These cells are capable of mitosis. Initially, the nucleus of orthochromatophilic erythroblasts (1) exhibits a concentrated, "checkerboard" chromatin pattern. Eventually, their nucleus decreases in size, becomes pyknotic, and is extruded from the cytoplasm, forming a biconcave cell with a bluish-pink cytoplasm called a reticulocyte or young erythrocyte. With special supravital staining, a delicate reticulum is seen in the reticulocyte cytoplasm because of the remaining polyribosomes (see Fig. 5-13). After polyribosomes are lost from the cytoplasm, the cells become mature **erythrocytes (9).** Erythrocytes (9) are small cells with a homogeneous acidophilic or pink cytoplasm.

Also visible in the bone marrow smear are different types of myelocytes and metamyelocytes of the granulocytic cell line. Myelocytes exhibit an eccentric nucleus with condensed chromatin and a less basophilic cytoplasm with few azurophilic granules. Different types of myelocytes exhibit varying number of granules. More mature myelocytes, such as the **neutrophilic myelocyte (14), eosinophilic myelocyte (15),** and the rare **basophilic myelocyte (11),** show an abundance of specific granules in their slightly acidophilic cytoplasm. The myelocyte is the last cell of the granulocytic line that is capable of mitosis, after which they mature into metamyelocytes.

The shape of the nucleus in the neutrophilic line changes from oval to indented, as seen in **neutrophil metamyelocytes (4).** Before complete maturation and segmentation of the nucleus into distinct lobes, the neturophils pass through a **band cell (10)** stage, in which the nucleus assumes a nearly uniform, curved rod or band shape.

Mature neutrophils (13) with segmented nuclei are also present in the bone marrow smear, as is a **mature eosinophil (7)** with specific pink granules filling its cytoplasm.

A section of a giant cell **megakaryocyte (17)** is visible. These cells measure approximately 80 to 100 m in diameter and have a large, slightly acidophilic cytoplasm that is filled with fine azurophilic granules. Cytoplasmic fragments derived from megakaryocytes are shed as **platelets (18).**

1 Orthochromatophilic erythroblasts (normoblasts)

2 Mitosis of orthochromatophilic erythroblast (normoblast)

3 Proerythroblast

4 Neutrophilic metamyelocyte

5 Eosinophilic metamyelocyte

6 Platelets

7 Mature eosinophil

8 Basophlic erythroblast

9 Mature erythrocytes

10 Neutrophil (band cell)

11 Basophilic myelocyte

12 Polychromatophilic erythroblast

13 Mature neutrophils

14 Neutrophilic myelocytes

15 Eosinophilic myelocyte

16 Basophlic erythroblast

17 Megakaryocyte

18 Platelets derived from megakaryocyte

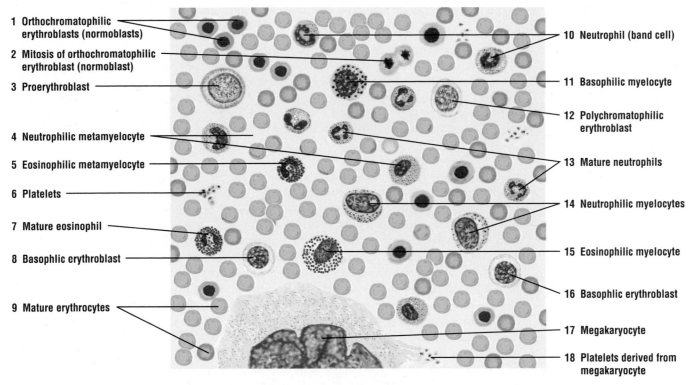

FIGURE 5.12 ■ Bone marrow smear: development of different blood cell types. Stain: Giemsa's stain. High magnification.

FIGURE 5.13 ■ Bone Marrow Smear: Selected Precursors of Different Blood Cells

This illustration shows, at a higher magnification, selected precursor cells of different blood cells that develop and mature in the red bone marrow.

A common stem cell gives rise to different hemopoietic cell lines, from which arise erythrocytes, granulocytes, lymphocytes, and megakaryocytes. Because of its ability to differentiate into all blood cells, this cell is called the pluripotential hemopoietic stem cell. Although this cell cannot be recognized microscopically, it resembles a large lymphocyte. In adults, the greatest concentration of pluripotential stem cells is found in the red bone marrow.

Development of Erythrocytes

In the erythrocytic cell line, the **pluripotential stem cell** differentiates into a **proerythroblast (1)**, which is a large cell with loose chromatin, one or two nucleoli, and a basophilic cytoplasm. The proerythroblast (1) then divides to produce a smaller cell called a **basophilic erythroblast (2)**, which has a rim of basophilic cytoplasm and a more condensed nucleus without visible nucleoli. In the next stage, a smaller cell called the **polychromatophilic erythroblast (3)** is produced. These cells show a decrease in basophilic ribosomes and an increase in the acidophilic hemoglobin content of their cytoplasm. As a result, staining these cells produces several colors in their cytoplasm. As differentiation continues, there is a further reduction in cell size, condensation of nuclear material, and a more uniform eosinophilc cytoplasm. At this stage, the cell is called an **orthochromatophilic erythroblast (normoblast) (4).** After extruding its nucleus, the orthochromatophilic erythroblast (4) becomes a **reticulocyte (5),** because a small number of ribosomes can be stained in its cytoplasm. After losing the ribosomes, the reticulocyte becomes a mature **erythrocyte (6).**

Development of Granulocytes

The **myeloblast (7)** is the first recognizable precursor in the granulocytic cell line. The myeloblast (7) is a small cell with a large nucleus, dispersed chromatin, three or more nucleoli, and a basophilic cytoplasm rim that lacks specific granules. As development progresses, the cell enlarges, acquires azurophilic granules, and becomes a **promyelocyte (8, 9)**. The chromatin in the oval nucleus is dispersed, and multiple nucleoli are evident. In more advanced promyelocytes, the cells become smaller, the nucleoli become inconspicuous, the number of azurophilic granules increases, and specific granules with different staining properties begin to appear in the perinuclear region. Promyelocytes (8, 9) divide to form smaller **myelocytes (10, 13, 14)**. The cytoplasm of myelocytes (10, 13, 14) is less basophilic and contains many azurophilic granules. Myelocytes differentiate into three kinds of granulocytes, which can only be recognized by the increased accumulation and staining of the specific granules in their cytoplasm, as seen in the **eosinophilic myelocyte (13)** with red or eosinophilic granules and the rare **basophilic myelocyte (14)** with blue or basophilic granules. Myelocytes develop into metamyelocytes.

The cytoplasm of the **neutrophilic metamyelocyte (11)** contains deep-staining azurophilic granules, lightly stained specific granules, and an indented, kidney-shaped nucleus. The **eosinophilic metamyelocytes (15)** are larger cells, and their specific cytoplasmic granules stain eosinophilic.

Megakaryoblasts (12) are large cells with a basophilic, homogeneous cytoplasm that is largely free of specific granules. The voluminous nucleus is ovoid or kidney-shaped, contains numerous nucleoli, and exhibits a loose chromatin pattern. Platelets are not formed at this stage.

During differentiation, megakaryoblasts (12) become very large. Their nucleus becomes convoluted, with multiple, irregular lobes that are interconnected by constricted regions. The chromatin becomes condensed and coarse, and nucleoli are not visible. In mature **megakaryocytes (17)**, the plasma membrane invaginates the cytoplasm and forms demarcation membranes. This delimits the areas of the megakaryocyte cytoplasm, which is then shed into the blood as small cell fragments in the form of **platelets (16).**

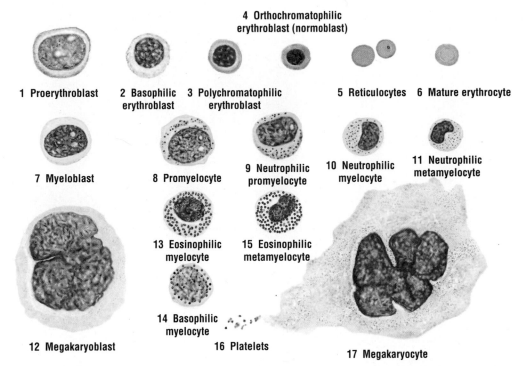

4 Orthochromatophilic erythroblast (normoblast)

1 Proerythroblast   2 Basophilic erythroblast   3 Polychromatophilic erythroblast   5 Reticulocytes   6 Mature erythrocyte

7 Myeloblast   8 Promyelocyte   9 Neutrophilic promyelocyte   10 Neutrophilic myelocyte   11 Neutrophilic metamyelocyte

13 Eosinophilic myelocyte   15 Eosinophilic metamyelocyte

14 Basophilic myelocyte

12 Megakaryoblast   16 Platelets   17 Megakaryocyte

FIGURE 5.13 ■ Bone marrow smear: selected precursor of different blood cells. Stain: Giemsa's stain. High magnification-oil immersion.

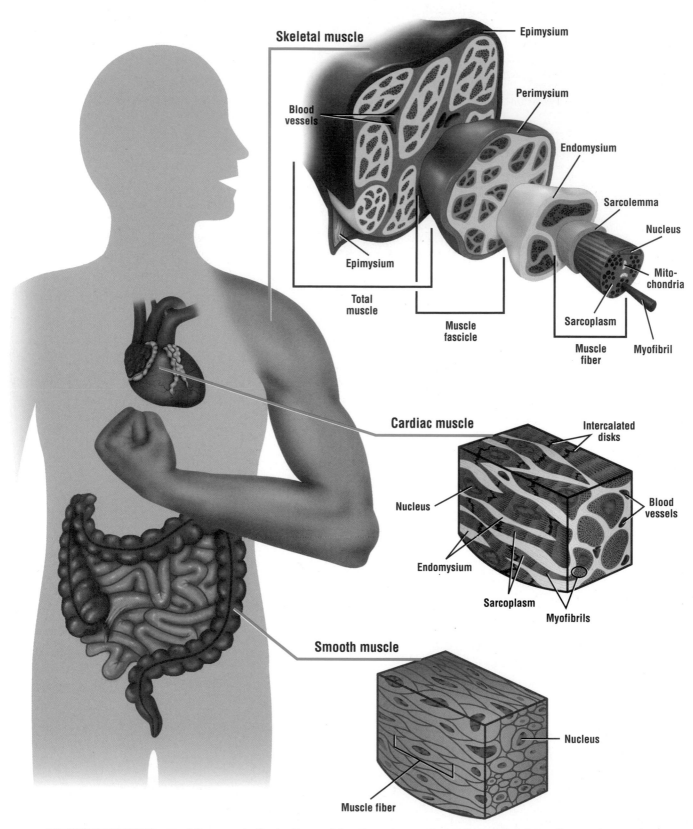

OVERVIEW FIGURE ■ Microscopic illustrations of the three types of muscles: skeletal, cardiac, and smooth.

CHAPTER 6

Muscle Tissue

There are three types of muscle tissues in the body: **skeletal muscle, cardiac muscle,** and **smooth muscle.** Each muscle type has structural and functional similarities as well as differences. All muscle tissues consist of elongated cells called **fibers.** The cytoplasm of muscle cells is called **sarcoplasm,** and the surrounding cell membrane or plasmalemma is called **sacrolemma.** Each muscle fiber sarcoplasm contains numerous **myofibrils,** which in turn contain two types of contractile protein filaments, **actin** and **myosin.**

Smooth Muscle

Smooth muscle has a wide distribution and is found in numerous organs. Smooth muscle fibers contain contractile actin and myosin filaments; however, they are not arranged in the regular, cross-striated patterns that are visible in both the skeletal and cardiac muscle fibers. As a result, these muscle fibers appear **smooth** or **nonstriated.** Smooth muscle fibers are also **involuntary muscles.** The fibers are small, spindle or fusiform in shape, and contain a single central **nucleus.**

Smooth muscle is often seen under a microscope as individual fibers or slender bundles called fascicles, and this type of tissue is predominantly found in the linings of **visceral hollow organs** and **blood vessels.** In the digestive tract, uterus, ureters, and other hollow organs, smooth muscles occur in large **sheets** or **layers.** Connective tissue surrounds individual muscle fibers as well as muscle layers. In the blood vessels, smooth muscle fibers are arranged in a circular pattern and control blood pressure by altering luminal diameters (see the overview figure).

Skeletal Muscle

Skeletal muscle fibers are long, **multinucleated cells** with peripheral nuclei. In their cytoplasm, the arrangement of the contractile protein actin and myosin filaments is very regular. As a result, these contractile filaments form distinct **cross-striation** patterns, which are seen under a microscope as light **I bands** and dark **A bands** in each muscle fiber. Because of these cross-striations, skeletal muscle is also called **striated muscle.**

Skeletal muscles are surrounded by a dense, irregular connective tissue layer called **epimysium.** From epimysium, a less dense, irregular connective tissue layer called **perimysium** extends inward and divides the interior of the muscle into bundles or **fascicles;** each fascicle is thus surrounded by perimysium. Thin connective tissue fibers called **endomysium** invest individual muscle fibers. Located in the different connective tissue sheaths are blood vessels, nerves, and lymphatics (see the overview figure).

Sensitive stretch receptors called **neuromuscular spindles** are located within nearly all skeletal muscles. These spindles consist of a connective tissue **capsule,** which contains modified muscle fibers called **intrafusal fibers** and numerous **nerve endings,** surrounded by a fluid-filled space.

Cardiac Muscle

Cardiac muscle is located primarily in the walls and septa of the **heart** and in the walls of the large vessels that are attached to the heart. Like skeletal muscle fibers, cardiac muscle fibers exhibit distinct **cross-striations,** because the actin and myosin filaments have a regular arrangement. In contrast to skeletal muscle fibers, cardiac muscle fibers exhibit one or two **central nuclei,** are shorter than skeletal muscle fibers, and are **branched.**

The terminal ends of adjacent cardiac muscle fibers show denser-staining, unique, end-to-end junctional complexes. These regions are special attachment sites called **intercalated disks.** Here, the opposing cell membranes contact each other and form **gap junctions.** Also, the intercalated disks are transverse lines that cross the cardiac cells at irregular intervals (see the overview figure).

FIGURE 6.1 ■ Smooth Muscle Layers of the Small Intestine (Transverse and Longitudinal Sections)

In the muscular region of the small intestine, smooth muscle fibers are arranged in two concentric layers: an inner circular layer and an outer longitudinal layer. Here, the muscle fibers are tightly packed, and the muscle fibers of one layer are arranged at right angles to the fibers of the adjacent layer.

The upper region of the illustration shows the smooth muscle fibers of the inner circular layer cut in longitudinal section. **Smooth muscle fibers (1, 7)** are spindle-shaped cells with tapered ends. The cytoplasm (sarcoplasm) of each muscle fiber stains dark. An elongated or ovoid **nucleus (7)** is in the center of each smooth muscle fiber.

The lower region of the illustration shows the muscles of the adjacent longitudinal layer cut in transverse section. Because the spindle-shaped cells are sectioned at different places along their length, the cells with their nuclei exhibit different shapes and sizes. Large **nuclei (5)** are seen only in those **smooth muscle fibers (5)** that have been sectioned through their center. Muscle fibers that were not sectioned through their center appear only as deeply stained areas of clear **cytoplasm (sarcoplasm) (3, lower leader; 9, lower leader)** or exhibit only a small portion of their nuclei.

In the small intestine, the smooth muscle layers are close to each other, with only a minimal amount of **connective tissue fibers** and **fibroblasts (2, 4, 8, 10)** between the two layers. Smooth muscle also has a rich blood supply, as evidenced by the numerous **capillaries (6, 11)** between individual fibers and layers.

FIGURE 6.2 ■ Smooth Muscle: Wall of the Small Intestine (Transverse and Longitudinal Sections)

A photomicrograph of the small intestine illustrates its muscular outer wall. The smooth muscle fibers are arranged in two layers: an **inner circular layer (7)** and an **outer longitudinal layer (8).** In the inner circular layer (7), a single **nucleus (1)** is visible in the center of the **cytoplasm (2)** of different fibers. In the outer longitudinal layer (8), when cut in transverse section, the **cytoplasm (5)** appears empty, and single **nuclei (6)** of individual muscle fibers are visible if the plane of section passes through them. Located between the two smooth muscle layers is a group of autonomic **neurons** of the **myenteric nerve plexus (3).** Small **blood vessels (4)** are seen between individual muscle fibers and muscle layers.

FUNCTIONAL CORRELATIONS

Smooth Muscle

Smooth muscle usually exhibits spontaneous, wave-like activity that passes in a slow, sustained contraction throughout the entire muscle. In this manner, smooth muscle produces a continuous contraction of low force and maintain **tonus** in hollow structures. In ureters, uterine tubes, and digestive organs, contraction of smooth muscle produces **peristaltic contractions,** which propel the contents along the lengths of these organs. In arteries and other blood vessels, smooth muscles regulate the luminal diameters.

Smooth muscle fibers also make close contacts with each other via specialized connections called **gap junctions.** These junctions allow rapid ionic communications between the smooth muscle fibers, resulting in coordinated activity in smooth muscle sheets or layers. Smooth muscles are **involuntary** muscles. They are innervated and regulated by nerves from postganglionic neurons, the cell bodies of which are loacted in the **sympathetic** and **parasympathetic divisions** of the **autonomic nervous system.** These innervations influence the rate and force of contractility. In addition, smooth muscle fibers contract and relax in response to nonneural stimulation, such as stretching or exposure to different hormones.

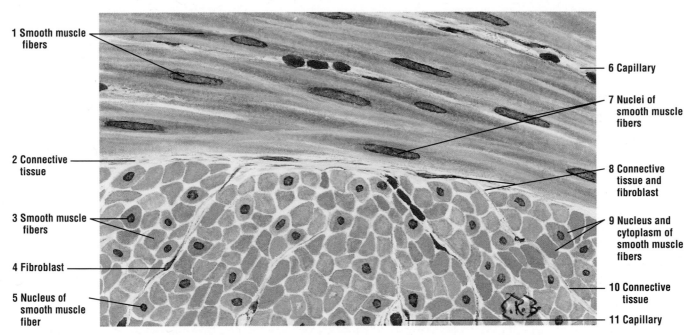

1 Smooth muscle fibers

2 Connective tissue

3 Smooth muscle fibers

4 Fibroblast

5 Nucleus of smooth muscle fiber

6 Capillary

7 Nuclei of smooth muscle fibers

8 Connective tissue and fibroblast

9 Nucleus and cytoplasm of smooth muscle fibers

10 Connective tissue

11 Capillary

FIGURE 6.1 ■ Smooth muscle layers of the small intestine. Stain: hematoxylin and eosin. High magnification.

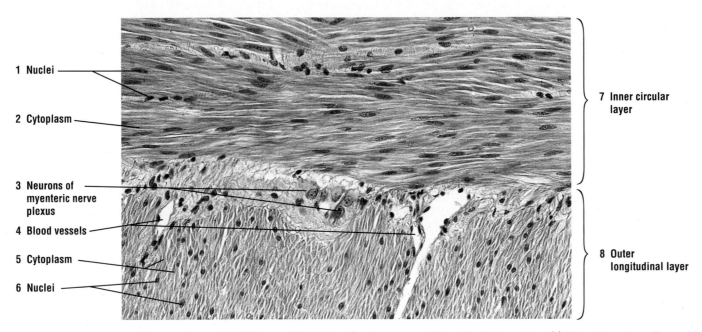

1 Nuclei

2 Cytoplasm

3 Neurons of myenteric nerve plexus

4 Blood vessels

5 Cytoplasm

6 Nuclei

7 Inner circular layer

8 Outer longitudinal layer

FIGURE 6.2 ■ Smooth muscle: wall of the small intestine (transverse and longitudinal sections). Stain: hematoxylin and eosin. 80×

FIGURE 6.3 ■ Skeletal (Striated) Muscles of the Tongue (Longitudinal and Transverse Sections)

Skeletal muscle fibers are much longer and larger in diameter than smooth muscle fibers. In the tongue, skeletal muscle fibers course in different directions. This illustration shows the tongue muscle fibers in both the longitudinal (upper region) and transverse (lower region) sections.

Each skeletal **muscle fiber (9, transverse section; 11, longitudinal section)** contains numerous nuclei; in other words, they are multinucleated. The **nuclei (1, 6)** are situated peripherally and immediately below the sarcolemma of each muscle fiber. (The sarcolemma is not illustrated.) Also, each skeletal muscle fiber shows **cross-striations (3),** which are visible as alternating dark or **A bands (3a)** and light or **I bands (3b).** With higher magnification, additional details of the cross-striations are illustrated in Figure 6-9.

Skeletal muscle fibers are aggregated into bundles or **fascicles (15)** and are surrounded by fibers of **connective tissue (5).** The connective tissue (5) sheath around each muscle fascicle is called **perimysium (12).** From each perimysium (12), thin partitions of connective tissue extend into each muscle fascicle (15) and invest individual muscle fibers (9, 11) with a connective tissue layer called **endomysium (4, 7).** Small **blood vessels (8)** and **capillaries (2, 14)** are present in the connective tissue (5) around each muscle fiber (9, 11).

Skeletal muscle fibers that are sectioned longitudinally (11) show light and dark cross-striations (3a, 3b). The muscle fibers that are sectioned transversely (9) exhibit cross-sections of **myofibrils (13)** and peripheral nuclei (6).

FIGURE 6.4 ■ Skeletal (Striated) Muscles of the Tongue (Longitudinal Section)

A higher-magnification photomicrograph of the tongue illustrates individual **skeletal muscle fibers (1)** and their **cross-striations (2).** Note the peripheral **nuclei (3)** and the tiny **myofibrils (6).** Surrounding each skeletal muscle fiber (1) is the thin layer of connective tissue called **endomysium (5).** Aggregates of muscle fibers, or fascicles, are invested by the thicker connective tissue layer called **perimysium (4).** Associated with the connective tissue (4) are the **adipose cells (7).**

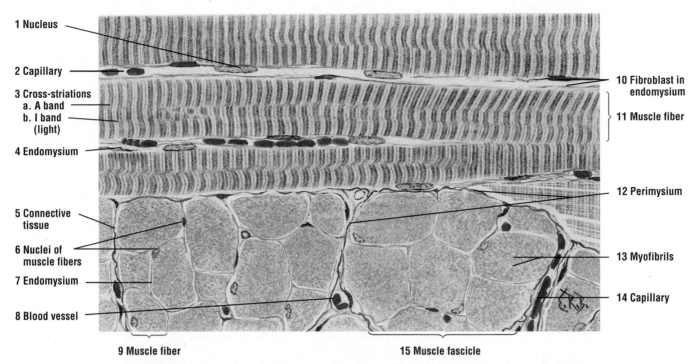

1 Nucleus
2 Capillary
3 Cross-striations
 a. A band
 b. I band
 (light)
4 Endomysium
5 Connective tissue
6 Nuclei of muscle fibers
7 Endomysium
8 Blood vessel
9 Muscle fiber

10 Fibroblast in endomysium
11 Muscle fiber
12 Perimysium
13 Myofibrils
14 Capillary
15 Muscle fascicle

FIGURE 6.3 ■ Skeletal (striated) muscles of the tongue. Stain: hematoxylin and eosin. High magnification.

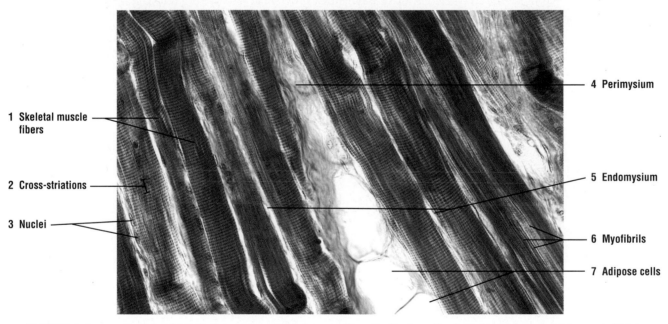

1 Skeletal muscle fibers
2 Cross-striations
3 Nuclei

4 Perimysium
5 Endomysium
6 Myofibrils
7 Adipose cells

FIGURE 6.4 ■ Skeletal (striated) muscles of the tongue (longitudinal section). Stain: Masson's trichrome. 130×

FIGURE 6.5 ■ Skeletal Muscle and Motor End Plates

A group of **skeletal muscle fibers (6, 7)** have been teased apart and stained to illustrate nerve terminations or myoneural junctions on individual muscle fibers. Note the characteristic **cross-striations (2, 8)** of the skeletal muscle fibers (7). The dark-stained, string-like structures between the separated muscle fibers (7) are the myelinated motor **nerves (3)** and their branches, the **axons (1, 5, 10).** The motor nerve (3) courses within the muscle, branches, and distrubutes its axons (1, 5, 10) to the individual muscle fibers (7). The axons (1, 5, 10) terminate on individual muscle fibers as specialized junctional regions called **motor end plates (4, 9).** The small, dark, round structures seen in each motor end plate (4, 9) are the terminal expansion of the axons (1, 5, 10). **Axons (1)** are also seen without motor end plates because of tissue preparation.

FUNCTIONAL CORRELATIONS

Skeletal Muscle and Motor End Plates

Skeletal muscles are **voluntary,** because the stimulation for their contraction and relaxation is under conscious control. Large motor nerves or axons innervate skeletal muscles. Near the skeletal muscle, the motor nerve branches, and a smaller axon branch individually innervates a single muscle fiber. As a result, skeletal muscle fibers contract only when they are stimulated by an axon. Also, each skeletal muscle fiber exhibits a specialized site where the axon terminates. This **neuromuscular junction** or **motor end plate** is the site where the impulse from the axon is transmitted to the skeletal muscle fiber.

The terminal end of each efferent axon contains numerous small **vesicles** that contain the neurotransmitter **acetylcholine.** Arrival of a nerve impulse, or an **action potential,** at the axon terminal causes the synaptic vesicles to fuse with the plasma membrane of the axon and release the acetylcholine into the **synaptic cleft,** a small gap between the axon terminal and cell membrane of the muscle fiber. The neurotransmitter then diffuses across the synaptic cleft, combines with **acetylcholine receptors** on the cell membrane of the muscle fiber, and stimulates the muscle to contract. An enzyme called **acetylcholinesterase,** located in the synaptic cleft near the surface of the muscle fiber cell membrane, inactivates or neutralizes the released acetylcholine. Inactivation of acetylcholine prevents further muscle stimulation and contraction until the next impulse arrives at the axon terminal.

1 Axon terminals

2 Cross-striations

3 Myelinated
  nerve

4 Motor end plates

5 Axons

6 Skeletal muscle
  fibers

7 Skeletal muscle
  fibers

8 Cross-striations

9 Motor end plates

10 Axons

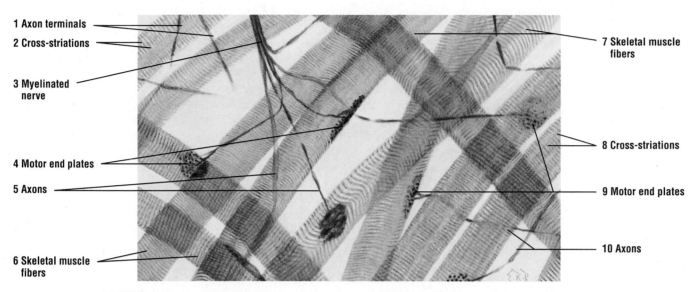

FIGURE 6.5 ■ Skeletal muscle and motor end plates. Stain: silver. High magnification.

FIGURE 6.6 ■ Skeletal Muscle and Muscle Spindle (Transverse Section)

A transverse section of an extraocular skeletal muscle shows individual **muscle fibers (2)** surrounded by connective tissue, the **endomysium (6).** In turn, the muscle fibers (2) are grouped into **fascicles (1)** that are surrounded by interfascicular connective tissue called **perimysium (4).** Located within the muscle fascicles (1) is a cross-section of a **muscle spindle (3).** Surrounding the muscle spindle (3) and the skeletal muscle fibers (2) are **arterioles (5)** in the perimysium (4).

The muscle spindle (3) is an encapsulated sensory organ. The connective tissue **capsule (8)** surrounding the muscle spindle (3) extends from the adjacent **perimysium (11)** and encloses several components of the spindle. The specialized muscle fibers located in the spindle and surrounded by the capsule (8) are called **intrafusal fibers (10)** [in contrast to the extrafusal **skeletal muscle fibers (7)** outside the spindle capsule (8)]. Small nerve fibers associated with the muscle spindles (3) are the myelinated and terminal unmyelinated **nerve fibers (axons) (9)** that are surrounded by the supportive neurolemmocytes (Schwann cells). Small blood vessels and an **arteriole (12)** from the perimysium (11) are found in and around the capsule of the muscle spindle (3).

FUNCTIONAL CORRELATIONS

Muscle Spindles

Muscle spindles are highly specialized **stretch receptors** that are located parallel to muscle fibers in nearly all skeletal muscles. Their main function is to detect changes in the length of muscle fibers. An increase in the length of muscle fibers stimulates the muscle spindle and sends **impulses** via the afferent axons into the spinal cord. These impulses result in a **stretch reflex** that immediately causes **contraction** of the **extrafusal muscle fibers,** thereby shortening the stretched muscle and producing movement. A decrease in skeletal muscle length stops the stimulation of the muscle spindle fibers and the conduction of its impulses to the spinal cord.

The simple stretch **reflex arc** illustrates the function of these receptors. Gently tapping the patellar tendon on the knee with a rubber mallet stretches the skeletal muscle and stimulates the muscle spindle. This action results in rapid muscle contraction of the stretched muscle and produces an involuntary response, or stretch reflex.

1 Fascicles

2 Skeletal muscle fibers

3 Muscle spindle

4 Perimysium

5 Arterioles

6 Endomysium

7 Extrafusal fibers

8 Capsule of muscle spindle

9 Nerve fibers with Schawann cells

10 Intrafusal fibers

11 Perimysium

12 Arteriole

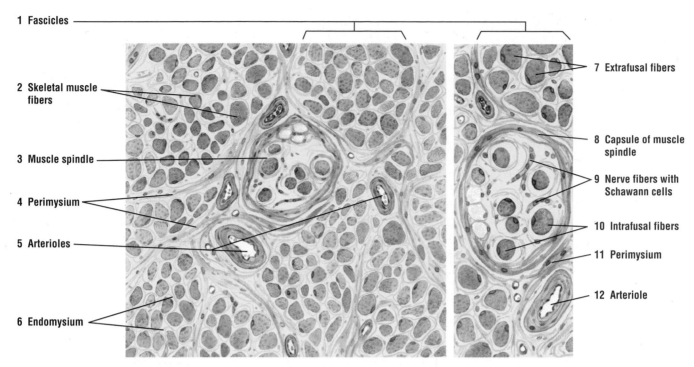

FIGURE 6.6 ■ Skeletal muscle and muscle spindle (transverse section). Frozen section stained with modified Van Giesen method (hematoxylin, picric acid-ponceau S). Left, medium magnification; right, high magnification. (Tissue samples courtesy of Dr. Mark DeSantis, WWAMI Medical Program, University of Idaho, Moscow, Idaho.)

FIGURE 6.7 ■ Cardiac Muscle

Cardiac muscle fibers exhibit some of the same features that are seen in skeletal muscle fibers. This illustration shows a section of a cardiac muscle cut in both the longitudinal (upper portion) and the transverse (lower portion) planes. The **cross-striations (2)** in cardiac muscle fibers closely resemble those in skeletal muscles, but the cardiac muscle fibers show **branching (5, 10)** without much change in their diameters. Also, each cardiac muscle fiber is shorter than a skeletal muscle fiber and contains a single, centrally located **nucleus (3, 7). Binucleate (two-nuclei) muscle fibers (8)** also occasionally are seen. The nuclei (7) are clearly visible in the center of each muscle fiber when they are cut in a transverse section. Around these nuclei (3, 7, 8) are the clear zones of nonfibrillar **perinuclear sarcoplasm (1, 13)**. In transverse sections, the perinuclear sarcoplasm (13) appears as a clear space if the section is not through the nucleus. Also visible in transverse sections are **myofibrils (14)** of individual cardiac muscle cells.

A distinguishing and characteristic feature of cardiac muscle fibers is the **intercalated disk (4, 9)**. These disks (4, 9) are dark-staining structures that are found at irregular intervals in the cardiac muscle, and they represent the specialized junctional complexes between adjacent cardiac muscle fibers.

The cardiac muscle has a vast blood supply. Numerous small blood vessels and **capillaries (6)** are found in the **connective tissue (11)** septa and the delicate **endomysium (12)** between individual muscle fibers.

Other examples of cardiac muscles are shown in Chapter 8.

FUNCTIONAL CORRELATIONS

Cardiac Muscle

Intercalated disks functionally couple all cardiac muscle fibers and rapidly spread stimuli for contraction of the heart muscle. The diffusion of ions through the pores in **gap junctions** between individual cardiac muscle fibers coordinates the heart functions and allows the cardiac muscle to act as a **functional syncytium,** thereby in turn allowing the stimuli for contraction to pass through the entire cardiac muscle.

Both the **parasympathetic division** and the **sympathetic division** of the autonomic nervous system innervate the heart. Nerve fibers from the parasympathetic division, by way of the vagus nerve, slow the heart and decrease the blood pressure. Nerve fibers from the sympathetic division produce the opposite effect, increasing both heart rate and blood pressure.

Additional information regarding cardiac muscle histology, heart pacemaker, Purkinje fibers, and heart hormones is presented in more detail in Chapter 8.

FIGURE 6.8 ■ Cardiac Muscle (Longitudinal Section)

A high-magnification photomicrograph illustrates a section of the cardiac muscle cut in the longitudinal plane. The **cardiac muscle fibers (2)** exhibit **cross-striations (4), branching (3),** and a single central **nucleus (5)**. The dark-staining **intercalated disks (1)** connect individual cardiac muscle fibers (2). Small **myofibrils (6)** are visible within each cardiac muscle fiber. Delicate strands of **connective tissue fibers (7)** surround the individual cardiac muscle fibers.

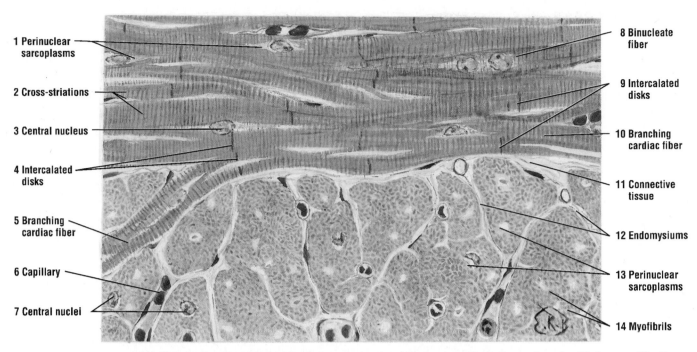

1 Perinuclear sarcoplasms
2 Cross-striations
3 Central nucleus
4 Intercalated disks
5 Branching cardiac fiber
6 Capillary
7 Central nuclei

8 Binucleate fiber
9 Intercalated disks
10 Branching cardiac fiber
11 Connective tissue
12 Endomysiums
13 Perinuclear sarcoplasms
14 Myofibrils

FIGURE 6.7 ■ Cardiac muscle (longitudinal and transverse sections). Stain: hematoxylin and eosin. High magnification.

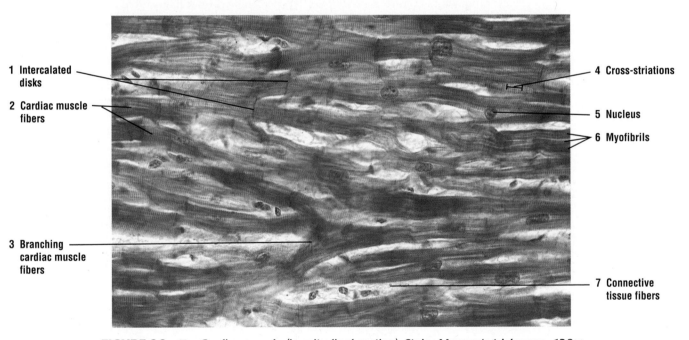

1 Intercalated disks
2 Cardiac muscle fibers
3 Branching cardiac muscle fibers

4 Cross-striations
5 Nucleus
6 Myofibrils
7 Connective tissue fibers

FIGURE 6.8 ■ Cardiac muscle (longitudinal section). Stain: Masson's trichrome. 130×

FIGURE 6.9 ■ Skeletal Muscle (Longitudinal Section)

A high-magnification illustration shows greater detail of individual skeletal muscle fibers. A cell membrane, or **sarcolemma (4)**, surrounds each skeletal **muscle fiber (2).** Note the peripheral location of the muscle fiber **nuclei (1, 15)** and their flattened appearance. Adjacent to the nuclei (1, 15) is the thin cytoplasm, or **sarcoplasm (6),** with its organelles. Each muscle fiber (2) consists of **individual myofibrils (13)** that are arranged longitudinally. Myofibrils (13) are best seen in cross-sections of the skeletal muscle fibers (see Fig. 6-3, label 13). Surrounding each skeletal muscle fiber (2) is a thin connective tissue, the **endomysium (14),** containing connective tissue cells called **fibrocytes (3, 11).** Blood vessels and **capillaries (12)** with blood cells are found in the endomysium (14).

At higher magnification, the cross-striations of skeletal muscle fibers are recognized as the light-staining **I bands (6)** and dark-staining **A bands (7).** Each A band (7) is bisected by the lighter H band and the darker **M line (8).** Crossing the central region of each I band is a distinct, narrow **Z line (9).** The cellular segments between the Z lines (9) represent a **sarcomere (10),** which is the structural and functional unit of striated muscles (both skeletal and cardiac). When the myofibrils (13) are seperated from the muscle fiber (2), the A and I bands as well as the Z lines remain visible. The close longitudinal arrangement of parallel myofibrils give the skeletal muscle fibers their striated appearance.

FIGURE 6.10 ■ Cardiac Muscle (Longitudinal Section)

Comparison of cardiac muscle fibers with skeletal muscles at higher magnification and using the same stain illustrates the similarities and differences between the two types of muscle tissue.

The **cross-striations (1)** are similar in both skeletal and cardiac muscle fibers, but they are less prominent in cardiac muscle fibers. The branching **cardiac fibers (9)** of the cardiac muscle are in contrast to the individual, elongated fibers of the skeletal muscle. The characteristic **intercalated disks (5, 7)** of cardiac muscle fibers and their irregular structure are more prominent at higher magnification. The intercalated disks (5, 7) appear either as straight bands (5) or staggered (7).

The large, oval **nuclei (3),** usually one per cell, occupy the central position of the cardiac fibers, in contrast to the numerous flattened and peripheral nuclei in each skeletal muscle fiber. Surrounding the nucleus of a cardiac muscle fiber is a prominent **perinuclear sarcoplasm (2, 10)** that is devoid of cross-striations and myofibrils.

The connective tissue **fibrobcytes (6, 8)** and fine connetive tissue fibers of the **endomysium (4)** surround the cardiac muscle fibers. **Capillaries** with **erythrocytes (11)** are normally seen in the endomysium (4, 6, 8).

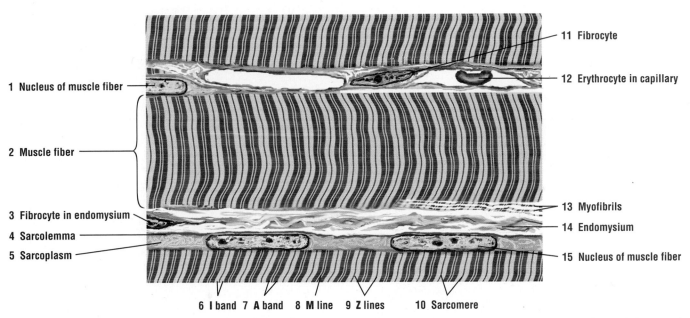

1 Nucleus of muscle fiber

2 Muscle fiber

3 Fibrocyte in endomysium

4 Sarcolemma

5 Sarcoplasm

11 Fibrocyte

12 Erythrocyte in capillary

13 Myofibrils

14 Endomysium

15 Nucleus of muscle fiber

6 I band   7 A band   8 M line   9 Z lines   10 Sarcomere

FIGURE 6.9 ■ Skeletal muscle fibers (longitudinal section). Stain: hematoxylin and eosin. Plastic section. High magnification.

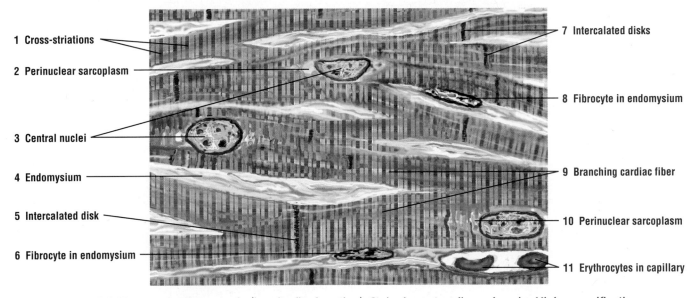

1 Cross-striations

2 Perinuclear sarcoplasm

3 Central nuclei

4 Endomysium

5 Intercalated disk

6 Fibrocyte in endomysium

7 Intercalated disks

8 Fibrocyte in endomysium

9 Branching cardiac fiber

10 Perinuclear sarcoplasm

11 Erythrocytes in capillary

FIGURE 6.10 ■ Cardiac muscle (longitudinal section). Stain: hematoxylin and eosin. High magnification.

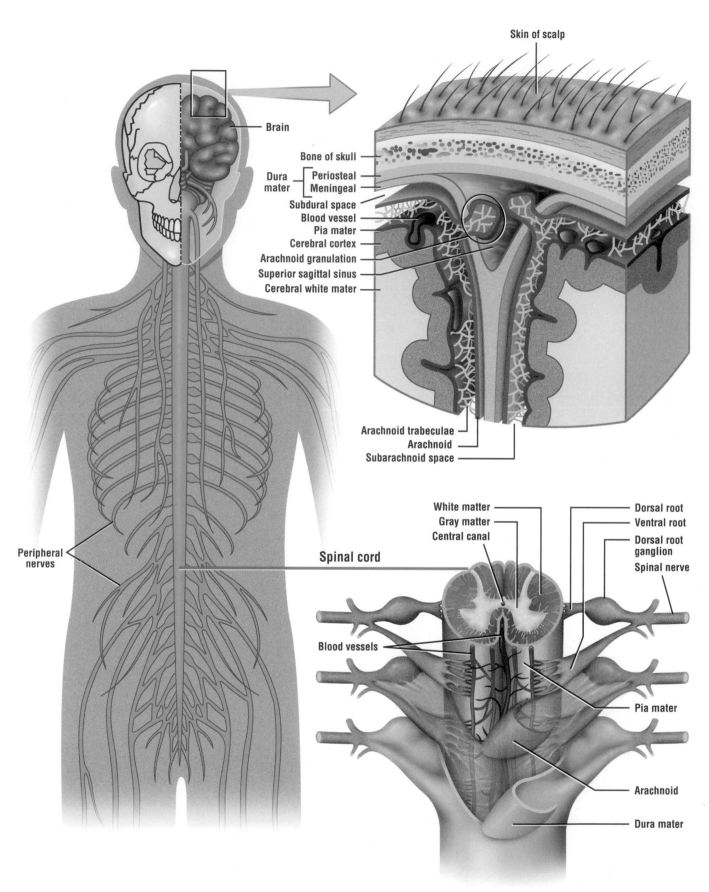

Skin of scalp

Brain

Bone of skull

Dura mater
- Periosteal
- Meningeal

Subdural space
Blood vessel
Pia mater
Cerebral cortex
Arachnoid granulation
Superior sagittal sinus
Cerebral white mater

Arachnoid trabeculae
Arachnoid
Subarachnoid space

Peripheral nerves

White matter
Gray matter
Central canal

Dorsal root
Ventral root
Dorsal root ganglion
Spinal nerve

Spinal cord

Blood vessels

Pia mater

Arachnoid

Dura mater

OVERVIEW FIGURE–CENTRAL NERVOUS SYSTEM ■ The central nervous system is composed of the brain and spinal cord. A section of the brain and spinal cord is illustrated here with their protective connective tissue layers called meninges (dura mater, arachoid, and pia mater).

120

CHAPTER 7

Nervous Tissue

SECTION 1 ■ Central Nervous System (Brain and Spinal Cord)

The mammalian nervous system is divided into two major parts, the **central nervous system (CNS)** and the **peripheral nervous system (PNS).** The CNS consists of the **brain** and the **spinal cord.** The components of the PNS—the cranial and spinal nerves—are located outside the CNS.

Protective Layers of the CNS

Because the nervous tissue is very delicate, bones, connective tissue layers, and a watery cerebrospinal fluid (CSF) surround and protect the brain and the spinal cord. Inferior to the cranial bones in the skull and the vertebral foramen in the vertebrae are the **meninges,** a connective tissue that consists of three layers: the dura mater, the arachnoid, and the pia mater (Overview Figure—Central Nervous System).

The most superficial meningeal layer is the **dura mater,** a tough, strong, thick layer of dense connective tissue fibers. Inferior to the dura mater is a more delicate connective tissue, the **arachnoid.** The dura mater and arachnoid surround the brain and spinal cord, respectively, on their external surfaces. The innermost meningeal layer is a delicate connective tissue, the **pia mater;** this layer contains numerous blood vessels and adheres directly to the surfaces of the brain and spinal cord.

Between the arachnoid and the pia mater is the **subarachnoid space.** Delicate, web-like strands of collagen and elastic fibers attach the arachnoid to the pia mater. Circulating in the subarachnoid space, the CSF bathes and protects the brain and spinal cord.

Cerebrospinal Fluid

The **cerebrospinal fluid (CSF)** is a clear, colorless fluid that cushions the brain and spinal cord and gives them buoyancy as a means of protection from physical injuries. The CSF fluid is continually produced by the **choroid plexuses** in the lateral, third, and fourth **ventricles** (or cavities) of the brain. Choroid plexuses are small, vascular extensions into the ventricles that are covered by epithelium. The CSF circulates through the ventricles and spinal cord (central canal) and around the outer surfaces of the brain and spinal cord in the subarachnoid space.

The CSF is important for homeostasis and brain metabolism. It brings nutrients to nourish brain cells, removes metabolites from brain cells that enter the CSF, and provides an optimal chemical environment for neuronal functions and impulse conduction. After circulation, the CSF is reabsorbed from the arachnoid space via the **arachnoid villi** into the venous blood of the superior sagittal sinus that drains the brain. Arachnoid villi are small, thin-walled, arachnoid extensions that project into the venous sinuses of the dura mater.

Morphology of a Typical Neuron

The structural and functional cells of the nervous tissue are the **neurons.** (The structure of a neuron and the type of neurons are shown in Overview Figure 7—Peripheral Nervous System.) Although neurons vary in size and shape, a general structure can be described. Each neuron consists of a **cell body** or **perikaryon,** numerous **dendrites,** and a single **axon.** The cell body of the neuron consists of cytoplasm containing numerous organelles, a nucleus, and a nucleolus. Projecting from the cell body are numerous cytoplasmic extensions, called dendrites, that are specialized to receive information from other dendrites, neurons, or axons. Axons conduct impulses away from neurons.

Neurons form a highly complex **intercommunicating network** of nerve cells that receive and conduct **impulses** along their axons to the CNS for analysis, integration, interpretation, and response. The appropriate response to a given stimulus from the neurons of the CNS is the activation of muscles (smooth or cardiac) and/or glands (endocrine or exocrine).

Types of Neurons in the CNS

The CNS contains three major types of neurons: multipolar, bipolar, and unipolar. This anatomic classification is based on the number of dendrites and axons that originate from the cell body.

- *Multipolar neurons.* These are the most common type in the CNS, and they include all **motor neurons** and **interneurons** of the brain and spinal cord. Projecting from the cell body of a multipolar neuron are numerous branched dendrites. On the opposite side of a multipolar neuron is a single axon.
- *Bipolar neurons.* These are not as common as multipolar neurons and are purely **sensory neurons.** In bipolar neurons, a single dendrite and a single axon are associated with the cell body. Bipolar neurons are found in the retina of the eye, in the organ of hearing in the inner ear, and in the olfactory epithelium in the upper region of the nose.
- *Unipolar neurons.* Most neurons in the adult organism that exhibit only one process leaving the cell body were initially bipolar during embryonic development. The unipolar neurons (formerly called **pseudounipolar neurons**) are also **sensory neurons.** Unipolar neurons are found in numerous craniosacral ganglia (located in the cranial and sacral regions of the spinal cord) of the body.

Myelin Sheath and Myelination of Axons

Highly specialized cells in both the CNS and the PNS move around the axon numerous times to build up successive layers of the cell membrane and form a lipid-rich, insulating sheath around the axon called a **myelin sheath.** Interspersed along the length of a myelinated axon are small gaps in the myelin sheath between individual cells that myelinate the axons. These gaps are called **neurofibrillar nodes** (of Ranvier). Axons in the CNS and PNS can be either myelinated or unmyelinated.

In the PNS, all axons are surrounded by **neurolemmocytes** (Schwann cells). Some axons are myelinated, whereas other axons are only embedded in the cytoplasm of neurolemmocytes and have no myelin sheath. The neurolemmocytes extend along the length of the peripheral axon, from its origin to its termination in the muscle or gland. Neurolemmocytes of the PNS are equivalent to the neuroglial cells, or **oligodendrocytes,** of the CNS, which myelinate CNS axons.

Smaller axons in the peripheral nerves, such as those in the nerves of the autonomic nervous system, are surrounded only by the neurolemmocyte cytoplasm. Such axons do not exhibit a myelin sheath and are called unmyelinated axons. The cytoplasm of a single neurolemmocyte may surround either a single axon or a group of axons.

White and Gray Matter

The brain and the spinal cord contain both gray matter and white matter. The **gray matter** of the CNS consists of neurons, their dendrites, and the supportive cells called **neuroglia.** This region represents the site of synapses between a multitude of neurons and dendrites. The size, shape, and mode of branching of these neurons are highly variable, however, and depend on which region of the CNS is being examined.

White matter in the CNS is devoid of neurons and consists primarily of myelinated axons. The myelin sheath around the axons imparts a white color to this region. (Conversely, the lack of myelin imparts a gray color to the gray matter of the CNS.) In addition to myelinated axons, white matter also contains some unmyelinated axons and the supportive neuroglial cells.

Supporting Cells in the CNS: Neuroglia

Neuroglia are the highly branched, supportive, nonneuronal cells in the CNS that are located between the neurons. These cells do not become stimulated or conduct impulses, and they are morphologically and functionally different from the neurons. They can be distinguished by their much smaller size and their dark-staining nuclei. The CNS contains approximately 10-fold more neuroglial cells than neurons. The four types of neuroglial cells are **astrocytes, oligodendrocytes, microglia,** and **ependymal cells.**

FIGURE 7.1 ■ Spinal Cord: Midthoracic Region (Transverse Section)

A transverse section of a spinal cord cut in the midthoracic region and stained with hematoxylin and eosin is illustrated. Although a basic structural pattern is seen throughout the spinal cord, the shape and structure of the cord vary at different levels (cervical, thoracic, lumbar, and sacral).

The thoracic region of the spinal cord differs from the cervical region illustrated in Figure 7-3. The thoracic spinal cord exhibits slender **posterior gray horns (6)** and smaller **anterior gray horns (10, 20)** with fewer **motor neurons.** The **lateral gray horns (8, 19),** on the other hand, are well developed in the thoracic region. These contain the **motor neurons** of the sympathetic division of the autonomic nervous system.

The remaining structures in the midthoracic region of the spinal cord closely correspond to the structures illustrated in the cervical cord region in Figure 7-3. These are the **posterior median sulcus (15), anterior median fissure (22), fasciculus gracilis (16),** and **fasciculus cuneatus (17)** (seen in the mid to upper thoracic region) of the **posterior white column (16, 17), lateral white column (7), central canal (9),** and **gray commissure (18).** Associated with the posterior gray horns (6) are axons of the **posterior roots (5),** and leaving the anterior gray horns (10, 20) are the **axons (21)** of the **anterior roots (11).**

Surrounding the spinal cord are the connective tissue layers of the meninges: the thick and fibrous outer **dura mater (2),** the thinner and middle **arachnoid (3),** and the delicate inner **pia mater (4),** which closely adheres to the surface of the spinal cord. Located in the pia mater (4) are numerous anterior and posterior **spinal blood vessels (1, 12)** of various sizes. Between the arachnoid (3) and the pia mater (4) is the **subarachnoid space (14).** Fine trabeculae in the subarachnoid space (14) connect the pia mater (4) with the arachnoid (3). In life, the subarachnoid space (14) is filled with CSF. Between the arachnoid (3) and the dura mater (2) is the **subdural space (13).** In this preparation, the subdural space (13) appears unusually large because of the artifactual retraction of the arachnoid during the specimen preparation.

FIGURE 7.2 ■ Spinal Cord: Anterior Gray Horn, Motor Neurons, and Adjacent Anterior White Matter

A higher magnification of a small section of the spinal cord illustrates the appearance of gray matter, white matter, neurons, neuroglia, and axons stained with hematoxylin and eosin. The cells in the anterior gray horn of the thoracic region of the spinal cord are **multipolar motor neurons (2, 6).** Their cytoplasm is characterized by a prominent vesicular **nucleus (7),** a distinct **nucleolus (7),** and coarse clumps of basophilic material called **Nissl substance (3).** Nissl substance extends into the **dendrites (5)** but not into the axons. One such neuron exhibits the root of an axon from the **axon hillock (4),** which is devoid of Nissl substance.

The nonneural **neuroglia (8),** seen here only as basophilic nuclei, are small in comparison to the prominent multipolar neurons (2, 6). Neuroglia (8) occupy the spaces between the neurons. The anterior white matter of the spinal cord contains myelinated axons of various sizes. Because of the histologic preparation of this section, the myelin sheaths appear as clear spaces around the dark-staining **axons (1).**

In certain neurons (2), the plane of section did not include the nucleus, and the cytoplasm appears enucleated (without nucleus).

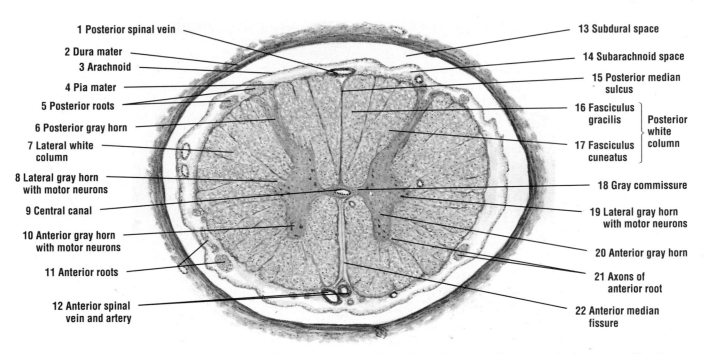

1 Posterior spinal vein
2 Dura mater
3 Arachnoid
4 Pia mater
5 Posterior roots
6 Posterior gray horn
7 Lateral white column
8 Lateral gray horn with motor neurons
9 Central canal
10 Anterior gray horn with motor neurons
11 Anterior roots
12 Anterior spinal vein and artery

13 Subdural space
14 Subarachnoid space
15 Posterior median sulcus
16 Fasciculus gracilis ⎫ Posterior
17 Fasciculus cuneatus ⎭ white column
18 Gray commissure
19 Lateral gray horn with motor neurons
20 Anterior gray horn
21 Axons of anterior root
22 Anterior median fissure

FIGURE 7.1 ■ Spinal cord: midthoracic region (transverse section). Stain: hematoxylin and eosin. Low magnification.

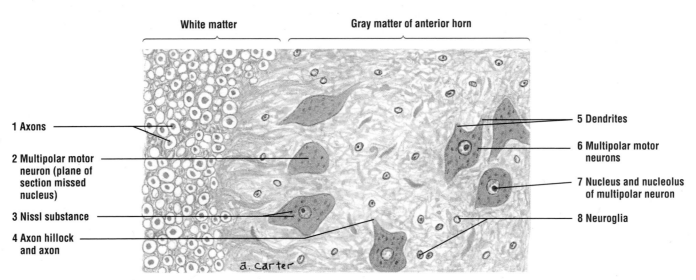

White matter   Gray matter of anterior horn

1 Axons
2 Multipolar motor neuron (plane of section missed nucleus)
3 Nissl substance
4 Axon hillock and axon

5 Dendrites
6 Multipolar motor neurons
7 Nucleus and nucleolus of multipolar neuron
8 Neuroglia

a. carter

FIGURE 7.2 ■ Spinal cord: anterior gray horn, motor neurons, and adjacent white matter. Stain: hematoxylin and eosin. Medium magnification.

FIGURE 7.3 ■ Spinal Cord: Midcervical Region (Transverse Section)

To illustrate the white matter and the gray matter of the spinal cord, a cross-section of the cord was prepared with the silver impregnation technique. After staining, the dark-brown, outer **white matter (3)** and the light-staining, inner **gray matter (4, 14)** are clearly visible. The white matter (3) consists primarily of ascending and descending myelinated nerve fibers or axons. In contrast, the gray matter contains the cell bodies of neurons and interneurons and their axons. The gray matter also exhibits a symmetrical H-shape, with the two sides connected across the midline of the spinal cord by the **gray commissure (15)**. The center of the gray commissure is located at the **central canal (16)** of the spinal cord.

The **anterior horns (6)** of the gray matter extend toward the front of the cord and are more prominent than the **posterior horns (2, 13)**. The anterior horns contain the cell bodies of the large **motor neurons (7, 17)**. Some **axons (8)** from the motor neurons of the anterior horns cross the white matter and exit the spinal cord as components of the **anterior roots (9, 21)** of the peripheral nerves. The posterior horns (2, 13) are the sensory areas and contain cell bodies of smaller neurons.

The spinal cord is surrounded by connective tissue meninges, consisting of an outer dura mater, a middle **arachnoid (5),** and an inner **pia mater (18)**. The spinal cord is also partially divided into right and left halves by a narrow, posterior (dorsal) groove, called the **posterior median sulcus (10)**, and by a deep, anterior (ventral) cleft, called the **anterior median fissure (19)**. In this illustration, the pia mater (18) is best seen in the anterior median fissure (19).

Between the posterior median sulcus (10) and the posterior horns (2, 13) of the gray matter are the prominent posterior columns of the white matter. In the midcervical region of the spinal cord, each dorsal column is subdivided into two fascicles: the posteromedial column, called the **fasciculus gracilis (11),** and the posterolateral column, called the **fasciculus cuneatus (1, 12)**.

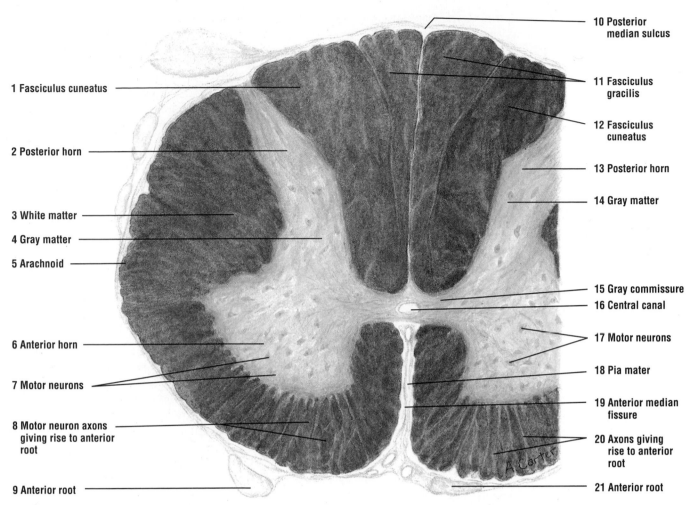

1 Fasciculus cuneatus

2 Posterior horn

3 White matter

4 Gray matter

5 Arachnoid

6 Anterior horn

7 Motor neurons

8 Motor neuron axons giving rise to anterior root

9 Anterior root

10 Posterior median sulcus

11 Fasciculus gracilis

12 Fasciculus cuneatus

13 Posterior horn

14 Gray matter

15 Gray commissure

16 Central canal

17 Motor neurons

18 Pia mater

19 Anterior median fissure

20 Axons giving rise to anterior root

21 Anterior root

FIGURE 7.3 ■ Spinal cord: midcervical region (transverse section). Stain: silver impregnation (Cajal's method). Low magnification.

FIGURE 7.4 ■ Spinal Cord: Anterior Gray Horn, Motor Neurons, and Adjacent Anterior White Matter

A small section of the white matter and the gray matter of the anterior horn of the spinal cord are illustrated at a higher magnification. The gray matter of the anterior horn contains large, **multipolar motor neurons (2, 3).** These neurons are characterized by numerous **dendrites (5, 6)** that extend in different directions from the perikaryon (cell bodies). In some neurons, the **nucleus (8)** is visible with its prominent **nucleolus (8).** In other neurons, the plane of section has missed the nucleus, and the perikaryon appears empty **(2).** In the vicinity of the motor neurons are **neuroglia (7),** the small, light-staining, supportive cells.

The white matter contains closely packed groups of myelinated axons. In cross-sections, the **axons (1)** appear dark-stained and surrounded by clear spaces, which are the remnants of the myelin sheaths. The axons of the white matter represent the ascending and descending tracts of the spinal cord. In contrast, the **axons (4)** of the anterior horn motor neurons aggregate into groups, pass through the white matter, and exit the spinal cord as the anterior (ventral) root fibers (see Fig. 7-3).

FUNCTIONAL CORRELATIONS

Neurons

Functionally, neurons are classified as **afferent** (sensory) neurons, **efferent** (motor) neurons, or **interneurons.** Sensory or afferent neurons conduct impulses from receptors in the internal organs or from the external environment to the CNS. Motor or efferent neurons convey impulses from the CNS to the effector muscles or glands in the periphery. Interneurons serve as intermediaries, connecting cells between the sensory and motor neurons in the CNS.

Neurons are highly specialized for **irritability, conductivity,** and **synthesis** of neuroactive substances, such as **neurotransmitters** and **neurohormones.** Following a mechanical or chemical stimulus, these neurons react (irritability) to the stimulus and transmit (conductivity) the information via axons to other neurons in different regions of the nervous system. Strong stimuli create a wave of excitation, or a nerve impulse (action potential), that is then propagated along the entire length of the axon (nerve fiber).

The main function of the neuronal dendrites is to receive information from other neurons or axons and then deliver that information to the cell body of the neuron. The main function of the axon is to conduct the received information away from the neuron to an interneuron, to another afferent or efferent neuron, or to an effector organ, such as a muscle or a gland. In addition to conducting impulses, axons also transport chemical substances that are synthesized within the neuron in small tubules, called **microtubules,** to the axon terminal or synapse, where they are released.

FIGURE 7.5 ■ Motor Neurons: Anterior Horn of the Spinal Cord

The large, multipolar **motor neurons (7)** of the CNS have a large central **nucleus (11),** a prominent **nucleolus (12),** and several radiating cell processes, called the **dendrites (10, 16).** A single, thin **axon (5, 14)** arises from a cone-shaped, clear area of the neuron, called the **axon hillock (6, 13).** The axons (5, 14) that leave the motor neurons (7) are thinner and much longer than the thicker but shorter dendrites (10, 16).

The cell body, or perikaryon, of the neuron is characterized by numerous clumps of coarse granules (basophilic masses) known as **Nissl bodies (4, 8).** Nissl bodies represent the granular endoplasmic reticulum of the neuron. When the plane of section misses the nucleus (4), only the dark-staining Nissl bodies (4) are seen in the perikaryon of the neuron. Nissl bodies (4, 8) extend into the dendrites (10, 16) but not into the axon hillock (6, 13) or the axon (5, 14). This feature distinguishes axons (5, 14) from dendrites (10, 16). The nucleus of the neuron (11) is outlined distinctly, and it stains light because of the uniform dispersion of chromatin. The nucleolus (12), in contrast, is prominent and dense, and the nucleolus stains dark. The **nuclei (2, 9)** of the surrounding **neuroglia (2, 9)** are stained prominently, whereas their cytoplasm remains unstained. Neuroglia (2, 9) are non-neural cells of the CNS; they provide structural and metabolic support for the neurons (7).

Surrounding the neurons (7) and the neuroglia (2, 9) are numerous blood vessels **(1, 3, 15)** of various sizes.

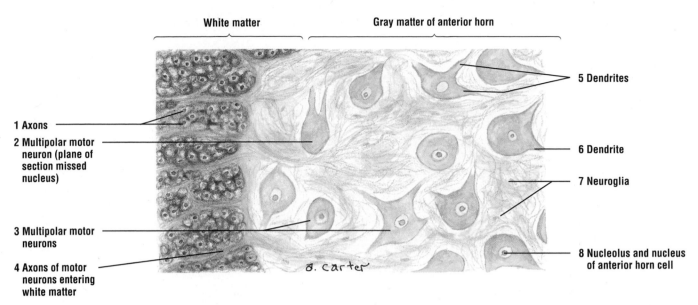

White matter

Gray matter of anterior horn

5 Dendrites

1 Axons

2 Multipolar motor neuron (plane of section missed nucleus)

6 Dendrite

7 Neuroglia

3 Multipolar motor neurons

4 Axons of motor neurons entering white matter

8 Nucleolus and nucleus of anterior horn cell

FIGURE 7.4 ■ Spinal cord: anterior gray horn, motor neurons, and adjacent anterior white matter. Stain: silver impregnation (Cajal's method). Medium magnification.

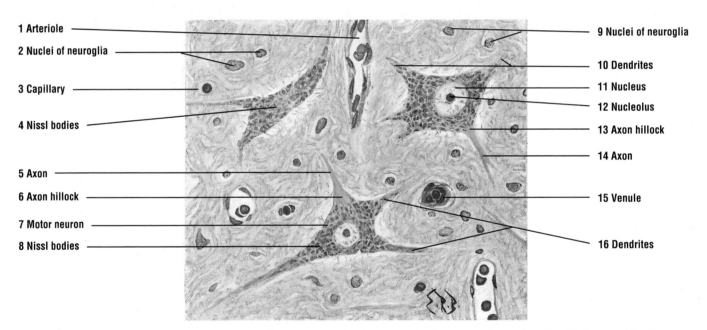

1 Arteriole

2 Nuclei of neuroglia

3 Capillary

4 Nissl bodies

5 Axon

6 Axon hillock

7 Motor neuron

8 Nissl bodies

9 Nuclei of neuroglia

10 Dendrites

11 Nucleus

12 Nucleolus

13 Axon hillock

14 Axon

15 Venule

16 Dendrites

FIGURE 7.5 ■ Motor neurons: anterior horn of the spinal cord. Stain: hematoxylin and eosin. High magnification.

FIGURE 7.6 ■ Neurofibrils and Motor Neurons in the Gray Matter of Anterior Horn of the Spinal Cord

This section of the anterior horn of the spinal cord was prepared by silver impregnation (Cajal's method) to demonstrate the distribution of neurofibrils in the gray matter and motor neurons. Fine **neurofibrils (2, 4)** are distributed throughout the **cell body (perikaryon) (4)** and **dendrites (2, 9)** of the **motor neurons (1, 10, 11).**

The silver impregnation technique does not allow axons and additional details of the motor neurons to be seen clearly. The nuclei of the **motor neurons (1, 11)** are yellow-stained, and their **nucleoli (5, 10)** are dark-stained. Not all motor neurons are sectioned through the middle. As a result, some motor neurons show only a **nucleus (1)** without a nucleolus, whereas others show only **peripheral cytoplasm (8)** without a nucleus.

Many **neurofibrils (6)** are also present in the **gray matter (3)** or intercellular areas. Some of these neurofibrils (3) belong to the axons of **anterior horn motor neurons (1, 11)** or to the adjacent **neuroglia (7)**, the **nuclei (7)** of which are visible throughout the gray matter (3) (see also Fig. 7-7).

The clear spaces around the neurons and their processes are artifacts caused by the chemical preparation of nervous tissue.

FIGURE 7.7 ■ Anterior Gray Horn of the Spinal Cord: Multipolar Motor Neurons, Axons, and Neuroglial Cells

This medium-magnification photomicrograph of the anterior gray horn of the spinal cord was prepared with silver stain to show the morphology of neurons and axons in the CNS. The large, multipolar **motor neurons (1)** of the gray horn exhibit numerous **dendrites (4)**. Each motor neuron (1) contains a distinct **nucleus (5)** and a prominent **nucleolus (6)**. Within the cytoplasm of the motor neurons (1) is the cytoskeleton, which consists of numerous **neurofibrils** (3) that course through the cell body and extend into the dendrites (4) and **axons (8).** Coursing past the motor neurons (1) are numerous axons of various sizes (8) from other nerve cells in the spinal cord. Surrounding the motor neurons (1) are numerous **nuclei** of **neuroglial cells (2)** and a **blood vessel (7)** containing blood cells.

As also seen in Figure 7-6, the clear spaces around the neurons and their processes are artifacts caused by tissue shrinkage during preparation of the spinal cord.

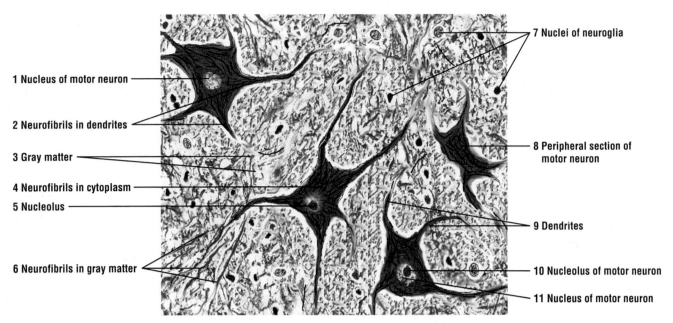

1 Nucleus of motor neuron

2 Neurofibrils in dendrites

3 Gray matter

4 Neurofibrils in cytoplasm

5 Nucleolus

6 Neurofibrils in gray matter

7 Nuclei of neuroglia

8 Peripheral section of motor neuron

9 Dendrites

10 Nucleolus of motor neuron

11 Nucleus of motor neuron

FIGURE 7.6 ■ Neurofibrils and motor neurons in the gray matter of the anterior horn of the spinal cord. Stain: silver impregnation (Cajal's method). High magnification.

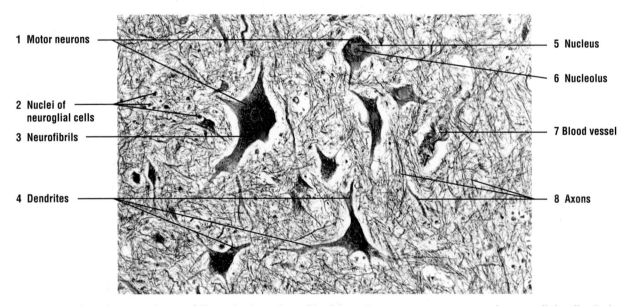

1 Motor neurons

2 Nuclei of neuroglial cells

3 Neurofibrils

4 Dendrites

5 Nucleus

6 Nucleolus

7 Blood vessel

8 Axons

FIGURE 7.7 ■ Anterior gray horn of the spinal cord: multipolar motor neurons, axons, and neuroglial cells. Stain: silver impregnation (Cajal's method). 80×

FIGURE 7.8 ■ Cerebral Cortex: Gray Matter

The different cell types that constitute the gray matter of the cerebral cortex are distributed in six layers, with one or more cell types being predominant in each layer (although some variations do exist). Horizontal and radial axons associated with neuronal cells in different layers give the cerebral cortex a laminated appearance. The different layers are labeled with Roman numerals on the right side of the figure.

The most superficial is the **molecular layer (I).** Overlying and covering the molecular layer (1) is the **pia mater (1),** one of the protective covering tissues of the brain. The peripheral portion of the molecular layer (1) is composed predominantly of **neuroglial cells (2)** and horizontal cells of Cajal. Their axons contribute to the horizontal fibers that are seen in the molecular layer (I).

The **external granular layer (II)** contains mainly different types of neuroglial cells and **small pyramidal cells (3).** Note that the pyramidal cells become progressively larger in the deeper layers of the cortex. The **dendrites of pyramidal cells (4, 7)** are directed toward the periphery of the cortex, whereas their axons extend downward (see Fig. 7-9, labels 4 and 10). In the **external pyramidal layer (III), medium-sized pyramidal cells (5)** predominate. The **internal granular layer (IV)** is a thin layer that contains mainly small **granule cells (6),** some pyramidal cells, and various neuroglia that form numerous complex connections with the pyramidal cells. The **internal pyramidal layer (V)** contains numerous neuroglial cells and **large pyramidal cells (8);** these are the largest cells in the motor area of the cerebral cortex. The deepest layer is the **multiform layer (VI),** which is adjacent to the **white matter (10)** of the cerebral cortex. The multiform layer (VI) contains intermixed cells of varying shapes and sizes, such as fusiform cells, granule cells, stellate cells, and cells of Martinotti. **Bundles of axons (9)** enter the white matter (10).

1 Pia mater with blood vessel

2 Neuroglial cells

3 Small pyramidal cells

4 Dendrites of pyramidal cells

5 Medium-sized pyramidal cells

6 Granule cells

7 Dendrites of pyramidal cells

8 Large pyramidal cells

9 Bundles of axons

10 White matter

I. Molecular layer

II. External granular layer

III. External pyramidal layer

IV. Internal granular layer

V. Internal pyramidal layer

VI. Multiform layer

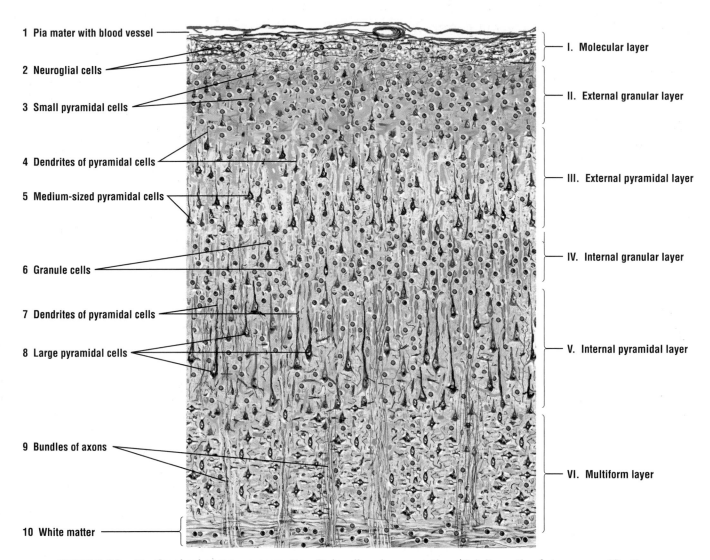

FIGURE 7.8 ■ Cerebral cortex: gray matter. Stain: silver impregnation (Cajal's method). Low magnification.

FIGURE 7.9 ■ Layer V of the Cerebral Cortex

A higher magnification of layer V of the cerebral cortex illustrates the large **pyramidal cells (3).** Note the typical large vesicular **nucleus (3)** with its prominent **nucleolus (3).** The silver stain also shows numerous **neurofibrils (9)** in the pyramidal cells (3). The most prominent cell processes are the apical **dendrites (7)** of the pyramidal cells (3), which are directed toward the surface of the cortex. The **axons (4, 10)** of the pyramidal cells (3) arise from the base of the cell body and pass into the white matter (see Fig. 7-8, label 10).

The intercellular area is occupied by **axons of neuroglial cells (2, 8)** in the cortex, small astrocytes, and blood vessels, including a **venule (5)** and **capillary (6).**

FIGURE 7.10 ■ Cerebellum (Transverse Section)

The **cerebellar cortex (1, 10)** exhibits numerous deeply convoluted folds, called **cerebellar folia (6)** (singular, folium), that are separated by **interfolial sulci (9)** (singular, sulcus). The cerebellar folia (6) are covered by thin connective tissue, the **pia mater (7),** that follows each folium (6) into the interfolial sulci (9). The detachment of pia mater (7) from the cerebellar cortex (1, 10) is an artifact resulting from tissue fixation and preparation.

The cerebellar cortex (1, 10) consists of an outer **gray matter (1, 10)** and an inner **white matter (5, 8).** Three distinct cell layers can be distinguished in the cerebellar cortex (1, 10): an outer **molecular layer (2),** with few cells and horizontally directed fibers; a central or middle **Purkinje cell layer (3);** and an inner **granular layer (4),** with numerous small cells that have intensely stained nuclei. The Purkinje cells (3) are pyriform or pyramidal in shape, with ramified dendrites that extend into the molecular layer (2).

The white matter (5, 8) forms the core of each cerebellar folium (6) and consists of myelinated nerve fibers or axons. The axons are the afferent and efferent fibers of the cerebellar cortex.

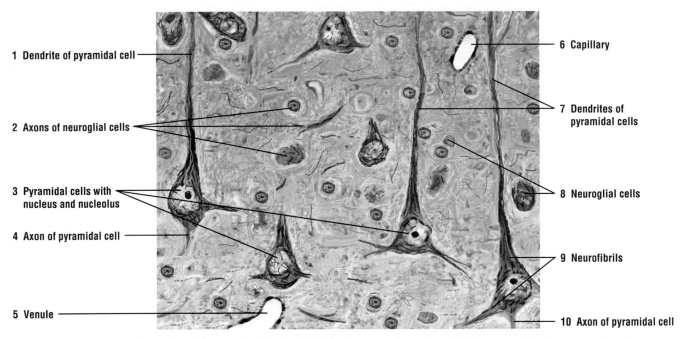

1 Dendrite of pyramidal cell

2 Axons of neuroglial cells

3 Pyramidal cells with nucleus and nucleolus

4 Axon of pyramidal cell

5 Venule

6 Capillary

7 Dendrites of pyramidal cells

8 Neuroglial cells

9 Neurofibrils

10 Axon of pyramidal cell

FIGURE 7.9 ■ Layer V of the cerebral cortex. Stain: silver impregnation (Cajal's method). High magnification.

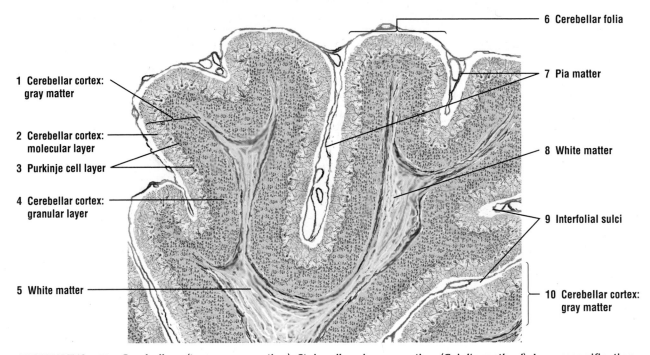

1 Cerebellar cortex: gray matter

2 Cerebellar cortex: molecular layer

3 Purkinje cell layer

4 Cerebellar cortex: granular layer

5 White matter

6 Cerebellar folia

7 Pia matter

8 White matter

9 Interfolial sulci

10 Cerebellar cortex: gray matter

FIGURE 7.10 ■ Cerebellum (transverse section). Stain: silver impregnation (Cajal's method). Low magnification.

FIGURE 7.11 ■ Cerebellar Cortex: Molecular Layer, Purkinje Cell Layer, and Granular Cell Layer

This illustration shows a small section of cerebellar cortex above the white matter at a higher magnification. The **Purkinje cells (3)** in the **Purkinje cell layer (7),** with their prominent nuclei and nucleoli, are arranged in a single row at the junction of the **molecular cell layer (6)** and the **granular cell layer (4).** The large, "flask-shaped" bodies of the Purkinje cells (3, 7) give off one or more thick **dendrites (2)** that extend through the molecular cell layer (6) to the cerebellar surface, giving rise to complex branching along their course. Thin axons leave the base of the Purkinje cells, pass through the granular cell layer (4), become myelinated, and enter the **white matter (5).**

The molecular cell layer (6) contains scattered **basket cells (1),** the unmyelinated axons of which normally course in a horizontal direction. Descending collaterals of more deeply placed basket cells (1) form connections around the Purkinje cells (3, 7) in a "basket-like" arrangement. Axons from the **granule cells (9)** in the granular cell layer (4) extend into the molecular layer and also course horizontally as unmyelinated **axons (11).**

In the granular cell layer (4) are numerous small granule cells (9), with dark-staining nuclei and a small amount of cytoplasm. Also scattered in the granular cell layer (4) are larger **Golgi type II cells (8),** with typical vesicular nuclei and more cytoplasm. Throughout the granular layer are small, irregularly dispersed, clear spaces, called the **glomeruli (10).** These regions contain only synaptic complexes.

FIGURE 7.12 ■ Fibrous Astrocytes and Capillary in the Brain

A section of the brain was prepared by Cajal's method to demonstrate the supportive neuroglial cells, called astrocytes. **Fibrous astrocytes (2, 5)** exhibit a small **cell body (5),** a large oval **nucleus (5),** and a dark-stained **nucleolus (5).** Extending from the cell body are long, thin, and smooth radiating **processes (4, 6)** that are found between the neurons and blood vessels. A **perivascular fibrous astrocyte (2)** surrounds a **capillary (8)** containing **red blood cells (erythrocytes).** From other fibrous astrocytes (2, 5), the long processes (4, 6) extend to and terminate on the capillary (8) as **perivascular end feet (3, 7).** Also seen are the nuclei of different **neuroglia (1)** of the brain.

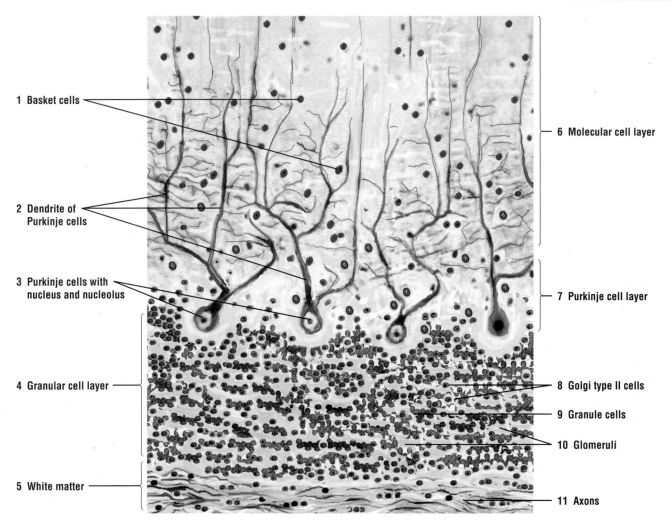

1 Basket cells

2 Dendrite of Purkinje cells

3 Purkinje cells with nucleus and nucleolus

4 Granular cell layer

5 White matter

6 Molecular cell layer

7 Purkinje cell layer

8 Golgi type II cells

9 Granule cells

10 Glomeruli

11 Axons

FIGURE 7.11 ■ Cerebellar cortex: molecular layer, Purkinje cell layer, and granular cell layer. Stain: silver impregnation (Cajal's method). High magnification.

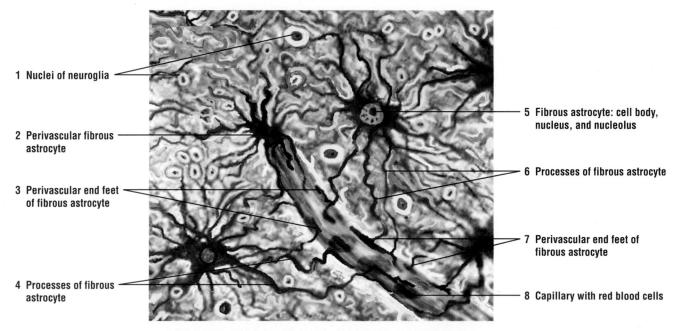

1 Nuclei of neuroglia

2 Perivascular fibrous astrocyte

3 Perivascular end feet of fibrous astrocyte

4 Processes of fibrous astrocyte

5 Fibrous astrocyte: cell body, nucleus, and nucleolus

6 Processes of fibrous astrocyte

7 Perivascular end feet of fibrous astrocyte

8 Capillary with red blood cells

FIGURE 7.12 ■ Fibrous astrocytes and capillary in the brain. Stain: silver impregnation (Cajal's method.) Medium magnification.

FIGURE 7.13 ▩ Oligodendrocytes of the Brain

This section of the brain was also prepared with Cajal's method to show the supportive neuroglial cells, called **oligodendrocytes (1, 4, 7).** In comparison with a **fibrous astrocyte (3),** the oligodendrocytes (1, 4, 7) are smaller and exhibit a few thin, short processes without excessive branching.

Oligodendrocytes (1, 4, 7) are found in both gray matter and white matter of the CNS. In the white matter, oligodendrocytes (1, 4, 7) form myelin sheaths around multiple axons and are analogous to the neurolemmocytes (Schwann cells) that myelinate only individual axons in the nerves of the PNS.

Two **neurons (2, 6)** are also illustrated to contrast their size with that of a fibrous astrocyte (3) and oligodendrocytes (1, 4, 7). A **capillary (5)** passes between the different cells.

FIGURE 7.14 ▩ Microglia of the Brain

This section of the brain was prepared with Hortega's method to show the smallest neuroglial cells, called the **microglia (2, 3).** The microglia (2, 3) vary in shape and often exhibit irregular contours. In addition, the small, deeply stained nucleus almost fills the entire cell. The cell processes of the microglia (2, 3) are few, short, and slender. Both the cell body and the processes of the microglia (2, 3) are covered with small spines. Two **neurons (1)** and a **capillary** containing **red blood cells (erythrocytes) (4)** provide a size comparison with the microglia (2, 3).

Microglia are found in both the white matter and the gray matter and are the main phagocytes of the CNS.

FUNCTIONAL CORRELATIONS

Neuroglia

Four types of neuroglial cells are recognized in the CNS: astrocytes, oligodendrocytes, microglia, and ependymal cells.

Astrocytes are the largest and most abundant neuroglial cells in the gray matter, and they consist of two types: fibrous astrocytes and protoplasmic astrocytes. In the CNS, both types of astrocytes are attached to the walls of the **capillaries** and to **neurons.** They support **metabolic exchange** between neurons and the capillaries of the CNS. In addition, the astrocytes control the **chemical environment** around neurons by clearing intercellular spaces of increased **potassium ion** levels and released **neurotransmitters,** such as **glutamate,** at active synaptic sites to maintain a proper ionic environment for their function. If these metabolic chemicals are not quickly removed from these sites, they can interfere with neuronal functions. Astrocytes remove glutamate and convert it to glutamine, which is then returned to the neurons. Astrocytes also contain reserves of glycogen, from which they release glucose and, in this manner, they contribute to the energy metabolism of the cerebral cortex.

Oligodendrocytes are smaller than astrocytes and have fewer cytoplasmic processes. Oligodendrocytes form **myelin sheaths** around the axons in the CNS. Because oligodendrocytes have several processes, a single oligodendrocyte can surround and myelinate several axons at the same time. In the PNS, a different type of supporting cell, called the **neurolemmocyte** (Schwann cell), myelinates the axons. In contrast to oligodendrocytes, neurolemmocytes can only form myelin sheaths around a single axon.

Microglia are the smallest neuroglial cells. The dark-staining microglia are believed to be part of the **mononuclear phagocyte system** of the CNS. Microglia are found throughout the CNS, and their main function is similar to that of the **macrophages** of the connective tissue. When nervous tissue is injured or damaged, microglia migrate to the region, proliferate, become phagocytic, and remove dead or foreign tissue.

Ependymal cells are simple cuboidal or low columnar epithelial cells that line the ventricles of the brain and the central canal in the spinal cord. Their apices contain both cilia and microvilli. Cilia facilitate movement of the CSF through the central canal, whereas microvilli may have some absorptive functions.

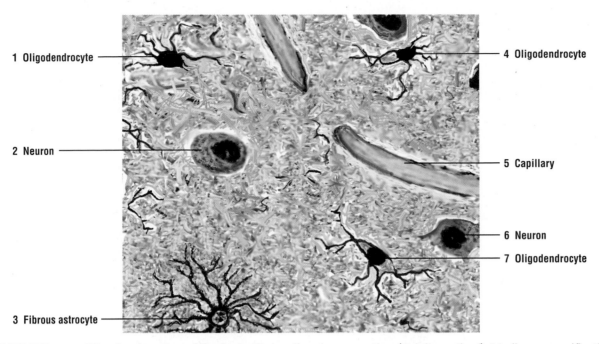

1 Oligodendrocyte

2 Neuron

3 Fibrous astrocyte

4 Oligodendrocyte

5 Capillary

6 Neuron

7 Oligodendrocyte

FIGURE 7.13 ■ Oligodendrocytes of the brain. Stain: silver impregnation (Cajal's method). Medium magnification.

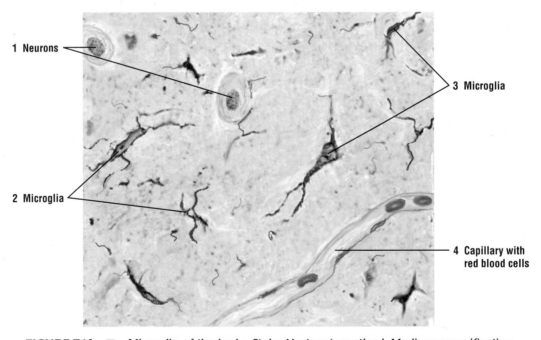

1 Neurons

2 Microglia

3 Microglia

4 Capillary with red blood cells

FIGURE 7.14 ■ Microglia of the brain. Stain: Hortega's method. Medium magnification.

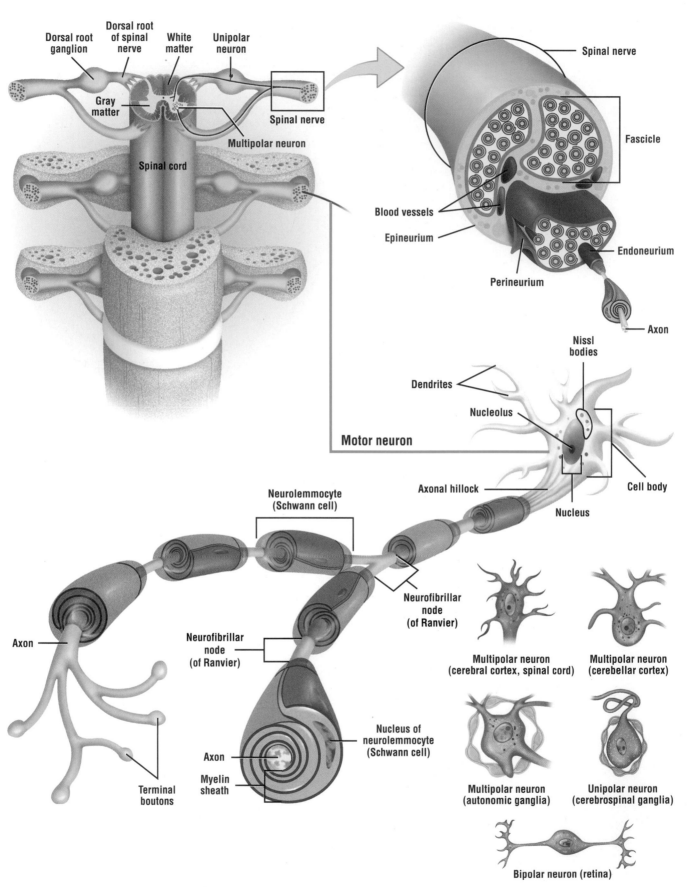

OVERVIEW FIGURE—PERIPHERAL NERVOUS SYSTEM ■ The peripheral nervous system is composed of the cranial and spinal nerves. A cross-section of the spinal cord is illustrated here with the characteristic features of the motor neuron and a cross-section of a peripheral nerve. Also illustrated are types of neurons located in different ganglia and organs outside of the central nervous system.

SECTION 2 ■ Peripheral Nervous System

The **peripheral nervous system (PNS)** consists of neurons, nerves, and axons that are located outside the CNS. These include **cranial nerves** from the brain and **spinal nerves** from the spinal cord, along with their associated ganglia. Ganglia (singular, ganglion) are small accumulations of neurons that are located outside the CNS and are surrounded by a connective tissue capsule. The nerves of the PNS contain both sensory and motor axons. These axons transmit information between the peripheral organs and the CNS. The neurons of the peripheral nerves are located either within or outside the CNS in different ganglia.

Connective Tissue Layers in the PNS

A peripheral nerve is composed of numerous axons of various sizes surrounded by several layers of connective tissue that partition the nerve into several nerve (axon) bundles, or **fascicles.** The outermost connective tissue layer is the **epineurium,** which consists of dense irregular connective tissue that completely surrounds the peripheral nerve. A thinner connective tissue layer, called the **perineurium,** extends into the nerve and surrounds numerous nerve fascicles. Within each fascicle are individual axons and their supporting cells, the neurolemmocytes (Schwann cells). Each axon is surrounded by a loose connective tissue layer of thin reticular fibers, called the **endoneurium.**

Supporting Cells in the PNS

The supportive cells in the PNS are the myelin-forming **neurolemmocytes (Schwann cells)** and the **satellite cells.** Satellite cells are small cells that surround the neuronal cells in paravertebral and peripheral ganglia. Paravertebral ganglia are an interconnected chain of ganglia that are located parallel to the vertebral column, near the junction of the dorsal and ventral roots of the spinal nerves. Peripheral ganglia are located distally from the vertebral column, near various visceral organs.

FIGURE 7.15 ■ Peripheral Nerves and Blood Vessels (Transverse Section)

In this illustration, several bundles of nerve axons (fibers), or **nerve fascicles (1),** and accompanying blood vessels have been sectioned in the transverse plane. Each nerve fascicle (1) is surrounded by a sheath of connective tissue, called the **perineurium (5),** that merges with the surrounding **interfascicular connective tissue (9).** Delicate connective tissue strands from the perineurium (5) surround individual nerve axons in a fascicle and form the innermost layer, or endoneurium (not visible in this figure and at this magnification).

Numerous nuclei are seen between individual nerve axons in the nerve fascicles (1). Most are the **nuclei** of **neurolemmocytes (Schwann cells) (2).** Neurolemmocytes (2) surround and myelinate the axons in the PNS. The myelin sheaths that surrounded the tiny **axons (3)** are seen as empty spaces because of the chemicals that are used in preparation of the tissue. Nuclei of **fibrocytes (4)** are also seen in the nerve fascicles of the endoneurium (see Fig. 7-18).

The arterial blood vessels in the interfascicular connective tissue (9) send branches into each nerve fascicle (1), where they branch into capillaries in the endoneurium. Different-size **arterioles (7, 12)** and **venules (11)** are found in the interfascicular connective tissue (8). In the larger arteriole (7) are visible red blood cells, an **internal elastic membrane (8),** and a muscular **tunica media (6).** Different-size **adipose cells (10)** are also present in the interfascicular connective tissue (9).

FIGURE 7.16 ■ Myelinated Nerve Fibers (Longitudinal and Transverse Sections)

Neurolemmocytes (Schwann cells) surround the axons of peripheral nerves and form a myelin sheath. To illustrate the myelin sheath, nerve fibers are fixed with an osmic acid; with this preparation, the lipid in the myelin sheath stains black. In this illustration, a portion of the peripheral nerve has been sectioned in a longitudinal plane (upper figure) and in the transverse plane (lower figure).

In the longitudinal plane (upper figure), the **myelin sheath (1)** appears as a thick, black band surrounding a lighter, central **axon (2).** At intervals of a few microns, the myelin sheath exhibits discontinuity between adjacent neurolemmocytes. These regions represent the **neurofibrillar nodes (of Ranvier) (4).**

A group of nerve fibers, or fascicle, is also illustrated. Each fascicle is surrounded by a light-appearing connective tissue layer, called the **perineurium (3, 5, 8).** In turn, each individual nerve fiber or axon is surrounded by a thin layer of connective tissue, called the **endoneurium (7, 10).** In the transverse plane (lower figure), different sizes of myelinated axons are seen. The **myelin sheath (9)** appears as a thick, black ring around the light, unstained **axon (12),** which in most fibers is seen in the center.

The connective tissue surrounding the fascicle exhibits a rich supply of **blood vessels (6, 11)** of different sizes.

FUNCTIONAL CORRELATIONS

Axon Myelination

The main function of the **neurolemmocytes** (Schwann cells) in the **PNS** is to form the insulating, lipid-rich **myelin sheaths** around the larger axons. The function of neurolemmocytes in the PNS is similar to that of the **oligodendrocytes** in the **CNS,** except that a single oligodendrocyte forms myelin sheaths around multiple axons.

Myelin sheaths are not continuous along the axon; rather, they are punctuated by gaps, called **neurofibrillar nodes** (of Ranvier). These nodes accelerate the conduction of **nerve impulses** (action potentials) along axons. In large, myelinated axons, nerve impulses are not propagated along the myelin sheath; instead, the nerve impulse or action potential jumps from node to node, resulting in a more efficient and faster conduction of the impulse. This type of impulse propagation in myelinated axons is called **saltatory conduction.**

Small, unmyelinated axons conduct nerve impulses at a much slower rate than larger, myelinated axons. In unmyelinated axons, even though they are surrounded by the cytoplasm of the neurolemmocyte, the impulse travels along the entire length of the axon; as a result, the conduction efficiency of the impulse and the velocity are reduced. Thus, the larger, myelinated axons have the highest velocity of impulse conduction. Also, the rate of impulse conduction depends directly on the axon size and the myelin sheath.

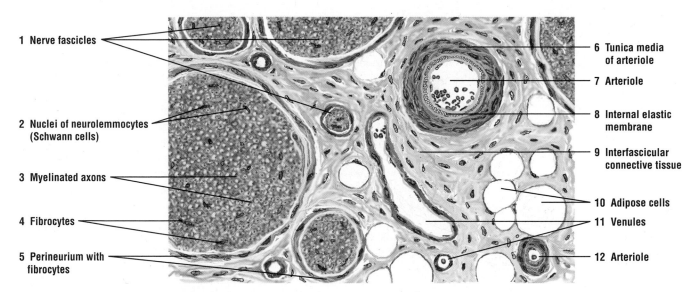

1 Nerve fascicles

2 Nuclei of neurolemmocytes (Schwann cells)

3 Myelinated axons

4 Fibrocytes

5 Perineurium with fibrocytes

6 Tunica media of arteriole

7 Arteriole

8 Internal elastic membrane

9 Interfascicular connective tissue

10 Adipose cells

11 Venules

12 Arteriole

FIGURE 7.15 ■ Peripheral nerves and blood vessels (transverse section). Stain: hematoxylin and eosin. Medium magnification.

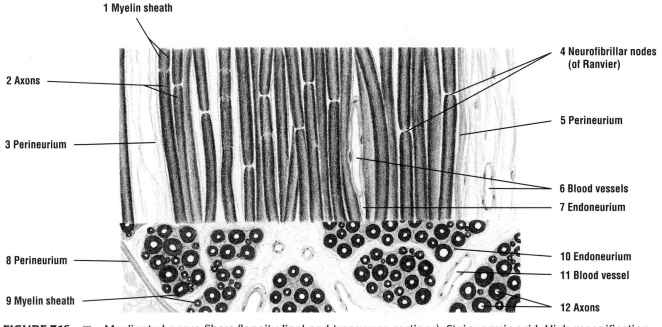

1 Myelin sheath

2 Axons

3 Perineurium

8 Perineurium

9 Myelin sheath

4 Neurofibrillar nodes (of Ranvier)

5 Perineurium

6 Blood vessels

7 Endoneurium

10 Endoneurium

11 Blood vessel

12 Axons

FIGURE 7.16 ■ Myelinated nerve fibers (longitudinal and transverse sections). Stain: osmic acid. High magnification.

FIGURE 7.17 ■ Sciatic Nerve (Longitudinal Section)

A longitudinal section of a sciatic nerve is illustrated at a low magnification. A small portion of the outer layer of dense connective tissue **epineurium (1)** that surrounds the entire nerve is visible. The deeper layer of the epineurium (1) contains numerous **blood vessels (5)** and **adipose cells (6).**

The connective tissue sheath directly inferior to the epineurium (1) that surrounds the bundles of nerve fibers, or **fascicles (3),** is the **perineurium (2).** Extensions of the epineurium (1) with **blood vessels (4)** between the fascicles (3) is the **interfascicular connective tissue (7).**

In a longitudinal section, the individual axons usually follow a characteristic, wavy pattern. Located among the wavy axons in the fascicle (3) are numerous **nuclei (8)** of neurolemmocytes (Schwann cells) and fibrocytes of the endoneurium connective tissue. Neurolemmocytes and fibrocytes cannot be differentiated at this magnification.

FIGURE 7.18 ■ Sciatic Nerve (Longitudinal Section)

A small portion of the sciatic nerve illustrated in Figure 7-17 is presented at higher magnification. The central **axons (1)** appear as slender threads that are stained lightly with hematoxylin and eosin. The surrounding myelin sheath has been dissolved by chemicals during histologic preparation, leaving a **neurokeratin network (6)** of protein. The myelin sheath, or cell membrane, of the **neurolemmocytes (Schwann cells) (4)** is not always distinguishable from the connective tissue **endoneurium (5)** that surrounds each axon. At the **neurofibrillar node (of Ranvier) (2),** the neurolemmocyte cell membrane (4) is seen as a thin, peripheral boundary that descends toward the axon.

Two **neurolemmocyte nuclei (4),** cut in different planes, are shown around the periphery of the myelinated axons (1). The **fibrocytes** of the connective tissue **endoneurium (3a)** and **perineurium (3b)** are also seen. The fibrocyte of the endoneurium (3a) is outside the myelin sheath, which is in contrast to the neurolemmocytes (4) that myelinate and/or surround the axons (1). However, it is often difficult to distinguish between the nuclei of neurolemmocytes (4) and the fibrocytes (3) of the endoneurium.

FIGURE 7.19 ■ Sciatic Nerve (Transverse Section)

A higher magnification of a transverse section of the sciatic nerve illustrated in Figure 7-17 shows the myelinated axons. The **axons (5)** appear as thin, dark, central structures that are surrounded by the dissolved remnants of myelin, the **neurokeratin network (2)** of protein with peripheral radial lines. The nuclei and cell membranes of the **neurolemmocytes (1)** are peripheral to the myelinated axons (5). The crescent shape of the neurolemmocytes (1), as they appear to encircle the axons (5), allows their identification.

The collagen fibers of the connective tissue endoneurium are faintly distinguishable, whereas the **fibrocytes** of the connective tissue **endoneurium (3a)** and **perineurium (3b, 6)** are seen clearly. Located in the **interfascicular connective tissue (4)** and draining the nerve fascicles is a small **venule (7).**

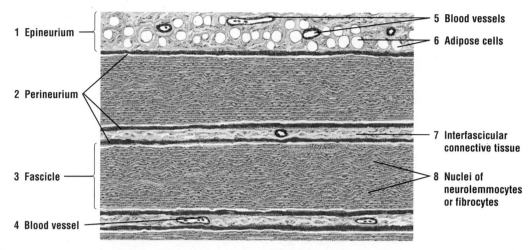

1 Epineurium

2 Perineurium

3 Fascicle

4 Blood vessel

5 Blood vessels

6 Adipose cells

7 Interfascicular connective tissue

8 Nuclei of neurolemmocytes or fibrocytes

FIGURE 7.17 ■ Sciatic nerve (longitudinal section). Stain: hematoxylin and eosin. Low magnification.

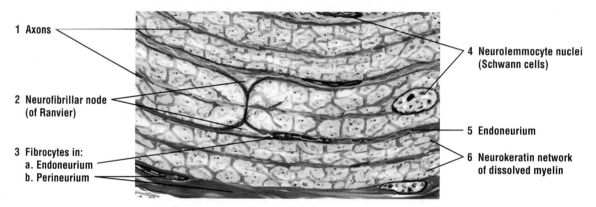

1 Axons

2 Neurofibrillar node (of Ranvier)

3 Fibrocytes in:
   a. Endoneurium
   b. Perineurium

4 Neurolemmocyte nuclei (Schwann cells)

5 Endoneurium

6 Neurokeratin network of dissolved myelin

FIGURE 7.18 ■ Sciatic nerve (longitudinal section). Stain: hematoxylin and eosin. High magnification (oil immersion).

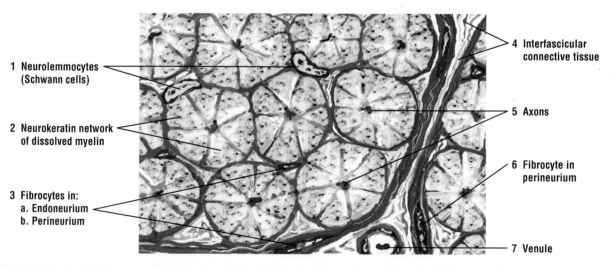

1 Neurolemmocytes (Schwann cells)

2 Neurokeratin network of dissolved myelin

3 Fibrocytes in:
   a. Endoneurium
   b. Perineurium

4 Interfascicular connective tissue

5 Axons

6 Fibrocyte in perineurium

7 Venule

FIGURE 7.19 ■ Sciatic nerve (transverse section). Stain: hematoxylin and eosin. High magnification (oil immersion).

FIGURE 7.20 ■ Peripheral Nerve: Neurofibrillar Nodes (of Ranvier) and Axons

A medium-magnification photomicrograph shows a peripheral nerve sectioned in a longitudinal plane. The myelin sheaths that normally surround the axons have been washed out in this preparation, and only **myelin spaces (7)** are seen. A centrally located **axon (2, 8)** can be seen in some of the nerve fibers that exhibited myelin sheaths. At regular intervals along the axon are indentations in the myelin sheaths. These represent the **neurofibrillar nodes (of Ranvier), (1, 9),** which in turn represent the edges of the myelin sheaths of two different neurolemmocytes that enclose the axon (2, 8). A possible **neurolemmocyte (Schwann cell) nucleus (3)** is associated with one of the axons (2, 8), and the thin, blue, connective tissue **endoneurium (6)** is shown surrounding some of the axons (2, 8). Outside the axons (2, 8) are a **capillary (4)** with red blood cells and **fibrocytes (5)** of the surrounding connective tissue layers.

FIGURE 7.21 ■ Dorsal Root Ganglion, with Dorsal and Ventral Roots, and Spinal Nerve (Longitudinal Section)

The dorsal root ganglia are aggregations of neurons outside the CNS. The **dorsal (posterior) root ganglion (7)** is situated on the **dorsal (posterior) nerve root (9)** of the spinal cord. Numerous round **unipolar neurons (2),** or sensory neurons, constitute the majority of the ganglion. Numerous **nerve fascicles (3)** pass between the unipolar neurons (2) and course either in the dorsal nerve root (9) or the **spinal nerve (5).** The nerve fascicles (3) represent the peripheral processes that are formed by the bifurcation of a single axon that emerges from each unipolar neuron (2).

Each dorsal root ganglion (7) is enclosed by an irregular **connective tissue layer (1)** that contains adipose cells, **nerves,** and **blood vessels (1, 6).** The connective tissue (1, 6) around the ganglion (7) merges with the connective tissue of the peripheral **spinal nerve (5),** the **epineurium (4).** The nerve fascicles in the **ventral (anterior) nerve root (11)** join the nerve fascicles (3) that emerge from the ganglion (7) to form the spinal nerve (5). The spinal nerve (5) is formed when the dorsal nerve root (9) and the ventral (anterior) nerve root (11) of the spinal cord unite.

On emerging from the spinal cord, the dorsal (9) and ventral roots (11) are surrounded by the delicate connective tissue, or the pia mater, and an **arachnoid sheath (8, 10)** of the spinal cord. These sheaths become continuous with the epineurium (4) of the spinal nerve (5). The connective tissue perineurium around the nerve fascicles (3) and the endoneurium around individual nerve fibers in the spinal nerve (5) or in the ganglion (7) are not distinguishable at this magnification.

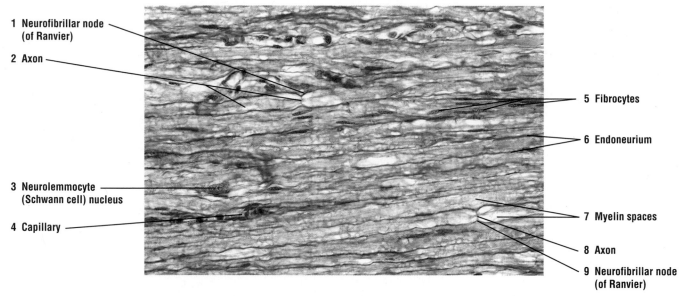

1 Neurofibrillar node (of Ranvier)

2 Axon

3 Neurolemmocyte (Schwann cell) nucleus

4 Capillary

5 Fibrocytes

6 Endoneurium

7 Myelin spaces

8 Axon

9 Neurofibrillar node (of Ranvier)

FIGURE 7.20 ■ Peripheral nerve: neurofibrillar nodes (of Ranvier) and axons. Stain: Masson's trichrome. 100×

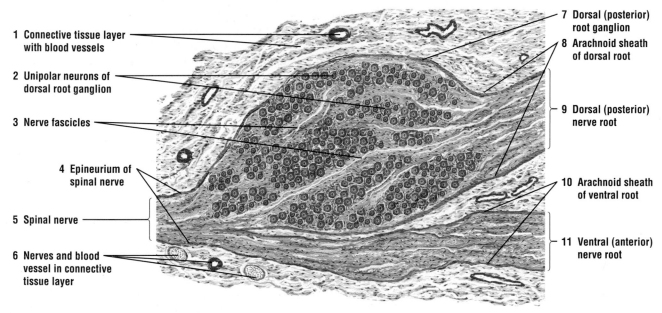

1 Connective tissue layer with blood vessels

2 Unipolar neurons of dorsal root ganglion

3 Nerve fascicles

4 Epineurium of spinal nerve

5 Spinal nerve

6 Nerves and blood vessel in connective tissue layer

7 Dorsal (posterior) root ganglion

8 Arachnoid sheath of dorsal root

9 Dorsal (posterior) nerve root

10 Arachnoid sheath of ventral root

11 Ventral (anterior) nerve root

FIGURE 7.21 ■ Dorsal root ganglion, with dorsal and ventral roots, and spinal nerve (longitudinal section). Stain: hematoxylin and eosin. Low magnification.

FIGURE 7.22 ▪ Cells and (Pseudo-)unipolar Neurons of a Dorsal Root Ganglion

The **unipolar neurons (1, 6)** of a dorsal (posterior) root ganglion are illustrated at higher magnification. When the plane of section passes through the middle of a neuron (1, 6), a pink-staining **cytoplasm (1b)** and a round **nucleus (1a),** with its characteristic, dark-staining **nucleolus (1a),** are visible. When the plane of section does not pass through the middle of unipolar neurons (1, 6) and misses their nuclei, only pink **cytoplasm of neurons (4)** is seen. Some of the unipolar neurons (1, 6) contain small clumps of brownish **lipofuscin pigment (9)** in their cytoplasm.

The cell body of each unipolar neuron (1, 6) is surrounded by two cellular capsules. The inner cell layer is within the perineuronal space and closely surrounds the unipolar neurons (1, 6); these are the smaller, flat, epithelium-like **satellite cells (3, 8).** The satellite cells (3, 8) have spherical nuclei, are of neuroectodermal origin, and are continuous with similar **neurolemmocytes (Schwann cells) (11)** that surround the unmyelinated and **myelinated axons (5, 10).** The satellite cells (3, 8) are surrounded by an outer layer of **capsule cells (7)** of the connective tissue. Between the unipolar neurons (1, 6) are numerous **fibrocytes (2)** that are randomly arranged in the surrounding connective tissue and that continue into the endoneurium between the axons (5).

With hematoxylin-and-eosin stain, small axons and individual connective tissue fibers are not clearly defined. Large, myelinated axons (5) are recognizable when sectioned longitudinally.

FIGURE 7.23 ▪ Multipolar Neurons, Surrounding Cells, and Nerve Fibers of a Sympathetic Ganglion

In contrast to the neurons of the dorsal root ganglion (see Fig. 7-22), the **neurons (3, 9)** of the sympathetic trunk are multipolar, smaller, and more uniform in size. As a result, the outlines of the neurons (3, 9) and their **dendritic processes (2, 11)** often appear irregular. Also, if the plane of section does not pass through the middle of the cell, only the **cytoplasm of the neuron (1, 10)** is visible. The sympathetic neurons (3, 9) also often exhibit **eccentric nuclei (9),** and binucleated cells are not uncommon. In older individuals, a brownish **lipofuscin pigment (12)** accumulates in the cytoplasm of numerous neurons (3, 9).

The **satellite cells (8)** surround the multipolar neurons (3, 9), but they are usually less numerous here than around the cells in the dorsal root ganglion. Also, the connective tissue capsule, with its capsule cells, may not be well defined. Surrounding the neurons (3, 9) are **fibrocytes (5)** of the intercellular connective tissue and different-size blood vessels, such as a **venule** with **red blood cells (6).** Unmyelinated and myelinated nerve **axons (4, 7)** aggregate into bundles and course through the sympathetic ganglion. The flattened nuclei on the peripheries of the myelinated axons are the **neurolemmocytes** (Schwann cells) **(4, 7).** These nerve fibers represent the preganglionic axons, postganglionic visceral efferent axons, and visceral afferent axons.

FIGURE 7.24 ▪ Dorsal Root Ganglion: Unipolar Neurons and Surrounding Cells

A medium-magnification photomicrograph of the dorsal root ganglion illustrates the spherical shape of the sensory **unipolar neurons (2).** The cytoplasm of these neurons contains a central **nucleus (6)** and a prominent, dense **nucleolus (5).** Surrounding the unipolar neurons (2) are smaller **satellite cells (1).** Other cells surrounding the satellite cells (1) and the unipolar neurons (2) are the connective tissue **fibrocytes (3).** Coursing through the dorsal root ganglion between the unipolar neurons (2) are numerous **bundles of sensory axons (4)** from the periphery.

The clear space around the neurons and the surrounding cells is an artifact caused by the tissue shrinkage that occurs during chemical preparation of the dorsal root ganglion.

FUNCTIONAL CORRELATIONS

Satellite Cells

Satellite cells are small, cuboidal cells that surround the neurons in different peripheral ganglia of the PNS. These cells provide **structural support** and **metabolic support** to the neurons that they surround. They insulate the neurons and provide for efficient metabolic exchange.

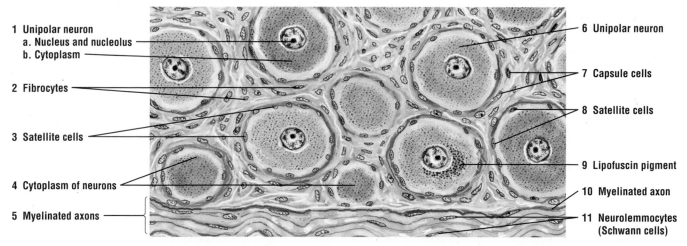

1 Unipolar neuron
   a. Nucleus and nucleolus
   b. Cytoplasm

2 Fibrocytes

3 Satellite cells

4 Cytoplasm of neurons

5 Myelinated axons

6 Unipolar neuron

7 Capsule cells

8 Satellite cells

9 Lipofuscin pigment

10 Myelinated axon

11 Neurolemmocytes
   (Schwann cells)

FIGURE 7.22 ■ Cells and unipolar neurons of a dorsal root ganglion. Stain: hematoxylin and eosin. High magnification.

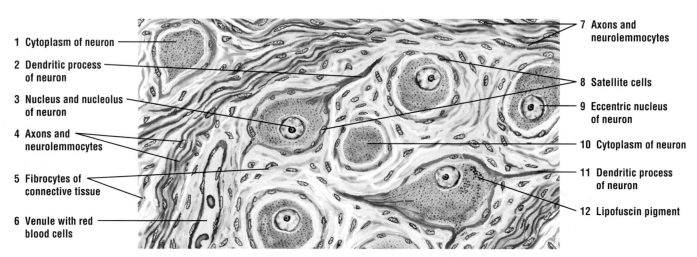

1 Cytoplasm of neuron

2 Dendritic process
   of neuron

3 Nucleus and nucleolus
   of neuron

4 Axons and
   neurolemmocytes

5 Fibrocytes of
   connective tissue

6 Venule with red
   blood cells

7 Axons and
   neurolemmocytes

8 Satellite cells

9 Eccentric nucleus
   of neuron

10 Cytoplasm of neuron

11 Dendritic process
   of neuron

12 Lipofuscin pigment

FIGURE 7.23 ■ Multipolar neurons, surrounding cells, and nerve fibers of sympathetic ganglion. Stain: hematoxylin and eosin. High magnification.

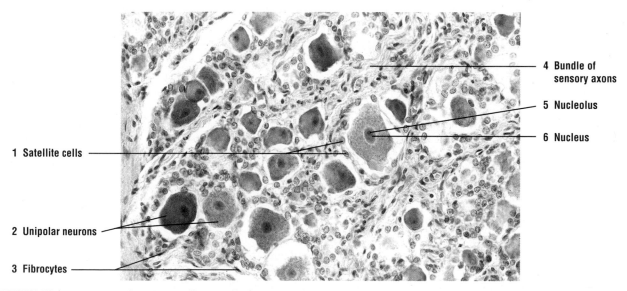

4 Bundle of
   sensory axons

5 Nucleolus

6 Nucleus

1 Satellite cells

2 Unipolar neurons

3 Fibrocytes

FIGURE 7.24 ■ Dorsal root ganglion: unipolar neurons and surrounding cells. Stain: hematoxylin and eosin. 100×

PART II

ORGANS

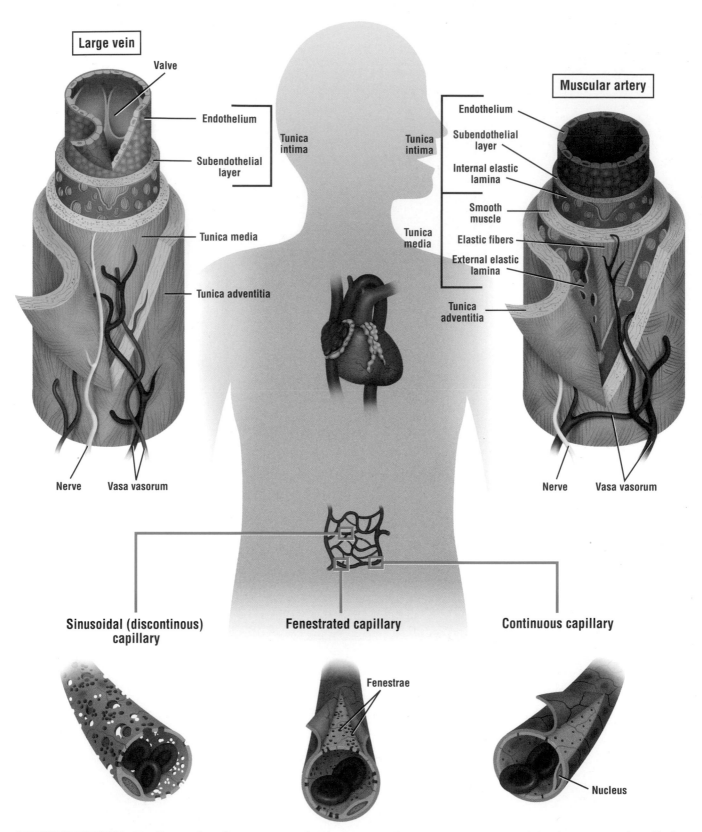

Large vein

Valve
Endothelium
Subendothelial layer
Tunica intima
Tunica media
Tunica adventitia
Nerve
Vasa vasorum

Muscular artery

Endothelium
Subendothelial layer
Internal elastic lamina
Tunica intima
Smooth muscle
Elastic fibers
External elastic lamina
Tunica media
Tunica adventitia
Nerve
Vasa vasorum

Sinusoidal (discontinous) capillary

Fenestrated capillary

Fenestrae

Continuous capillary

Nucleus

OVERVIEW FIGURE ■ Comparison (transverse sections) of a muscular artery, large vein, and the three types of capillaries.

CHAPTER 8

Circulatory System

The Blood Vascular System

The mammalian **blood vascular system** consists of the heart, major arteries, arterioles, capillaries, venules, and veins. The main function of this system is to deliver oxygenated blood to cells and tissues and to return venous blood to the lungs for gaseous exchange. The histology of the heart muscle was described in detail in Chapter 6 as one of the four main tissues. In this chapter, heart histology is illustrated only as part of the cardiovascular system.

Types of Arteries

The human body contains three types of arteries: elastic arteries, muscular arteries, and arterioles. Arteries that leave the heart to distribute oxygenated blood exhibit progressive branching. With each branching, the luminal diameters of the arteries gradually decrease, until the smallest vessel, the capillary, is formed.

Elastic arteries are the largest blood vessels in the body. They include the **pulmonary trunk** and **aorta** with its major branches: the brachiocephalic, common carotid, subclavian, vertebral, pulmonary, and common iliac arteries. The walls of these vessels are composed primarily of elastic connective tissue fibers. These fibers provide great resilience and flexibility during blood flow. The large elastic arteries branch and become medium-sized **muscular arteries,** the most numerous vessels in the body. In contrast to the walls of elastic arteries, those of muscular arteries contain greater amounts of **smooth muscle fiber. Arterioles** are the smallest branches of the arterial system, and their walls consist of one to five layers of smooth muscle fibers. Arterioles deliver blood to the **capillaries,** which are microscopic blood vessels that connect arterioles with the smallest veins or venules.

Structure of Arteries

The wall of a typical artery contains three concentric layers, or **tunics.** The innermost layer is the **tunica intima.** This layer consists of a simple squamous epithelium, called the **endothelium** in the vascular system, and the underlying **subendothelial connective tissue.** The middle layer is the **tunica media,** which is composed primarily of smooth muscle fibers. The outermost layer is the **tunica adventitia,** which is composed primarily of connective tissue fibers.

The walls of some muscular arteries also exhibit two thin, wavy bands of elastic fibers. The **internal elastic lamina** is located adjacent to the tunica intima; this layer is not seen in some small vessels. The **external elastic lamina** is located on the periphery of the muscular tunica media and is seen primarily in large muscular arteries (see the overview figure).

Veins

Capillaries unite to form larger blood vessels, called **venules,** that usually accompany arterioles. The venous blood initially flows into smaller **postcapillary venules** and then into veins of increasing size. The veins are arbitrarily classified as small, medium, and large. Compared with arteries, veins typically are more numerous and have thinner walls, larger diameters, and greater structural variation.

Small- and medium-sized veins, particularly in the extremities, have **valves.** Because of the low blood pressure in the veins, blood flow to the heart in the veins is slow and can even back up.

The presence of valves in veins assists the flow of venous blood by preventing backflow. When blood flows toward the heart, pressure in the veins forces the valves to open. As the blood begins to flow backward, the valve flaps close the lumen and prevent backflow of blood. Venous blood between the valves in the extremities flows toward the heart because of the contraction of muscles that surround the veins. Valves are absent in the veins of the central nervous system, inferior and superior vena cava, and viscera.

The walls of the veins, like those of the arteries, also exhibit three layers or tunics; however, the muscular layer is much less prominent. The **tunica intima** in large veins exhibits a prominent endothelium and subendothelial connective tissue. In large veins, the muscular **tunica media** is thin. The **tunica adventitia** is the thickest and best-developed layer of the three tunics. Longitudinal bundles of smooth muscle fibers are common in the connective tissue of this layer (see the overview figure).

Vasa Vasorum

The walls of larger arteries and veins are too thick to receive nourishment through direct diffusion from their lumina. As a result, these walls are supplied by their own small blood vessels, called the **vasa vasorum** ("vessels of the vessel"). The vasa vasorum exchange nutrients and metabolites with cells in the tunica adventitia and tunica media.

Types of Capillaries

Capillaries are the smallest blood vessels. Their average diameter is approximately 8 m, which is about the size of an **erythrocyte** (red blood cell). The human body contains three types of capillaries: continuous capillaries, fenestrated capillaries, and sinusoids. These structural variations allow different types of metabolic exchange between the blood and the surrounding tissues.

Continuous capillaries are the most common type. They are found in muscle, connective tissue, nervous tissue, and exocrine glands. In these capillaries, the **endothelial cells** are joined and form an uninterrupted, solid endothelial lining.

Fenestrated capillaries are characterized by large openings, or **fenestrations** (pores), in the cytoplasm of endothelial cells for rapid exchange of molecules between blood and tissues. Fenestrated capillaries are found in endocrine organs, small intestine, and kidney glomeruli.

Sinusoidal (discontinuous) capillaries are blood vessels that exhibit irregular, tortuous paths. Their much wider diameters slow the flow of blood. Endothelial cell junctions are rare in sinusoidal capillaries, and wide gaps exist between individual endothelial cells. Also, because a **basement membrane** underlying the endothelium is either incomplete or absent, direct exchange of molecules occurs between blood contents and cells. Sinusoidal capillaries are found in the liver, spleen, and bone marrow (see the overview figure).

The Lymph Vascular System

The **lymphatic system** consists of lymph capillaries and lymph vessels. This system starts as blind-ending tubules or lymphatic capillaries in the connective tissue of different organs. Lymphatic capillaries collect excess **interstitial fluid (lymph)** from tissues, and they return it to the venous blood via the larger **lymph vessels,** the thoracic duct, and the right lymphatic duct. Also, to allow greater permeability, the endothelium in lymph capillaries and vessels is extremely thin. The structure of larger lymph vessels is similar to that of veins, except that their walls are much thinner.

Lymph movement in the lymphatic vessels is similar to that of blood movement; that is, the contraction of surrounding muscles forces the lymph to move forward. Also, the lymph vessels contain more valves to prevent backflow of the collected lymph. Lymph vessels are found in all tissues except the central nervous system, cartilage, bone and bone marrow, thymus, placenta, and teeth.

FIGURE 8.1 ■ Blood and Lymphatic Vessels in the Connective Tissue

This composite figure illustrates a section of irregular connective tissue with nerve fibers, blood and lymphatic vessels, and adipose tissue. To illustrate structural differences, the vessels have been sectioned in the transverse, longitudinal, or oblique planes.

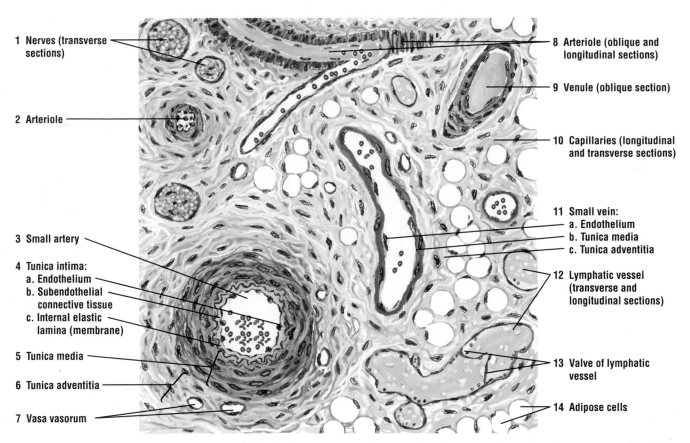

1 Nerves (transverse sections)

2 Arteriole

3 Small artery

4 Tunica intima:
   a. Endothelium
   b. Subendothelial connective tissue
   c. Internal elastic lamina (membrane)

5 Tunica media

6 Tunica adventitia

7 Vasa vasorum

8 Arteriole (oblique and longitudinal sections)

9 Venule (oblique section)

10 Capillaries (longitudinal and transverse sections)

11 Small vein:
   a. Endothelium
   b. Tunica media
   c. Tunica adventitia

12 Lymphatic vessel (transverse and longitudinal sections)

13 Valve of lymphatic vessel

14 Adipose cells

FIGURE 8.1 ■ Blood and lymphatic vessels in the connective tissue. Stain: hematoxylin and eosin. Low magnification.

A **small artery (3)** is shown in the lower left corner. In contrast to **veins (11),** an artery has a relatively thick wall and a small lumen. In cross-section, the wall of a small artery (3) exhibits the following layers:

a. The **tunica intima (4)** is the innermost layer. It is composed of **endothelium (4a),** a **subendothelial (4b)** layer of connective tissue, and an **internal elastic lamina (membrane) (4c),** which separates the tunica intima (4) from the next layer, the tunica media.

b. The **tunica media (5)** is composed predominantly of circular smooth muscle fibers. A loose network of fine elastic fibers is interspersed among the smooth muscle cells.

c. The **tunica adventitia (6)** is the connective tissue layer that surrounds the vessel. This layer contains small nerves and blood vessels. In the tunica adventitia (6), the blood vessels are collectively called the **vasa vasorum (7),** or "blood vessels of the blood vessel."

When arteries acquire approximately 25 or more layers of smooth muscle fibers in the tunica media, they are called muscular or distributing arteries. Elastic fibers become more numerous in the tunica media but remain present as thin fibers and networks.

A **venule (9)** and **small vein (11)** are also illustrated. Note the relatively thin wall and large lumen. The thin wall, however, appears to have many cell layers when cut in an **oblique** section **(9).** In cross-section, the wall of the vein exhibits the following layers:

a. The **tunica intima** is composed of **endothelium (11a)** and an extremely thin layer of fine collagen and elastic fibers, which blend with the connective tissue of the tunica media.

b. The **tunica media (11b)** consists of a thin layer of circularly arranged smooth muscle that is loosely embedded in connective tissue. The tunica media (11b) is much thinner in veins than it is in arteries (5).

c. The **tunica adventitia (11c)** contains a wide layer of connective tissue. In veins, the tunica adventitia (11c) is thicker than the tunica media (11b).

Two arterioles cut in different planes are also illustrated. **Arterioles (2, 8)** have a thin, internal elastic lamina and a layer of smooth muscle fibers in the tunica media. One **arteriole (8)** is shown cut in the longitudinal plane with a branching **capillary (10).** When an arteriole (8) is cut at an oblique angle, only the circular smooth muscle layer of the tunica media is seeen. Also visible are **capillaries (10)** sectioned in longitudinal and oblique planes and small **nerves (1)** sectioned in transverse planes.

Lymphatic vessels (12, 13) are recognized by the thinnest walls. When the lymphatic vessel is cut in a longitudinal plane, the flaps of a **valve (13)** are seen in their lumen. Many veins in the arms and legs have similar valves in their lumina.

Numerous **adipose cells (14)** are found in the surrounding connective tissue.

FUNCTIONAL CORRELATIONS

Lymphatic Capillaries and Vessels

The main function of the **lymphatic system** is to passively collect excess tissue fluid and proteins, called **lymph,** from the intercellular spaces of the connective tissue and return it to the venous blood. Lymph is a clear fluid and an **ultrafiltrate** of the blood plasma. Numerous **lymph nodes** are located along the route of the lymph vessels. In the maze of lymph node channels, the collected lymph is filtered of cells and/or particulate matter. Lymph that flows through the lymph nodes is also exposed to numerous macrophages, which engulf foreign microorganisms as well as other suspended matter. Lymph vessels bring to the systemic bloodstream **lymphocytes; fatty acids** are absorbed through the capillary lymph vessels called **lacteals,** in the small intestine; and **immunoglobulins** (antibodies) are produced in the lymph nodes.

FIGURE 8.2 ■ Muscular Artery and Vein (Transverse Section)

The walls of blood vessels contain elastic tissue that allows the vessel to expand and contract. In this illustration, a muscular **artery (1)** and **vein (4)** have been cut in a transverse plane and prepared with an elastic stain to illustrate the distribution of elastic fibers in their walls. The elastic fibers stain black, and the collagen fibers light yellow.

The wall of the artery (1) is much thicker and contains more smooth muscle fibers than the wall of the vein (4). The innermost layer, or tunica intima, of the artery (1) is stained dark because of the thick **internal elastic lamina (membrane) (1a).** The thick middle layer of the muscular artery, the **tunica media (1b),** contains several layers of smooth muscle fibers, arranged in a circular pattern, and thin, dark strands of **elastic fibers (1b).** On the periphery of the tunica media (1b) is the less conspicuous **external elastic lamina (1c).** Surrounding the artery is the connective tissue **tunica adventitia (1d),** which contains both light-staining **collagen fibers (2)** and dark-staining **elastic fibers (3).**

The wall of the vein (4) also contains the **tunica intima (4a), tunica media (4b),** and **tunica adventitia (4c)** layers. However, these three layers are not as thick in the vein (4) as they are in the wall of the artery (1).

Surrounding both vessels are a **capillary (5), arteriole (7), venule (6),** and **adipose tissue (8).** Present in the lumina of both vessels (1, 4) are numerous erythrocytes and leukocytes.

FIGURE 8.3 ■ Artery and Vein in Connective Tissue of the Vas Deferens

This phtomicrograph illustrates the structural differences between a **small artery (1)** and a **small vein (6)** in dense irregular **connective tissue (5).** The small artery (1) has a relatively thick muscular wall and a small lumen. The arterial wall consists of the **tunica intima (2),** which is composed of an inner layer of **endothelium (2a),** a layer of **subendothelial connective tissue (2b),** and an **internal elastic lamina (membrane) (2c).** This membrane (2c) separates the tunica intima (2) from the **tunica media (3),** which consists predominantly of circular smooth muscle fibers. Surrounding the tunica media (3) is a connective tissue layer, the **tunica adventitia (4).**

Adjacent to the small artery (1) is a small vein (6) with a much larger lumen that is filled with blood cells. The wall of the vein (6) is much thinner compared to that of the artery (1), but it also consists of a **tunica intima (7)** that is composed of **endothelium (7a);** a thin layer of circular smooth muscle, the **tunica media (8);** and a layer of connective tissue, the **tunica adventitia (9).**

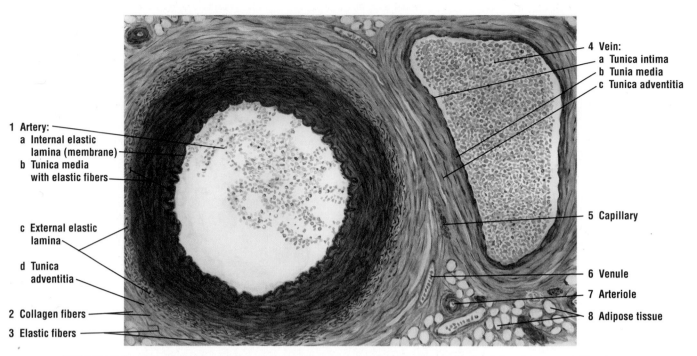

1 Artery:
a Internal elastic lamina (membrane)
b Tunica media with elastic fibers

c External elastic lamina

d Tunica adventitia

2 Collagen fibers
3 Elastic fibers

4 Vein:
a Tunica intima
b Tunia media
c Tunica adventitia

5 Capillary

6 Venule
7 Arteriole
8 Adipose tissue

FIGURE 8.2 ■ Muscular artery and vein (transverse section). Stain: elastic stain. Low magnification.

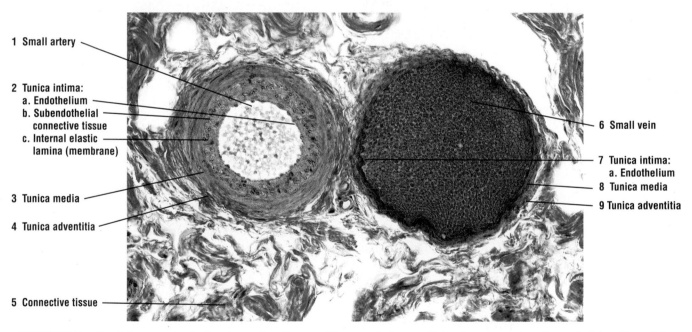

1 Small artery

2 Tunica intima:
a. Endothelium
b. Subendothelial connective tissue
c. Internal elastic lamina (membrane)

3 Tunica media

4 Tunica adventitia

5 Connective tissue

6 Small vein

7 Tunica intima:
a. Endothelium
8 Tunica media
9 Tunica adventitia

FIGURE 8.3 ■ Artery and vein in connective tissue of the vas deferens. Stain: iron hematoxylin and alcian blue. 64×

FIGURE 8.4 ■ Wall of an Elastic Artery: Aorta (Transverse Section)

The wall of the aorta is similar in morphology to that of the artery illustrated in Figure 8-3. In contrast to muscular arteries, **elastic fibers (4)** constitute the bulk of the **tunica media (6),** and in elastic arteries, **smooth muscle fibers (10)** are less abundant.. The size and arrangement of the elastic fibers (4) in the tunica media (6) are demonstrated with the elastic stain. Other tissues in the wall of the aorta, such as fine elastic fibers and smooth muscle fibers (10), either stain lightly or remain colorless.

The simple squamous **endothelium (1)** and the **subendothelial connective tissue (2)** in the **tunica intima (5)** are indicated but remain unstained. The membrane that is visible is the **internal elastic lamina (3).**

The **tunica adventitia (7),** which is somewhat less stained with elastic stain, is a narrow, peripheral zone of **connective tissue (8).** Venules (9a, 11) of different size and an **arteriole (9b)** of the **vasa vasorum (9)** supply the connective tissue (8) of the tunica adventitia (7). In large blood vessels, such as the aorta and pulmonary arteries, the tunica media (6) occupies most of the vessel wall, whereas the tunica adventitia (7) is reduced to a proportionately smaller area, as illustrated in this figure.

FIGURE 8.5 ■ Wall of a Large Vein: Portal Vein (Transverse Section)

In contrast to the wall of a large elastic artery (see Fig. 8-4), the wall of a large vein is characterized by thick, muscular **tunica adventitia (6)** in which the **smooth muscle fibers (7)** show a longitudinal orientation. In a transverse section of the portal vein, the smooth muscle fibers (7) are segregated into bundles and are seen mainly in cross-section, surrounded by the connective tissue of the tunica adventitia (6). An **arteriole (8a),** two **venules (8b),** and a **capillary (8c)** in a longitudinal section of the **vasa vasorum (8)** are visible in the connective tissue of the tunica adventitia (6).

In contrast to the thick tunica adventitia (6), the **tunica media (5)** is thinner. The **smooth muscle fibers (3)** exhibit a circular orientation. In other large veins, the tunica media (5) may be extremely thin and compact.

The **tunica intima (4)** is part of the **endothelium (1)** and is supported by a small amount of **subendothelial connective tissue (2).** In addition, large veins may exhibit an internal elastic lamina but it is not as well developed as in the arteries.

FUNCTIONAL CORRELATIONS

Blood Vessels

The **elastic arteries** transport blood from the heart and along the systemic vascular path. The increased number of **elastic fibers** in their walls allows the elastic arteries to greatly expand in diameter during **systole** (heart contraction), when a large volume of blood is ejected from the ventricles into their lumina. During **diastole** (heart relaxation), the expanded elastic walls recoil on the blood in their lumina and force it to move forward through the vascular channels. As a result, a less variable systemic blood pressure is maintained, and blood flows more evenly through the body during heartbeats.

In contrast to elastic arteries, **muscular arteries** control blood flow and blood pressure through **vasoconstriction** or **vasodilation** of their lumina. Vasoconstriction and vasodilation, because of a high proportion of **smooth muscle fibers** in the arterial walls, are controlled by unmyelinated axons of the **sympathetic division** of the **autonomic nervous system.** Similarly, by autonomic constriction or dilation of their arterial lumina, the smooth muscle fibers in the smaller muscular arteries or arterioles regulate blood flow into the capillary beds.

Terminal arterioles give rise to the smallest blood vessels, called **capillaries.** Because of their very thin walls, capillaries are sites for the exchange of gases, metabolites, nutrients, and waste products between blood and tissues.

In **veins,** blood pressure is lower than in the arteries. As a result, venous blood flow is **passive.** In the head and trunk, venous blood flow primarily results from negative pressures in the thorax and abdominal cavities that in turn result from respiratory movements. Venous blood return from the extremities is aided by surrounding **muscle contractions.**

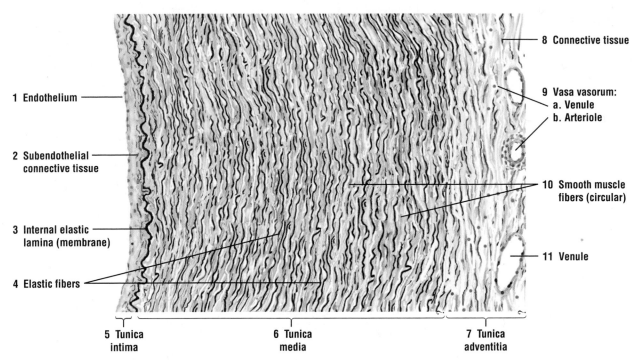

1 Endothelium

2 Subendothelial connective tissue

3 Internal elastic lamina (membrane)

4 Elastic fibers

5 Tunica intima

6 Tunica media

7 Tunica adventitia

8 Connective tissue

9 Vasa vasorum:
  a. Venule
  b. Arteriole

10 Smooth muscle fibers (circular)

11 Venule

FIGURE 8.4 ■ Wall of an elastic artery: aorta (transverse section). Stain: elastic stain. Low magnification.

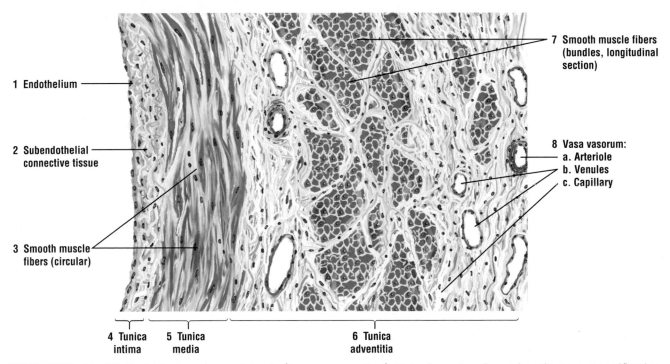

1 Endothelium

2 Subendothelial connective tissue

3 Smooth muscle fibers (circular)

4 Tunica intima

5 Tunica media

6 Tunica adventitia

7 Smooth muscle fibers (bundles, longitudinal section)

8 Vasa vasorum:
  a. Arteriole
  b. Venules
  c. Capillary

FIGURE 8.5 ■ Wall of a large vein: portal vein (transverse section). Stain: hematoxylin and eosin. Low magnification.

FIGURE 8.6 ■ Heart: Left Atrium, Atrioventricular Valve, and Left Ventricle (Longitudinal Section)

The wall of the heart consists of three layers: an inner endocardium, a middle myocardium, and an outer epicardium. The endocardium consists of a simple squamous endothelium and a thin subendothelial connective tissue. Deeper to the endocardium is the subendocardial layer of connective tissue, in which are found small blood vessels and Purkinje fibers. The subendocardial layer attaches to the endomysium of the cardiac muscle fibers. The myocardium is the thickest layer and consists of cardiac muscle fibers. The epicardium consists of a simple squamous mesothelium and an underlying subepicardial layer of connective tissue. The subepicardial layer contains coronary blood vessels, nerves, and adipose tissue.

A longitudinal section through the left side of the heart illustrates a portion of the **atrium (1),** the **cusps** of the **atrioventricular (mitral) valve (5),** and a section of the **ventricle (19).** The **endocardium (1, 9)** lines the cavities of the atrium and ventricle. Below the endocardium (1, 9) is the **subendocardial connective tissue (2).** The **myocardium (3, 19)** in both the atrium (3) and ventricle (19) consists of cardiac muscle fibers.

The outer **epicardium (13, 16)** of the atrium (13) and ventricle (16) is continuous and covers the heart externally with mesothelium. A layer of **subepicardial connective tissue (17)** contains connective tissue, **adipose tissue (15),** and numerous **coronary veins (15),** which vary in amount in different regions of the heart. The epicardium (13, 16) also extends into the coronary (atrioventricular) sulcus and interventricular sulcus of the heart.

Between the atrium (1) and ventricle (19) is a layer of dense fibrous connective tissue, called the **annulus fibrosus (4).** A biscuspid (mitral) atrioventricular valve separates the atrium (1) from the ventricle (19). The **cusps** of the **atrioventricular (mitral) valve (5)** are formed by a double membrane of the **endocardium (6)** and a dense **connective tissue core (7)** that is continuous with the annulus fibrosus (4). On the ventral surface of each cusp (5) are insertions of connective tissue cords, called **chorda tendineae (8),** that extend from the cusps of the valve (5) and attach to a **papillary muscle (11)** that projects from the ventricle wall. The inner surface of the ventricle also contains prominent muscular (myocardial) ridges, called **trabeculae carneae (10),** that give rise to the papillary muscles (11). The papillary muscles (11), via the chorda tendineae (8), hold and stabilize the cusps in the atrioventricular valves of the right and left ventricles during ventricular contractions.

The **Purkinje fibers (18),** or impulse-conducting fibers, are located in the subendocardial connective tissue (2). They are distinguished by their larger size and lighter-staining properties compared with cardiac fibers. The Purkinje fibers are illustrated in greater detail and higher magnification in Figures 8-7 and 8-9.

A large blood vessel of the heart, the **coronary artery (12),** is found in the **subepicardial connective tissue (17).** Below the coronary artery is the **coronary sinus (14),** a blood vessel that drains the heart. Entering the coronary sinus (14) is a **coronary vein (14)** with its valve. Smaller **coronary veins (15)** are seen in the subepicardial connective tissue (17) and in the connective tissue septa in the myocardium (19).

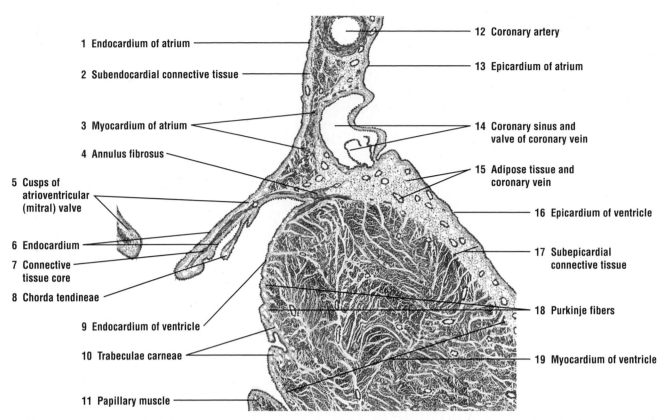

1 Endocardium of atrium

2 Subendocardial connective tissue

3 Myocardium of atrium

4 Annulus fibrosus

5 Cusps of atrioventricular (mitral) valve

6 Endocardium

7 Connective tissue core

8 Chorda tendineae

9 Endocardium of ventricle

10 Trabeculae carneae

11 Papillary muscle

12 Coronary artery

13 Epicardium of atrium

14 Coronary sinus and valve of coronary vein

15 Adipose tissue and coronary vein

16 Epicardium of ventricle

17 Subepicardial connective tissue

18 Purkinje fibers

19 Myocardium of ventricle

FIGURE 8.6 ■ Heart: left atrium, atrioventricular valve, and left ventricle (longitudinal section). Stain: hematoxylin and eosin. Low magnification.

FIGURE 8.7 ■ Heart: Right Ventricle, Pulmonary Trunk, and Pulmonary Valve (Longitudinal Section)

A section of the right ventricle and a lower portion of **pulmonary trunk (5)** are illustrated. As in other blood vessels, the pulmonary trunk (5) is lined by endothelium of the **tunica intima (5a).** The **tunica media (5b)** constitutes the thickest portion of the wall of the pulmonary trunk (5); however, its thick, elastic laminae are not seen at this magnification. The thin connective tissue, or **tunica adventitia (5c)**, merges with the surrounding **subepicardial connective tissue (2)**, which contains **adipose tissue (2)** and **coronary arterioles and venules (3).**

The **pulmonary trunk (5)** arises from the **annulus fibrosus (8).** One cusp of its **semilunar (pulmonary) valve (6)** is illustrated. Similar to the atrioventricular valve (see Fig. 8-6), the semilunar valve (6) of the pulmonary trunk (5) is covered with **endocardium (6).** A **connective tissue core (7)** from the **annulus fibrosus (8)** extends into the base of the semilunar valve (6) and forms its central core.

The thick **myocardium (4)** of the right ventricle is lined internally by **endocardium (9).** The endocardium (9) extends over the pulmonary valve (6) and the annulus fibrosus (8), and it blends in with the tunica intima (5a) of the pulmonary trunk (5).

The pulmonary trunk (5) is lined by the **subepicardial connective tissue** and **adipose tissue (2),** which in turn is covered by **epicardium (1).** Both of these layers cover the external surface of the right ventricle. **Coronary arterioles and venules (3)** are seen in the subepicardial connective tissue (2).

FIGURE 8.8 ■ Heart: Contracting Cardiac Muscle Fibers and Impulse-Conducting Purkinje Fibers

This figure illustrates a section of the heart stained with Mallory-azan. With this preparation, the blue-stained collagen fibers accentuate the **subendocardial connective tissue (9)** that surrounds the **Purkinje fibers (6, 10).** The characteristic features of Purkinje fibers (6, 10) are demonstrated in both longitudinal and transverse planes of section. In the transverse plane (6), Purkinje fibers exhibit fewer peripheral myofibrils, leaving a perinuclear zone of comparatively clear sarcoplasm. A nucleus is seen in some transverse sections; in others, a central area of clear sarcoplasm is seen, with the plane of section bypassing the nucleus.

The Purkinje fibers (6, 10) are located under the **endocardium (7),** which represents the endothelium of the heart cavities. The Purkinje fibers (6, 10) differ from typical **cardiac muscle fibers (1, 3).** In contrast to cardiac muscle fibers (1, 3), Purkinje fibers (6, 10) are larger in size and show less intense staining.

The cardiac muscle fibers (1, 3) are connected to each other via the prominent **intercalated disks (4).** Intercalated disks are not observed in Purkinje fibers (6, 10). Instead, Purkinje fibers (6, 10) are connected to each other via desmosomes and gap junctions and eventually merge with cardiac muscle fibers (1, 3).

The heart musculature has a rich blood supply. Seen in this illustration are a **capillary (8),** an **arteriole (5),** and a **venule (2).**

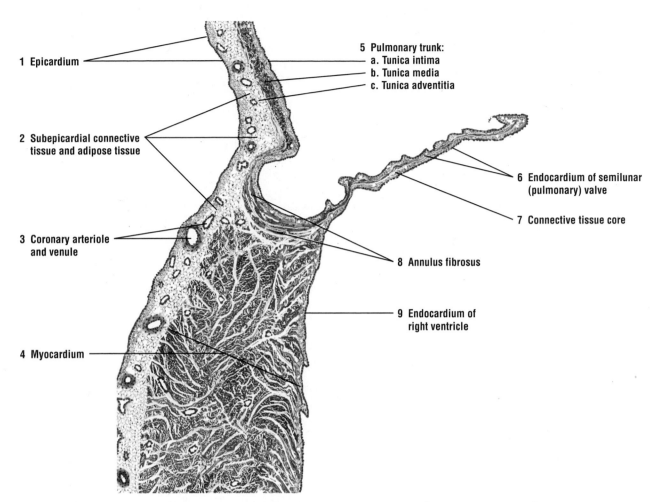

1 Epicardium

2 Subepicardial connective tissue and adipose tissue

3 Coronary arteriole and venule

4 Myocardium

5 Pulmonary trunk:
  a. Tunica intima
  b. Tunica media
  c. Tunica adventitia

6 Endocardium of semilunar (pulmonary) valve

7 Connective tissue core

8 Annulus fibrosus

9 Endocardium of right ventricle

FIGURE 8.7 ■ Heart: right ventricle, pulmonary trunk, and pulmonary valve (longitudinal section). Stain: hematoxylin and eosin. Low magnification.

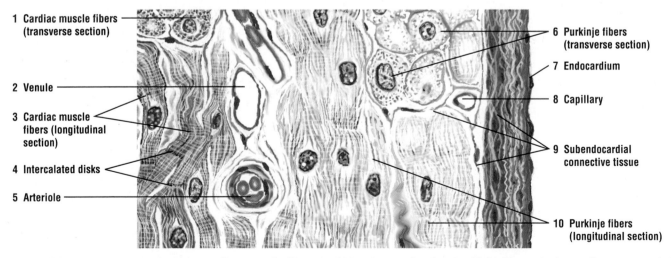

1 Cardiac muscle fibers (transverse section)

2 Venule

3 Cardiac muscle fibers (longitudinal section)

4 Intercalated disks

5 Arteriole

6 Purkinje fibers (transverse section)

7 Endocardium

8 Capillary

9 Subendocardial connective tissue

10 Purkinje fibers (longitudinal section)

FIGURE 8.8 ■ Heart: contracting cardiac muscle fibers and impulse-conducting Purkinje fibers. Stain: Mallory-azan. High magnification.

FIGURE 8.9 ■ Heart Wall: Purkinje Fibers

A photomicrograph of the ventricular heart wall illustrates the **endocardium (3)** of the heart chamber, the **subendocardial connective tissue (4),** and the underlying **Purkinje fibers (5).** In comparison to the adjacent, red-stained **cardiac muscle fibers (1),** the Purkinje fibers **(5)** are larger in size and exhibit less intense staining. Also, the Purkinje fibers **(5)** exhibit fewer myofibrils, which are peripherally distributed and leave a perinuclear zone of clear sarcoplasm. Purkinje fibers **(5)** gradually merge with the cardiac muscle fibers **(1).** Surrounding both the Purkinje fibers **(5)** and the cardiac muscle fibers **(1)** are bundles of **connective tissue fibers (2).**

FUNCTIONAL CORRELATIONS

Pacemaker of the Heart and Impulse Conduction

Cardiac muscle is **involuntary;** it contracts rhythmically and automatically. The **impulse-generating** and **impulse-conducting** portions of the heart are the specialized or modified cardiac muscle fibers located in the **sinoatrial (SA) node** and the **atrioventricular (AV) node** in the right atrium of the heart. The modified muscle fibers in these nodes undergo spontaneous depolarization, which sends a wave of stimulation throughout the myocardium of the heart. Because the fibers in the SA node depolarize and repolarize faster than those in the AV node, the SA node sets the pace for the heartbeat and is, therefore, the **pacemaker.**

Intercalated disks bind all cardiac muscle fibers as stimulatory impulses from the SA node are conducted via **gap junctions** to atrial musculature, causing their contraction. Impulses from the SA node travel through the heart musculature via the **internodal pathway** to stimulate the AV node in the interatrial septum. From the AV node, the impulses spread along a bundle of specialized conducting cardiac fibers, called the **atrioventricular bundle (of His),** located in the interventricular septum. The atrioventricular bundle divides into right and left bundle branches. Approximately halfway down the interventricular septum, the atrioventricular bundle becomes the **Purkinje fibers,** which branch in the myocardium and transmit stimulation throughout the ventricles.

The pacemaker activities of the heart are also influenced by nerve fibers from the **autonomic nervous system** and by certain **hormones.** Although the nerves of the autonomic system that innervate the myocardium of the heart do not affect initiation of the rhythmic activity of the nodes, they do affect the heart rate. Stimulation by the sympathetic nerves accelerates the heart rate, whereas stimulation by the parasympathetic nerves decreases the heart rate.

Purkinje Fibers

Purkinje fibers are thicker and larger than cardiac muscle fibers, and they contain a greater amount of **glycogen.** They also contain fewer contractile filaments. Purkinje fibers are part of the conducting system of the heart and are recognized in the **endocardium** on either side of the interventricular septum as separate tracts. Purkinje fibers deliver continuous waves of stimulation from atrial nodes to the rest of the heart musculature via the **gap junctions,** producing ventricular contractions (systole) and ejection of blood from both ventricular chambers.

Atrial Natriuretic Hormone

Certain cardiac muscle fibers in the atria exhibit dense granules in their cytoplasm. These granules contain **atrial natriuretic hormone,** a chemical that is released in response to atrial distension. The main function of atrial natriuretic hormone is to decrease blood pressure by regulating blood volume. This action is accomplished by inhibiting the release of renin by the specialized cells in the kidney and of aldosterone from the adrenal gland cortex. The overall effects alter the heart function and produce decreased blood volume and blood pressure.

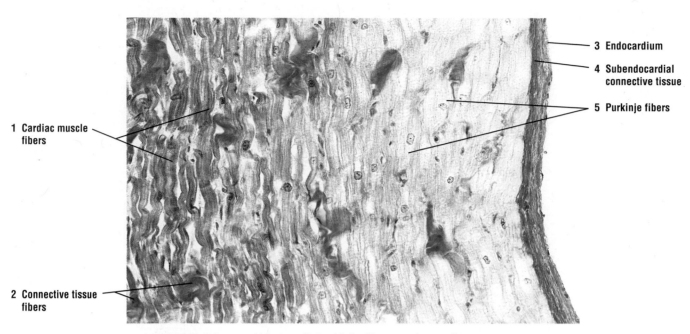

1 Cardiac muscle fibers

2 Connective tissue fibers

3 Endocardium

4 Subendocardial connective tissue

5 Purkinje fibers

FIGURE 8.9 ■ Heart wall: Purkinje fibers. Stain: Mallory-azan. 64×

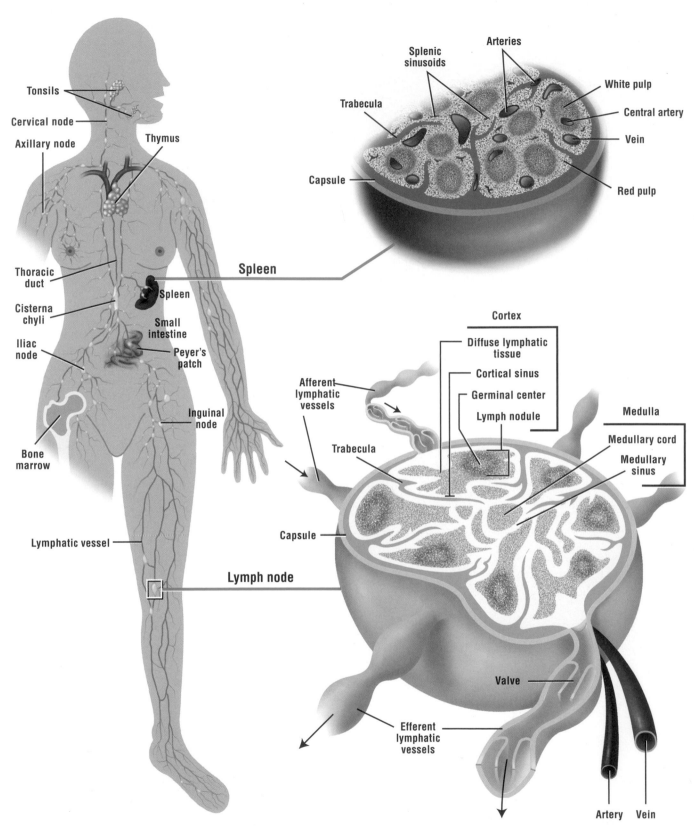

OVERVIEW FIGURE ■ Location and distribution of the lymphoid organs and lymphatic channels in the body. Internal contents of the lymph node and spleen are illustrated in greater detail.

CHAPTER 9

Lymphoid System

The **lymphoid system** includes all the cells, tissues, and organs in the body that contain aggregates of immune cells, called **lymphocytes.** Cells of the immune system, especially lymphocytes, are distributed throughout the body as single cells; as isolated accumulations of cells; as distinct, nonencapsulated lymphatic nodules in the loose connective tissue of different organs; or as encapsulated individual lymphoid organs. The major lymphoid organs are the lymph nodes, tonsils, thymus, and spleen. Because bone marrow produces lymphocytes, it is considered to be a lymphoid organ and part of the lymphoid system.

The lymphoid system performs numerous functions. It collects excess interstitial fluid into lymphatic capillaries, transports absorbed lipids from the small intestine, and responds immunologically to invading foreign substances.

Lymphoid Organs: Lymph Nodes and Spleen

The overview figure for this chapter illustrates the general structures of two encapsulated lymphoid organs, the **lymph node** and the **spleen.** A connective tissue **capsule** surrounds the lymph node and sends its **trabeculae** into the interior. Lymph enters the lymph node via **afferent lymphatic vessels** that penetrate the capsule on the convex surface.

Each lymph nodes contains an outer **cortex** and an inner **medulla.** A network of reticular fibers and spherical, nonencapsulated aggregations of lymphocytes, called **lymphoid nodules,** characterize the cortex. Some lymphoid nodules exhibit lighter-staining central areas, called **germinal centers.** The medulla consists of **medullary cords** and **medullary sinuses.** Medullary cords are networks of reticular fibers that are filled with plasma cells, macrophages, and lymphocytes separated by capillary-like channels, called medullary sinuses. Lymph flows through the medullary sinuses and exits the lymph node on the opposite side via the **efferent lymphatic vessels** (see the overview figure).

The spleen is a large lymphoid organ with a rich blood supply. A connective tissue capsule surrounds the spleen and divides its interior into incomplete compartments, called the splenic pulp. **White pulp** consists of dark-staining lymphoid aggregations, or **lymphatic nodules,** that surround a blood vessel, called the **central artery.** White pulp is located within the blood-rich **red pulp,** which in turn consists of **splenic cords** and **splenic sinusoids.** Splenic cords contain networks of reticular fibers in which macrophages, lymphocytes, plasma cells, and different blood cells are found. Splenic sinuses are interconnected blood channels that drain splenic blood into larger sinuses that eventually leave the spleen via the splenic vein (see the overview figure).

Types of Lymphoid Cells: T lymphocytes and B lymphocytes

All components of the lymphoid system are an essential part of the **immune system.** A vital function of this system is to resist—and to eliminate from the body—disease-causing **pathogens,** such as bacteria, viruses, and parasites, by specifically reacting against them in an **immune response.** Because pathogens can enter the body at different points, the lymphoid system has a wide distribution.

Lymphocytes are the cells that carry out the immune response. Different types of lymphocytes are present in various organs of the body. Morphologically, all types of lymphocytes appear very similar, but functionally, they are very different. When lymphocytes are properly stimulated, **B lymphocytes,** or **B cells,** and **T lymphocytes,** or **T cells,** are produced. These two subclasses of lymphocytes are distinguished based on where they differentiate and mature into immunocompetent cells and on the types of receptors that are present on their cell membranes. These two functionally distinct types of lymphocytes are found in blood, lymph, lymphoid tissues, and lymphoid organs. Like all blood cells, both types of lymphocytes originate from precursor **hemopoietic stem cells** in the **bone marrow** and then enter the bloodstream.

The T lymphocytes arise from lymphocytes that are carried from the bone marrow to the **thymus gland,** where they mature and acquire **immunocompetence** before migrating to peripheral lymphoid tissues and organs. The thymus gland produces mature T lymphocytes early in life. After their stay in this gland, T lymphocytes are distributed throughout the body in blood, and they populate lymph nodes, the spleen, and lymphoid aggregates or nodules in connective tissue. In these regions, the T lymphocytes carry out immune responses when stimulated. On encountering an antigen, T lymphocytes destroy it, either by cytotoxic action or by activating B lymphocytes.

The T lymphocytes can be differentiated into four main types: helper T lymphocytes, cytotoxic T lymphocytes, memory T lymphocytes, and suppressor T lymphocytes. When encountering an antigen, **helper T lymphocytes** assist other lymphocytes by secreting immune chemicals, called **cytokines.** Cytokines are protein hormones that stimulate proliferation, secretion, differentiation, and maturation of B lymphocytes into plasma cells, which then produce immune proteins, called **antibodies. Cytotoxic T lymphocytes** specifically recognize antigenically different cells, such as virus-infected cells, foreign cells, or malignant cells. On activation and binding to the target cells, cytotoxic T lymphocytes produce protein molecules, called **perforins,** that perforate or puncture the target cell membranes, causing cell death. Cytotoxic T lymphocytes also destroy foreign cells by inducing **apoptosis,** or programmed cell death. **Memory T lymphocytes** are the long-lived progeny of T lymphocytes. They respond rapidly to the same antigens in the body, and they stimulate production of cytotoxic T lymphocytes. Memory T lymphocytes are the counterparts of memory B lymphocytes. **Suppressor T lymphocytes** decrease or inhibit the functions of helper T lymphocytes and cytotoxic T lymphocytes.

The **B lymphocytes** mature and become immunocompetent in bone marrow. After maturation, blood carries B lymphocytes to the nonthymic lymphoid tissues, such as lymph nodes, the spleen, and connective tissue. The B lymphocytes are able to recognize a particular type of antigen because of the presence of **antigen receptors** on the surface of their cell membrane. Immunocompetent B lymphocytes become activated when they encounter a specific antigen that binds to the B lymphocyte's surface antigen receptor. The response of B lymphocytes to an antigen, however, is more intense when antigen-presenting cells, such as **helper T lymphocytes,** present that antigen to the B lymphocytes. Helper T lymphocytes secrete a cytokine, called **interleukin-2,** that induces increased proliferation and differentiation of antigen-activated B lymphocytes. Numerous progeny of activated B lymphocytes enlarge, divide, proliferate, and differentiate into **plasma cells,** which then secrete large amounts of antibodies specific to the antigen that triggered the plasma cell formation. Antibodies react with the antigens and initiate a complex process that eventually destroys the foreign substance that activated the immune response. Other activated B lymphocytes do not become plasma cells; instead, they persist in lymphoid organs as **memory B lymphocytes.** These memory cells produce a more rapid immunologic response should the same antigen reappear.

In addition to T lymphocytes and B lymphocytes, cells called macrophages, natural killer cells, and antigen-presenting cells perform important functions in immune responses. **Natural killer cells** attack virally infected cells and cancer cells. **Antigen-presenting cells,** which are found in most tissues, phagocytose and process antigens and then present the antigen to T lymphocytes, inducing their activation.

Basic Types of Immune Responses

The presence of foreign cells or antigens in the body stimulates a highly complex series of reactions. These result in either production of antibodies that bind to the antigens or stimulation of cells that destroy foreign cells. Two types of closely related immune responses take place in the body, both of which are triggered by antigens.

In the **cell-mediated immune response,** T lymphocytes proliferate into cytotoxic T lymphocytes, which then destroy foreign microorganisms, parasites, or virus-infected cells. The T lymphocytes may also attack indirectly, by activating B lymphocytes or **macrophages** of the immune system. The T lymphocytes provide specific immune protection without secreting antibodies.

In the **humoral immune response,** exposure of B lymphocytes to an antigen transforms some of the B lymphocytes into plasma cells, which secrete specific antibodies into blood and lymph. These antibodies then bind to, inactivate, and/or destroy the specific foreign substance or antigen. The activation and proliferation of B lymphocytes against most antigens require the cooperation of helper T lymphocytes that respond to the same antigen and the production of certain cytokines.

FIGURE 9.1 ■ Lymph Node (Panoramic View)

The lymph node consists of dense masses of lymphocyte aggregations intermixed with dilated lymphatic sinuses that contain lymph and supported by a framework of fine reticular fibers. Here, a lymph node has been sectioned in half to show the outer, dark-staining **cortex (4)** and the inner, light-staining **medulla (10)**.

The lymph node is surrounded by a **pericapsular adipose tissue (1)** that contains numerous blood vessels, shown here as an **arteriole** and **venule (9)**. A dense connective tissue **capsule (2)** also surrounds the lymph node. From the capsule (2), **connective tissue trabeculae (6)** extend into the node, initially between the lymphatic nodules and then ramifying throughout the medulla (10) for variable distance. The trabecular connective tissue (6) also contain the major, **trabecular blood vessels (5, 8)** of the lymph node.

Afferent lymphatic vessels with **valves (7)** course in the connective tissue capsule (2) of the lymph node and, at intervals, penetrate the capsule to enter a narrow space, called the **subcapsular sinus (3, 15)**. From here, the sinuses (cortical sinuses) extend along the trabeculae (6) to pass into the **medullary sinuses (11)**.

The cortex (4) of the lymph node contains numerous lymphocyte aggregations, called **lymphatic nodules (16)**. When the lymphatic nodules (16) are sectioned through the center, lighter-staining areas become visible. These lighter-staining areas are the **germinal centers (17)** of the lymphatic nodules (16), and they represent the active sites of lymphocyte proliferation.

In the medulla (10) of the lymph node, the lymphocytes are arranged as irregular cords of lymphatic tissue, called **medullary cords (14)**. Medullary cords (14) contain macrophages, plasma cells, and small lymphocytes. The dilated medullary sinuses (11) drain the lymph from the cortical region of the lymph node and course between the medullary cords (14) toward the hilus of the organ.

The concavity of the lymph node represents the **hilus (12)**. Nerves, blood vessels, and veins that supply and drain the lymph node are located in the hilus (12). **Efferent lymphatic vessels (13)** drain the lymph from the medullary sinuses (11) and exit the lymph node in the hilus (12).

1 Pericapsular adipose tissue

2 Capsule

3 Subcapsular sinus

4 Cortex

5 Trabecular blood vessels

6 Connective tissue trabeculae

7 Afferent lymphatic vessels with valves

8 Trabecular blood vessels

9 Arteriole and venule

10 Medulla

11 Medullary sinuses

12 Hilus

13 Efferent lymphatic vessels

14 Medullary cords

15 Subcapsular sinus

16 Lymphatic nodules

17 Germinal centers of lymphatic nodules

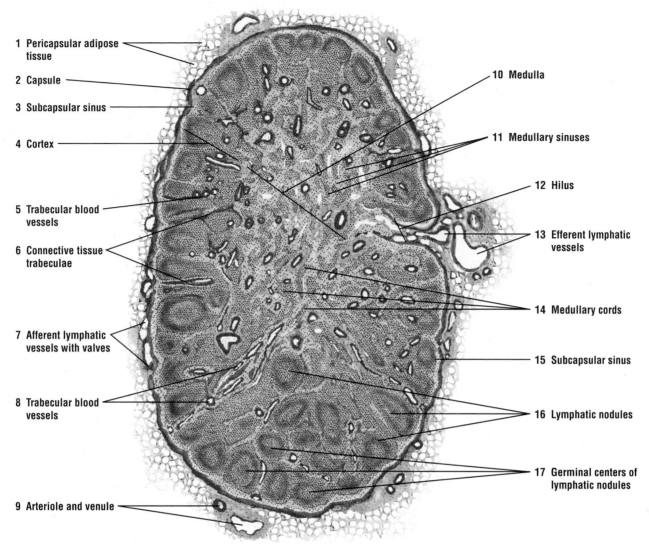

FIGURE 9.1 ▨ Lymph node (panoramic view). Stain: hematoxylin and eosin. Medium magnification.

FIGURE 9.2 ■ Lymph Node Capsule, Cortex, and Medulla (Sectional View)

A small section of a cortical region of the lymph node is illustrated at higher magnification.

A layer of **connective tissue (1)** with a **venule** and **arteriole (11)** surround the lymph node **capsule (3).** Visible in the connective tissue (1) is an afferent **lymphatic vessel (2)** lined with endothelium and containing a **valve (2).** Arising from the inner surface of the capsule (3), the **connective tissue trabeculae (5, 14)** extend through the cortex and medulla. Associated with the connective tissue trabeculae (5, 14) are numerous **trabecular blood vessels (16).**

The cortex of the lymph node is separated from the connective tissue capsule (3) by the **subcapsular (marginal) sinus (4, 12).** The cortex consists of **lymphatic nodules (13)** situated adjacent to each other but incompletely separated by internodular connective tissue trabeculae (5, 14) and **trabecular (cortical) sinuses (6).** In this illustration, two complete lymphatic nodules (13) are illustrated. When sectioned through the middle, the lymphatic nodules exhibit a central, lighter-staining **germinal center (7, 15)** surrounded by the darker-staining, peripheral portion of the nodule (13). In the germinal centers (7, 15) of the lymphatic nodules (13), the cells are more loosely aggregated, and the developing lymphocytes have larger and lighter-staining nuclei with more cytoplasm.

The deeper portion of the lymph node cortex is the **paracortex (8, 17).** A thymus-dependent zone, this area is primarily occupied by T lymphocytes. It is also a transition area from the lymphatic nodules (7, 13) to the **medullary cords (9, 19)** of the lymph node medulla. The medulla consists of anastomosing cords of lymphatic tissue, the medullary cords (9, 19), interspersed with **medullary sinuses (10, 18)** that drain the lymph from the node into the efferent lymphatic vessels at the hilus (see Fig. 9-1).

Fine reticular connective tissue provides the main structural support for the lymph node and forms the core of the lymphatic nodules (13) in the cortex, the medullary cords (9, 19), and all the medullary sinuses (10, 18) in the medulla. Relatively few lymphocytes are seen in the medullary sinuses (10, 18); thus, it is possible to distinguish the reticular framework of the node. In the lymphatic nodules (13) and the medullary cords (9, 19), the lymphocytes are so abundant that the fine reticulum is obscured unless it is specifically stained (see Fig. 9-5). Most of the lymphocytes are small, with large, deep-staining nuclei and condensed chromatin, and they exhibit either a small amount of cytoplasm or none at all.

FUNCTIONAL CORRELATIONS

Lymph Nodes

Lymph nodes are important components of the defense mechanism. They are distributed throughout the body along the paths of **lymphatic vessels** and are most prominent in the **inguinal** and **axillary regions.** Their major functions are **lymph filtration** and **phagocytosis** of bacteria or foreign substances from the lymph. Trapped within the reticular fiber network of each node are fixed or free macrophages that destroy any foreign substances. Thus, as lymph is filtered, the nodes participate in localizing and preventing the spread of infection into the general circulation and other organs.

Lymph nodes also produce, store, and recirculate **B lymphocytes** and **T lymphocytes.** The B lymphocytes congregate in the **lymphatic nodules** of lymph nodes, whereas the T lymphocytes are concentrated below the nodules, in the deep **cortical** or **paracortical regions.** Lymph nodes are also the sites of **antigenic recognition** and **antigenic activation** of B lymphocytes, which give rise to **plasma cells** and **memory B lymphocytes.**

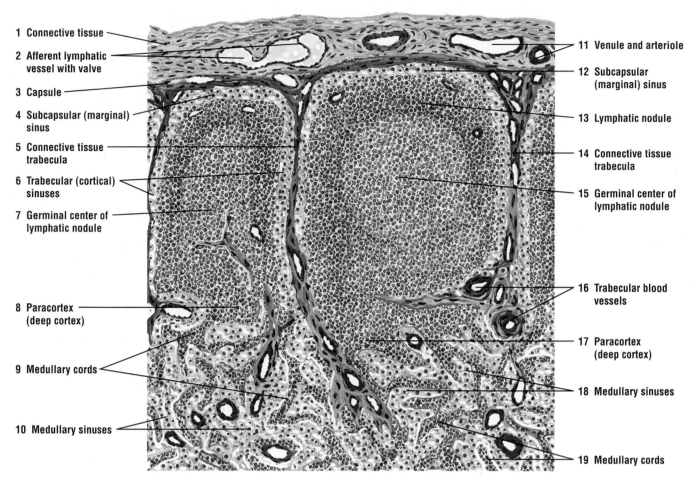

1 Connective tissue

2 Afferent lymphatic vessel with valve

3 Capsule

4 Subcapsular (marginal) sinus

5 Connective tissue trabecula

6 Trabecular (cortical) sinuses

7 Germinal center of lymphatic nodule

8 Paracortex (deep cortex)

9 Medullary cords

10 Medullary sinuses

11 Venule and arteriole

12 Subcapsular (marginal) sinus

13 Lymphatic nodule

14 Connective tissue trabecula

15 Germinal center of lymphatic nodule

16 Trabecular blood vessels

17 Paracortex (deep cortex)

18 Medullary sinuses

19 Medullary cords

FIGURE 9.2   ■ Lymph node capsule, cortex, and medulla (sectional view). Stain: hematoxylin and eosin. Medium magnification.

FIGURE 9.3 ■ Cortex and Medulla of a Lymph Node

This low-power photomicrograph illustrates the cortex and medulla of the lymph node. A loose connective tissue **capsule (4)** with blood vessels and **adipose cells (7)** covers the lymph node. Inferior to the capsule (4) is the **subcapsular (marginal) sinus (5),** which overlies the darker-staining and peripheral lymph node **cortex (3).** In the cortex (3) are numerous **lymphatic nodules (1, 6),** some of which contain a lighter-staining **germinal center (2).**

The central region of the lymph node is the lighter-staining **medulla (9).** This region is characterized by the dark-staining **medullary cords (12)** and the light-staining lymphatic channels, or **medullary sinuses (11).** The medullary sinuses (11) drain the lymph that enters the lymph node through the afferent lymphatic vessels in the capsule (see Fig. 9-2) and converges toward the hilum of the lymph node (see Fig. 9-1). In the hilum are numerous **arteries (8)** and veins. The lymph leaves the lymph node via the **efferent lymphatic vessels** with **valves (10)** at the hilum.

FIGURE 9.4 ■ Lymph Node: Subcortical Sinus and Lymphatic Nodule

This figure illustrates, at higher magnification and in greater detail, a portion of the lymph node with the connective tissue **capsule (3), trabecula (4),** and **subcapsular sinus (1)** that continue on both sides of the trabecula (4), as the **trabecular sinuses (12),** into the interior of the lymph node.

The reticular connective tissue of the lymph node, or the **reticular cells (8, 11),** are seen in different regions of the node. Reticular cells (8, 11) are visible in the subcapsular sinus (1), trabecular sinuses (12), and **germinal center (9)** of the **lymphatic nodule (14).** Numerous free **macrophages (2, 6, 16)** are also seen in the subcapsular sinus (1), trabecular sinuses (12), and germinal center (9) of the lymphatic nodule (14).

A lymphatic nodule with a small section of its **peripheral zone (14)** and a germinal center (9) with developing lymphocytes are also visible. **Endothelial cells (5, 13)** line the sinuses (1, 12) and form an incomplete cover over the surface of the lymphatic nodules (14).

The peripheral zone of the lymphatic nodule (14) stains dense because of the accumulations of **small lymphocytes (7).** The small lymphocytes (7) are characterized by dark-staining nuclei, condensed chromatin, and little or no cytoplasm. Small lymphocytes (7) are also present in the subcapsular sinus (1) and trabecular sinuses (12).

The germinal center (9) of the lymphatic nodule (14) contains **medium-sized lymphocytes (10).** These cells are characterized by larger, lighter-staining nuclei and more cytoplasm than in the small lymphocytes (7). The nuclei of medium-sized lymphocytes (10) exhibit variations in size and density of chromatin. The largest lymphocytes, with less condensed chromatin, are derived from **lymphoblasts (17).** Small numbers of lymphoblasts (17) are visible in the germinal center (9) of the lymphatic nodules (14) as large, round cells with a broad band of cytoplasm and a large vesicular nucleus having one or more nucleoli. **Lymphoblasts undergoing mitosis (15)** produce other lymphoblasts and medium-sized lymphocytes (10). With successive mitotic divisions of lymphoblasts (15), the chromatin condenses, and the cells decrease in size, resulting in the formation of small lymphocytes (7).

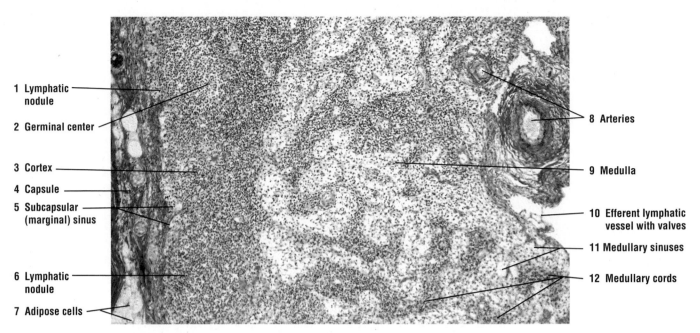

1 Lymphatic nodule
2 Germinal center
3 Cortex
4 Capsule
5 Subcapsular (marginal) sinus
6 Lymphatic nodule
7 Adipose cells

8 Arteries
9 Medulla
10 Efferent lymphatic vessel with valves
11 Medullary sinuses
12 Medullary cords

FIGURE 9.3 ■ Cortex and medulla of a lymph node. Stain: Mallory-azan. 25×

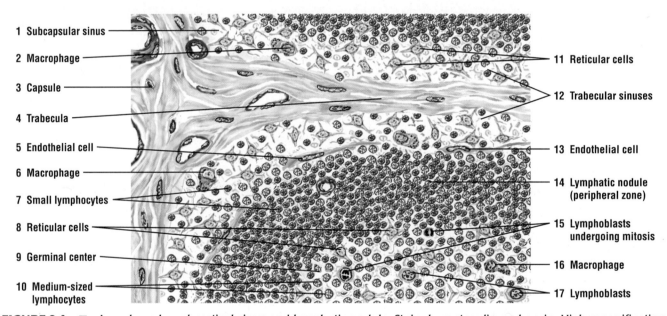

1 Subcapsular sinus
2 Macrophage
3 Capsule
4 Trabecula
5 Endothelial cell
6 Macrophage
7 Small lymphocytes
8 Reticular cells
9 Germinal center
10 Medium-sized lymphocytes

11 Reticular cells
12 Trabecular sinuses
13 Endothelial cell
14 Lymphatic nodule (peripheral zone)
15 Lymphoblasts undergoing mitosis
16 Macrophage
17 Lymphoblasts

FIGURE 9.4 ■ Lymph node: subcortical sinus and lymphatic nodule. Stain: hematoxylin and eosin. High magnification.

FIGURE 9.5 ■ Lymph Node: Subcapsular Sinus, Trabecular Sinus, and Supporting Reticular Fibers

A section of a lymph node has been stained with the silver method to illustrate the intricate arrangement of the supporting **reticular fibers (6, 9)** of a lymph node. The thicker and denser collagen fibers in the connective tissue **capsule (3)** stain pink. Both the capsule and the rest of the lymph node are supported by delicate reticular fibers (6, 9) that stain black and form a fine meshwork throughout the organ.

The various zones illustrated in Figure 9-2 with hematoxylin-and-eosin stain are readily recognizable with the silver stain. A connective tissue **trabecula (4)** from the capsule (3) penetrates the interior of the lymph node between two **lymphatic nodules (8, 12).** Inferior to the capsule (3) are **subcapsular (marginal) sinuses (1, 7)** that continue on each side of the trabecula (4), as the **trabecular sinuses (2, 5),** into the medulla of the node and eventually exit through the efferent lymph vessels in the hilum.

FIGURE 9.6 ■ Thymus Gland (Panoramic View)

The thymus gland is a lobulated lymphoid organ that is enclosed by a connective tissue **capsule (1)** from which arise connective tissue **trabeculae (2, 10).** The trabeculae (2, 10) extend into the interior of the organ, and they subdivide the thymus gland into numerous incomplete **lobules (8).** Each lobule consists of a dark-staining, outer **cortex (3, 13)** and a lighter-staining, inner **medulla (4, 12).** Because the lobules are incomplete, the medulla shows continuity between the neighboring lobules (4, 12). **Blood vessels (5, 14)** pass into the thymus gland via the connective tissue capsule (1) and the trabeculae (2, 10).

The cortex (3, 13) of each lobule contains densely packed lymphocytes that do not form lymphatic nodules. In contrast, the medulla (4, 12) contains fewer lymphocytes but more epithelial reticular cells (see Fig. 9-7). The medulla also contains numerous **thymic (Hassall's) corpuscles (6, 9)** that characterize the thymus gland.

The histology of the thymus gland varies with age. The thymus gland attains its greatest development shortly after birth. By the time of puberty, it begins to involute or show signs of gradual regression/degeneration. Consequently, lymphocyte production declines, and the thymic (Hassall's) corpuscles (6, 9) become more prominent. In addition, the parenchyma, or cellular portion of the gland, is gradually replaced by loose **connective tissue (10)** and **adipose cells (7, 11).** The thymus gland depicted in this illustration exhibits adipose tissue accumulation and initial signs of involution associated with increasing age.

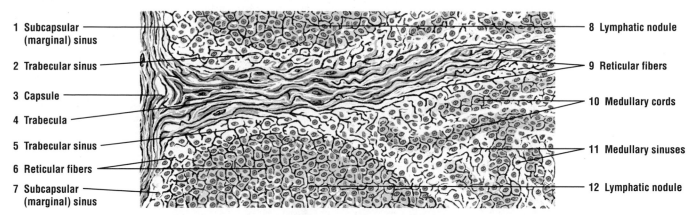

1 Subcapsular (marginal) sinus

2 Trabecular sinus

3 Capsule

4 Trabecula

5 Trabecular sinus

6 Reticular fibers

7 Subcapsular (marginal) sinus

8 Lymphatic nodule

9 Reticular fibers

10 Medullary cords

11 Medullary sinuses

12 Lymphatic nodule

FIGURE 9.5 ■ Lymph node: subcapsular sinus, trabecular sinus, and supporting reticular fibers. Stain: Silver stain. Medium magnification.

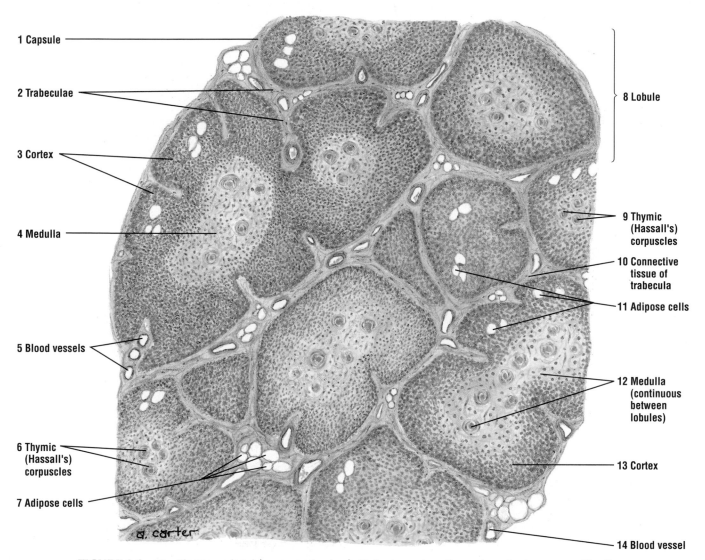

1 Capsule

2 Trabeculae

3 Cortex

4 Medulla

5 Blood vessels

6 Thymic (Hassall's) corpuscles

7 Adipose cells

8 Lobule

9 Thymic (Hassall's) corpuscles

10 Connective tissue of trabecula

11 Adipose cells

12 Medulla (continuous between lobules)

13 Cortex

14 Blood vessel

FIGURE 9.6 ■ Thymus gland (panoramic view). Stain: hematoxylin and eosin. Low magnification.

FIGURE 9.7 ■ Thymus Gland (Sectional View)

A small section of the cortex and medulla of a thymus gland lobule is illustrated at higher magnification.

The thymic lymphocytes in the **cortex (1, 5)** form dense aggregations. In contrast, the **medulla (3)** contains few lymphocytes but more **epithelial reticular cells (7, 10).**

The **thymic (Hassall's) corpuscles (8, 9)** are oval structures consisting of round or spherical aggregations (whorls) of flattened epithelial cells. The thymic corpuscles also exhibit calcification or **degeneration centers (9)** that stain pink or eosinophilic. The functional significance of these corpuscles remains unknown.

Blood vessels (6) and **adipose cells (4)** are present in both the thymic lobules and in a connective tissue **trabecula (2).**

FIGURE 9.8 ■ Cortex and Medulla of a Thymus Gland

A low-magnification photomicrograph shows a portion of a thymus gland lobule. A **connective tissue trabecula (1)** subdivides the gland into incomplete lobules. Each lobule consists of the darker-staining **cortex (2)** and the lighter-staining **medulla (3).** A characteristic **thymic (Hassall's) corpuscle (4)** is present in the center of the medulla.

FUNCTIONAL CORRELATIONS

Thymus Gland

The **thymus gland** performs an important role during early childhood in **immune system development.** Undifferentiated **lymphocytes** are carried from bone marrow by the bloodstream to the thymus gland. Here, the lymphocytes proliferate and differentiate into mature **immunocompetent T lymphocytes, helper T lymphocytes,** and **cytotoxic T lymphocytes,** whereby they acquire their surface receptors for the recognition of antigens.

Mature T lymphocytes leave the thymus gland via the bloodstream and populate the **lymph nodes, spleen,** and other thymus-dependent **lymphatic tissues.** The thymus gland involutes after puberty, and the production of T lymphocytes decreases. However, because T lymphocyte progeny have been established, immunity is maintained without the need for new T lymphocytes. Most T lymphocytes develop in the cortex of the thymus gland. These developing lymphocytes are prevented from coming into contact with bloodborne antigens by a physical **blood-thymus barrier. Macrophages** outside the capillaries ensure that substances transported in the blood vessels do not interact with the developing T lymphocytes in the cortex and induce an autoimmune response against the body's own cells or tissues.

The thymus gland also contains **epithelial reticular cells.** These cells secrete hormones that are necessary for the proliferation, differentiation, and maturation of T lymphocytes and for the expression of their surface markers. These hormones are **thymulin, thymopoietin, thymosin,** and **thymic humoral factor.**

If the thymus gland is removed from a newborn, the lymphoid organs will not receive the immunocompetent T lymphocytes, and the individual will not acquire the immunological competence to fight pathogens. Thus, death may occur early in life because of complications from an infection.

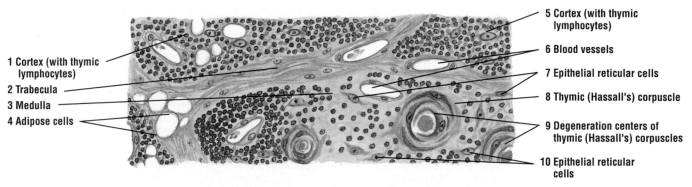

1 Cortex (with thymic
lymphocytes)

2 Trabecula

3 Medulla

4 Adipose cells

5 Cortex (with thymic
lymphocytes)

6 Blood vessels

7 Epithelial reticular cells

8 Thymic (Hassall's) corpuscle

9 Degeneration centers of
thymic (Hassall's) corpuscles

10 Epithelial reticular
cells

FIGURE 9.7 ■ Thymus gland (sectional view). Stain: hematoxylin and eosin. High magnification.

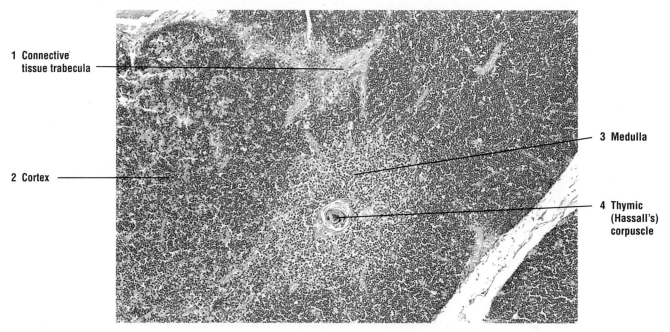

1 Connective
tissue trabecula

2 Cortex

3 Medulla

4 Thymic
(Hassall's)
corpuscle

FIGURE 9.8 ■ Cortex and medulla of a thymus gland. Stain: hematoxylin and eosin. 30×

FIGURE 9.9 ■ Spleen (Panoramic View)

The spleen is surrounded by a dense connective tissue **capsule (1)** from which arise connective tissue **trabeculae (3, 5, 11)** that extend deep into the interior. The main trabeculae enter the spleen at the hilus and extend throughout the organ. Located within the trabeculae (3, 5, 11) are **trabecular arteries (5b)** and **trabecular veins (5a).** Trabeculae that are sectioned in the transverse plane (11) appear round or nodular and may contain blood vessels.

The spleen is characterized by numerous aggregations of **lymphatic nodules (4, 6).** These nodules constitute the **white pulp (4, 6)** of the organ. The lymphatic nodules (4, 6) also contain **germinal centers (8, 9)** that decrease in number with age. Passing through each lymphatic nodule (4, 6) is a blood vessel, called the **central artery (2, 7, 10),** that is located in the periphery of the nodule. Central arteries (2, 7, 10) are branches of trabecular arteries (5b) that become ensheathed with lymphatic tissue as they leave the connective tissue trabeculae (3, 5, 11). This periarterial lymphatic sheath also forms the lymphatic nodules (4, 6) that constitute the white pulp (4, 6) of the spleen.

Surrounding the lymphatic nodules (4, 6) and intermeshed with the connective tissue trabeculae (3, 5, 11) is a diffuse cellular meshwork that makes up the bulk of the organ. This meshwork collectively forms the splenic or **red pulp (12, 13).** In fresh preparations, red pulp is red because of its extensive vascular tissue. The red pulp (12, 13) also contains **pulp arteries (14), venous sinuses (13),** and **splenic cords (of Billroth) (12).** The splenic cords (12) appear as diffuse strands of lymphatic tissue between the venous sinuses (13), and they form a spongy meshwork of reticular connective tissue. This is usually obscured by the density of other tissue.

The spleen does not exhibit a distinct cortex and a medulla as seen in lymph nodes. However, lymphatic nodules (4, 6) are found throughout the spleen. In addition, the spleen contains venous sinuses (13), in contrast to the lymphatic sinuses that are found in the lymph nodes. The spleen also does not exhibit subcapsular or trabecular sinuses. The capsule (1) and trabeculae (3, 5, 11) in the spleen are thicker than those around the lymph nodes, and they contain some smooth muscle cells.

FIGURE 9.10 ■ Spleen: Red and White Pulp

A higher magnification of a section of the spleen illustrates the red and white pulp and the associated connective tissue trabeculae, blood vessels, venous sinuses, and the splenic cords.

The large **lymphatic nodule (3)** represents the white pulp of the spleen. Each nodule normally exhibits a peripheral zone, the periarterial lymphatic sheath, with densely packed small lymphocytes. The **central artery (4)** in the lymphatic nodule (3) has a peripheral or an eccentric position. Because the artery occupies the center of the periarterial lymphatic sheath, it is called the central artery. The cells in the periarterial lymphatic sheath are mainly T lymphocytes. A **germinal center (5)** may not always be present. In the more lightly stained germinal center (5) are B lymphocytes, many medium-sized lymphocytes, some small lymphocytes, and lymphoblasts.

The red pulp contains the **splenic cords** (of Billroth) **(1, 8)** and **venous sinuses (2, 9)** that course between the cords. The splenic cords (1, 8) are thin aggregations of lymphatic tissue containing small lymphocytes, associated cells, and various blood cells. Venous sinuses (2, 9) are dilated vessels that are lined with modified endothelium of elongated cells that appear cuboidal in transverse sections.

Also present in the red pulp are the **pulp arteries (10).** These represent the branches of the central artery (4) after it leaves the lymphatic nodule (3). Capillaries and pulp veins (venules) are also present.

Connective tissue trabeculae with a **trabecular artery (6)** and **trabecular vein (7)** are evident. These vessels have endothelial tunica intima and muscular tunica media. The tunica adventitia is not apparent, because the connective tissue of the trabeculae surrounds the tunica media.

1 Capsule

2 Central artery

3 Trabeculae

4 Lymphatic nodule
  (white pulp)

9 Germinal center

10 Central artery

5 Trabecular:
  a. Vein
  b. Artery

11 Trabeculae

12 Splenic cords
  (in red pulp)

13 Venous sinuses
  (in red pulp)

6 Lymphatic nodule
  (white pulp)

7 Central artery

8 Germinal center

14 Pulp arteries

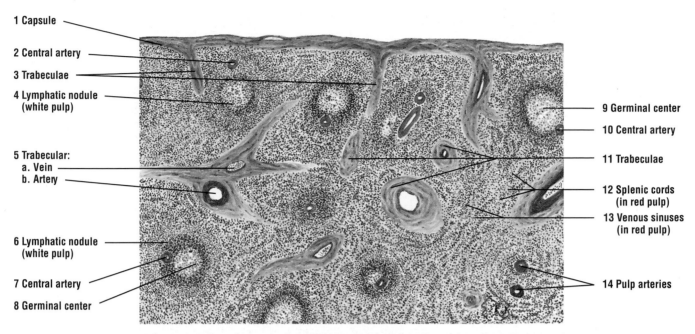

FIGURE 9.9 ■ Spleen (panoramic view). Stain: hematoxylin and eosin. Low magnification.

1 Splenic cord

2 Venous sinus

3 Lymphatic nodule

4 Central artery

5 Germinal center

6 Trabecular artery

7 Trabecular vein

8 Splenic cords

9 Venous sinuses

10 Pulp arteries

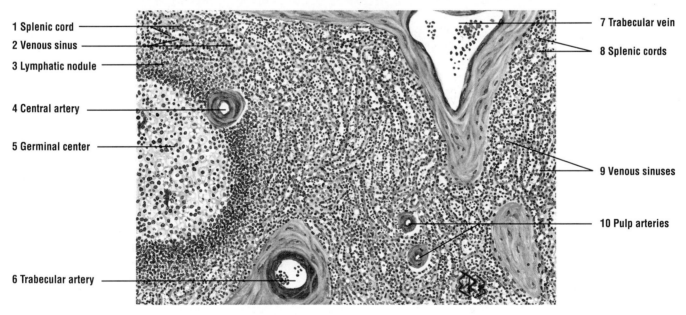

FIGURE 9.10 ■ Spleen: red and white pulp. Stain: hematoxylin and eosin. Medium magnification.

FIGURE 9.11 ■ Red and White Pulp of the Spleen

A low-magnification photomicrograph illustrates a section of the spleen. A dense irregular **connective tissue capsule (1)** covers the organ. From the capsule (1), **connective tissue trabeculae (3)** with blood vessels extend into the interior. The spleen is composed of white pulp and red pulp. **White pulp (2)** consists of lymphocytes and aggregations of **lymphatic nodules (2a)**. Within the lymphatic nodule (2a) are the **germinal center (2b)** and a **central artery (2c)** that is located off-center. Surrounding the lymphatic nodules (2) of the white pulp is the **red pulp (4)**, which is primarily composed of **venous sinuses (4a)** and **splenic cords (4b)**.

FUNCTIONAL CORRELATIONS

The Spleen

The **spleen** is the largest lymphoid organ of all and has an extensive blood supply. It filters blood and is the site of immune responses to bloodborne antigens. The spleen consists of red pulp and white pulp.

Red pulp consists of a dense network of reticular fibers that contain numerous erythrocytes, lymphocytes, plasma cells, macrophages, and other granulocytes. Its main function is to filter antigens, microorganisms, platelets, and aged or abnormal erythrocytes from the blood.

White pulp consists mainly of **lymphatic tissue.** Lymphatic cells that surround the **central arteries** of the white pulp are primarily **T lymphocytes,** whereas the lymphatic nodules contain mainly **B lymphocytes. Antigen-presenting cells** and **macrophages** reside within the white pulp. These cells detect trapped bacteria and antigens, and they initiate immune responses against them. As a result, T lymphocytes and B lymphocytes interact, activate, proliferate, and perform their immune response.

Macrophages in the spleen also break down **hemoglobin** of worn-out **erythrocytes.** Iron from hemoglobin is recycled and returned to the **bone marrow,** where it is reused during the synthesis of new hemoglobin by developing erythrocytes. The **heme** from the hemoglobin is further degraded and then excreted into **bile** by the liver cells.

During fetal life, the spleen is a **hemopoietic organ,** producing **granulocytes** and **erythrocytes.** This hemopoietic capability, however, ceases after birth. The spleen also serves as an important **reservoir** for blood. Because it has a sponge-like microstructure, much blood can be stored in its interior; when needed, the stored blood is returned from the spleen to the general circulation. Although the spleen performs various important functions in the body, this organ is not essential for life.

FIGURE 9.12 ■ Palatine Tonsil

The paired palatine tonsils consist of aggregates of lymphatic nodules in the oral cavity. The palatine tonsils are not surrounded by a connective tissue capsule. As a result, the surface of the palatine tonsil is covered by a protective **stratified squamous nonkeratinized epithelium (1, 6)** that covers the rest of the oral cavity. Each tonsil is invaginated by deep grooves, called **tonsillar crypts (3, 9),** that are also lined by stratified squamous nonkeratinized epithelium (1, 6).

Below the epithelium (1, 6) in the underlying connective tissue are numerous **lymphatic nodules (2)** that are distributed along the lengths of the tonsillar crypts (3, 10). The lymphatic nodules (2) frequently merge with each other and usually exhibit lighter-staining **germinal centers (7).**

A dense connective tissue underlies the palatine tonsil and forms its **capsule (4, 10).** The connective tissue **trabeculae (8),** some with **blood vessels (8),** arise from the capsule (4, 10) and pass toward the surface of the tonsil between the lymphatic nodules (2).

Below the connective tissue capsule (10) are sections of **skeletal muscle (5)** fibers.

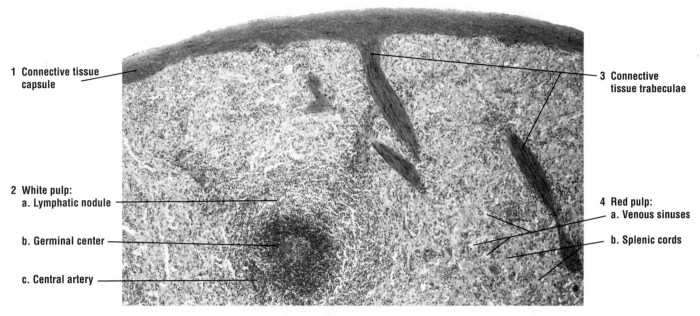

1 Connective tissue capsule

2 White pulp:
  a. Lymphatic nodule
  b. Germinal center
  c. Central artery

3 Connective tissue trabeculae

4 Red pulp:
  a. Venous sinuses
  b. Splenic cords

FIGURE 9.11 ■ Red and white pulp of the spleen. Stain: Mallory-azan. 21×

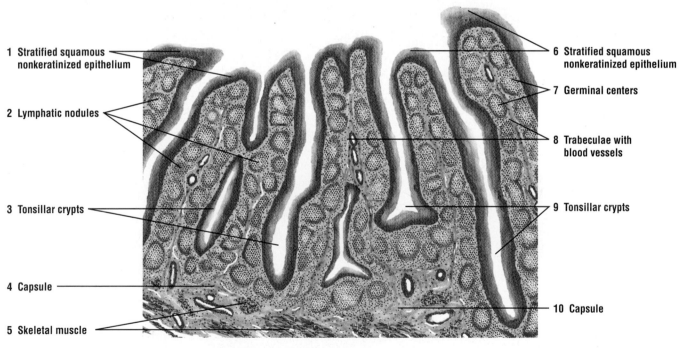

1 Stratified squamous nonkeratinized epithelium

2 Lymphatic nodules

3 Tonsillar crypts

4 Capsule

5 Skeletal muscle

6 Stratified squamous nonkeratinized epithelium

7 Germinal centers

8 Trabeculae with blood vessels

9 Tonsillar crypts

10 Capsule

FIGURE 9.12 ■ Palatine tonsil. Stain: hematoxylin and eosin. Low magnification.

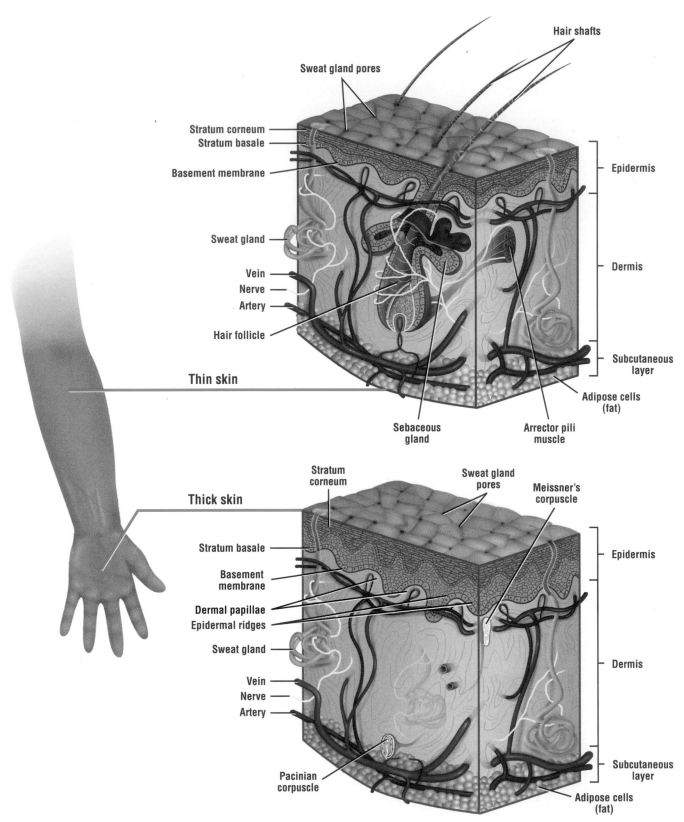

Hair shafts

Sweat gland pores

Stratum corneum

Stratum basale

Basement membrane

Epidermis

Sweat gland

Vein

Nerve

Artery

Dermis

Hair follicle

Thin skin

Subcutaneous layer

Adipose cells (fat)

Sebaceous gland

Arrector pili muscle

Stratum corneum

Sweat gland pores

Meissner's corpuscle

Thick skin

Stratum basale

Basement membrane

Epidermis

Dermal papillae

Epidermal ridges

Sweat gland

Vein

Nerve

Artery

Dermis

Pacinian corpuscle

Subcutaneous layer

Adipose cells (fat)

OVERVIEW FIGURE ■ Comparison between thin skin in the arm and thick skin in the palm, including contents of the connective tissue dermis.

CHAPTER 10

Integumentary System

Skin and its derivatives and appendages form the **integumentary system.** In humans, skin derivatives include nails, hair, and several types of sweat and sebaceous glands. Skin, or **integument,** consists of two distinct regions, the superficial epidermis and a deep dermis. The superficial **epidermis** is nonvascular and lined by **keratinized stratified squamous epithelium** with distinct cell types and cell layers. Inferior to the epidermis is the vascular **dermis,** which is characterized by dense irregular connective tissue. Beneath the dermis is the **hypodermis,** or the **subcutaneous layer** of connective tissue and adipose tissue that forms the fascia seen in gross anatomy.

Epidermis: Thick Versus Thin Skin

The basic histology of skin is similar in different regions of the body, except regarding the thickness of the epidermis. **Palms** and **soles** are constantly exposed to increased wear, tear, and abrasion. As a result, the epidermis in these regions, especially the outermost stratified keratinized layer, is thick. Skin in these regions is called **thick skin.** Thick skin also contains numerous **sweat glands,** but it lacks hair follicles, sebaceous glands, and smooth muscle fibers.

The remainder of the body is covered skin called **thin skin.** In these regions, the epidermis is thinner and its cellular composition simpler than that of thick skin. Thin skin contains **hair follicles, sebaceous glands,** and **sweat glands.** Attached to the connective tissue sheath of hair follicles and the connective tissue of the dermis are smooth muscle fibers, called **arrector pili.** Also associated with the hair follicles are numerous sebaceous glands (see the overview figure).

Dermis: Papillary and Reticular Layers

Dermis is the connective tissue layer that binds to the epidermis. The junction of the dermis with the epidermis is irregular. The superficial layer of the dermis forms numerous raised projections, called **dermal papillae,** that interdigitate with evaginations of epidermis, called **epidermal ridges.** This region of skin is the **papillary layer** of the dermis. This layer is filled with loose irregular connective tissue and connective tissue fibers, capillaries, blood vessels, fibroblasts, macrophages, and other loose connective tissue cells.

The deeper layer of dermis, called the **reticular layer,** is thicker and contains dense irregular connective tissue. It is characterized by connective tissue fibers and fewer cells than are found in the papillary layer. No distinct boundary is seen between the two dermal layers. Also, dermis blends inferiorly with the **hypodermis,** or the **subcutaneous layer,** which contains the superficial fascia and adipose tissue.

The connective tissue of the dermis is highly vascular, and it contains numerous blood vessels, lymph vessels, and nerves. Certain regions of skin exhibit **arteriovenous anastomoses,** which are used for temperature regulation. Here, blood passes directly from arteries into veins. In addition, the dermis contains numerous sensory receptors. **Meissner's corpuscles** are located closer to the surface of skin in dermal papillae, whereas **Pacinian corpuscles** are found deeper in the connective tissue of the dermis (see the overview figure).

FUNCTIONAL CORRELATIONS

Epidermal Cells

Four types of cells are found in the epidermis of skin. The dominant cells, called **keratinocytes,** are arranged in distinct and recognizable layers. Keratinocytes divide, grow, migrate up, and undergo **keratinization** or **cornification,** and form a protective layer for skin. The other three types of epidermal cells—melanocytes, Langerhans cells, and Merkel cells—are interspersed among the keratinocytes.

Epidermal Layers

Five epidermal layers are found in the human body: the stratum basale (germinativum), stratum spinosum, stratum granulosum, stratum lucidum, and stratum corneum.

Stratum Basale (Germinativum)

The **stratum basale** is the deepest, or basal, layer in epidermis. It consists of a single layer of columnar to cuboidal cells that rest on a **basement membrane** separating the dermis from the epidermis. The cells are attached to one another by cell junctions, called **desmosomes,** and to the underlying basement membrane by **hemidesmosomes.** Cells in the stratum basale serve as stem cells for the epidermis; thus, much increased mitotic activity is seen in this layer. The cells divide and mature as they migrate up toward the superficial layers. All cells in the stratum basale contain **intermediate keratin filaments** that increase in number as the cells move upward.

Stratum Spinosum

As the cells move upward in the epidermis, a second cell layer, called the **stratum spinosum,** forms. This layer consists of four to six rows of cells. In routine histologic preparations, cells in this layer shrink. As a result, the developed intercellular spaces between cells appear to form numerous cytoplasmic extensions, or spines, that project from their surfaces. The spines represent the sites where desmosomes are anchored to bundles of keratin filaments, or **tonofilaments,** and to neighboring cells. Tonofilaments provide resistance to abrasion of the epidermis.

Stratum Granulosum

Cells above the stratum spinosum become filled with dense basophilic **keratohyalin granules** and form the third layer, called the **stratum granulosum.** Three to five layers of flattened cells form the stratum granulosum. Keratohyalin granules are the source of the soft keratin in skin. These granules are not surrounded by a membrane and are associated with bundles of keratin filaments. In addition, the cytoplasm of these cells contains **lamellar granules** formed by lipid bilayers. The lamellar granules are discharged into the intercellular spaces of the stratum granulosum as layers of **lipid** and seal the skin.

Stratum Lucidum

In thick skin only, **stratum lucidum** is translucent and barely visible; it lies just superior to the stratum granulosum. The stratum lucidum contains tightly packed cells that lack nuclei or organelles and are dead. The flattened cells in this layer contain densely packed keratin filaments.

Stratum Corneum

The **stratum corneum** is the fifth and most superficial layer of skin. All nuclei and organelles have disappeared from these cells. Stratum corneum primarily consists of flattened, dead cells that are filled with soft **keratin filaments.** The keratinized, superficial cells from this layer are continually shed, or **desquamated,** and replaced by new cells arising from the deep stratum basale.

FIGURE 10.1 ■ Thin Skin: Epidermis and Contents of the Dermis

This illustration depicts a section of thin skin from the general body surface, where wear and tear are minimal. To differentiate between the cellular and connective tissue components of skin, a special stain was used. With this stain, the collagen fibers of the connective tissue components stain blue, and the cellular components stain bright red.

Skin consists of two principal layers, the **epidermis (10)** and the **dermis (14).** The epidermis (10) is the superficial cellular layer with different cells types. The dermis (14), which is located directly below the epidermis (10), contains connective tissue fibers and cellular components of epidermal origin.

In thin skin, the epidermis (10) exhibits a stratified squamous epithelium and a thin layer of keratinized cells, called the **stratum corneum (1).** The most superficial cells in the stratum corneum (1) are constantly shed, or desquamated, from the surface. Also, the stratum corneum (1) of thin skin is much thinner compared to that of thick skin. In this illustration, a few rows of polygonal-shaped cells are visible in the epidermis (10). These cells form the layer **stratum spinosum (2).**

The narrow zone of irregular, lighter-staining connective tissue directly below the epidermis (10) is the **papillary layer (11)** of the dermis (14). The papillary layer (11) indents the base of the epidermis to form the **dermal papillae (3).** The deeper **reticular layer (12)** comprises the bulk of the dermis (14) and consists of dense irregular connective tissue. A small portion of **hypodermis (13),** of the superficial region of the underlying subcutaneous **adipose tissue (9),** is also illustrated.

Skin appendages, such as the **sweat gland (7)** and the **hair follicle (8),** develop from the epidermis (10) and are located in the dermis (14). The sweat gland is illustrated in greater detail in Figure 10-4. The expanded terminal portion of the hair follicle (8) observed here in longitudinal section is the hair **bulb (8a).** The base of the hair bulb (8a) is indented by the connective tissue to form a **dermal papilla (8b).** Within each dermal papilla (8b) is a capillary network vital for sustaining the hair follicle. Attached to hair follicles (8) are thin strips of smooth muscle, called the **arrector pili muscles (5).** Also associated with hair follicles are numerous **sebaceous glands (6).**

In the reticular layer of the dermis (14) are cross-sections of a coiled portion of the **sweat gland (7).** The elongated portions of the sweat gland (7) that continue to the skin surface are the excretory **ductal portions (4, 7a)** of the sweat glands. The more circular and deeper-lying parts of the sweat gland are the **secretory portions (7b)** of the sweat gland.

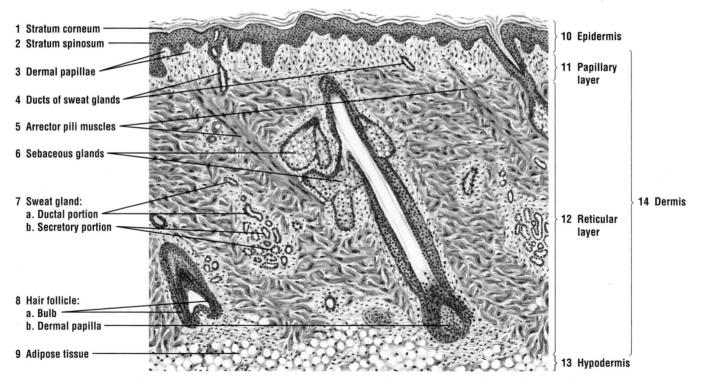

1 Stratum corneum
2 Stratum spinosum
3 Dermal papillae
4 Ducts of sweat glands
5 Arrector pili muscles
6 Sebaceous glands
7 Sweat gland:
　a. Ductal portion
　b. Secretory portion
8 Hair follicle:
　a. Bulb
　b. Dermal papilla
9 Adipose tissue
10 Epidermis
11 Papillary layer
12 Reticular layer
13 Hypodermis
14 Dermis

FIGURE 10.1 ■ Thin skin: epidermis and contents of the dermis. Stain: Masson's trichrome (blue stain). Low magnification.

FIGURE 10.2 ■ Skin: Scalp

This low-magnification section of thin skin from the scalp was prepared with routine histologic stain. It illustrates the epidermis, the dermis, and some of the skin derivatives in the deeper connective tissue layers. The epidermis stains darker than the underlying connective tissue of the dermis. In the epidermis, the following cell layers are seen: the **stratum corneum (1),** with desquamating superficial cells; the **stratum spinosum (2);** and the basal cell layer, or the **stratum basale (3),** with brown **melanin (pigment) granules (3).**

The connective tissue **dermal papillae (4)** indent the underside of the epidermis. The thin connective tissue papillary layer of the dermis is located immediately under the epidermis. The thicker connective tissue **reticular layer (12)** of the dermis extends from just below the epidermis to the **subcutaneous layer with adipose tissue (8).** Located inferior to the subcutaneous layer (8) are **skeletal muscle fibers (9),** which are sectioned here in both transverse and longitudinal planes.

Hair follicles (13) in the skin of the scalp are numerous, closely packed, and oriented at an angle to the surface. A complete hair follicle in longitudinal section is illustrated in this figure. Parts of other hair follicles (13), sectioned in different planes, are also visible. When the hair follicle (13) is cut in a transverse plane, the following structures are visible: the cuticle, the **internal root sheath (13a),** the **external root sheath (13b),** the **connective tissue sheath (13c),** the **hair bulb (13d),** and the connective tissue dermal **papilla (13e).** The hair passes upward through the follicle (13) to the skin surface. Numerous **sebaceous glands (11)** surround each hair follicle (13). The sebaceous follicles are aggregates of clear cells that are connected to a duct that opens into the hair follicle (see Fig. 10-4).

The **arrector pili muscles (5, 10)** are smooth muscles aligned at an oblique angle to the hair follicles (13). The arrector pili muscles (5, 10) attach to the papillary layer of the dermis and to the connective tissue sheath (13c) of the hair follicle (13). The contraction of arrector pili muscles (5, 10) causes the hair shaft to move into a more vertical position.

Deep in the dermis or subcutaneous layer (8) are the basal portions of the highly coiled **sweat glands (6).** Sections of the sweat gland (6) that exhibit lightly stained columnar epithelium are the **secretory portion (6b)** of the gland. The secretory portion (6b) is distinct from the **excretory ducts (6a),** which are lined by stratified cuboidal epithelium of smaller, darker-stained cells. Each sweat gland excretory duct (6a) is coiled deep in the dermis but straightens out in the upper dermis, and it follows a spiral course through the epidermis to the surface of the skin (see Fig. 10-5).

Skin contains many **blood vessels (14)** and has a rich sensory innervation. The sensory receptors for pressure and vibration are the **Pacinian corpuscles (7)** in the subcutaneous tissue (8). The Pacinian corpuscles (7) are illustrated in greater detail and at higher magnification in Figure 10-10.

FUNCTIONAL CORRELATIONS

Other Skin Cells

In addition to keratinocytes, the epidermis contains three other cell types: melanocytes, Langerhans cells, and Merkel cells. Unless skin is prepared with special stains, these cells normally are not distinguishable (e.g., in sections prepared with hematoxylin and eosin).

Melanocytes are located in the basal layer of the epidermis, and they synthesize the pigment **melanin.** Melanin granules within melanocytes migrate to their cytoplasmic extensions, from which they are transferred to cells in the stratum basale and stratum spinosum. Melanin imparts a dark color to the skin, and exposure of skin to sunlight promotes increased synthesis of melanin. The function of melanin is to protect the skin from the damaging effects of ultraviolet radiation.

Langerhans cells are found mainly in the stratum spinosum. They participate in the body's immune responses. Langerhans cells recognize, phagocytose, and process foreign **antigens** and then present them to T lymphocytes for an immune response. Thus, these cells function as **antigen-presenting cells.**

A small number of **Merkel cells** are found in the basal layer of the epidermis, and they are most abundant in the fingertips. Because these cells are closely associated with afferent **unmyelinated axons,** they are believed to function as **mechanoreceptors** to detect pressure.

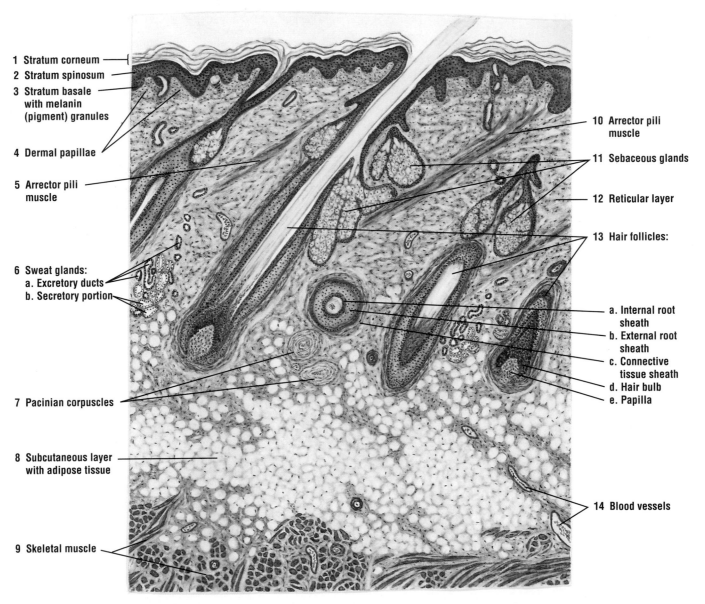

1 **Stratum corneum**

2 **Stratum spinosum**

3 **Stratum basale with melanin (pigment) granules**

4 **Dermal papillae**

5 **Arrector pili muscle**

6 **Sweat glands:**
   a. Excretory ducts
   b. Secretory portion

7 **Pacinian corpuscles**

8 **Subcutaneous layer with adipose tissue**

9 **Skeletal muscle**

10 **Arrector pili muscle**

11 **Sebaceous glands**

12 **Reticular layer**

13 **Hair follicles:**

   a. Internal root sheath
   b. External root sheath
   c. Connective tissue sheath
   d. Hair bulb
   e. Papilla

14 **Blood vessels**

FIGURE 10.2 ■ Skin: scalp. Stain: hematoxylin and eosin. Low magnification.

FIGURE 10.3 ■ Hairy Thin Skin of the Scalp: Hair Follicles and Surrounding Structures

This low-power photomicrograph illustrates a section of the thin skin of the scalp. In the **epidermis (1)**, the **stratum corneum (1a), stratum granulosum (1b),** and **stratum spinosum (1c)** layers are thinner than the same layers in the thick skin. In the dense irregular connective tissue of the **dermis (4)** are **hair follicles (3)** and associated **sebaceous glands (2, 5)**. An **arrector pili muscle (6)** extends from the deep connective tissue around the hair follicle (3) to the connective tissue of the papillary layer of the dermis (1).

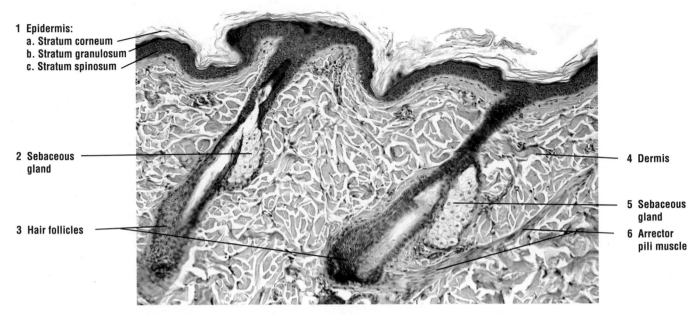

1 **Epidermis:**
   a. **Stratum corneum**
   b. **Stratum granulosum**
   c. **Stratum spinosum**

2 **Sebaceous gland**

3 **Hair follicles**

4 **Dermis**

5 **Sebaceous gland**

6 **Arrector pili muscle**

FIGURE 10.3 ■ Hairy thin skin of the scalp: hair follicles and surrounding structures. Stain: hematoxylin and eosin. 40×

FIGURE 10.4 ■ Hair Follicle with Surrounding Structures

This figure illustrates a longitudinal section of a hair follicle and its surrounding glands and structures. The different layers of the hair follicle are identified on the right. The hair follicle is surrounded by an outer **connective tissue sheath (15)** of the **dermis (7)**. Under the connective tissue sheath (15) is an **external root sheath (14)** that is composed of several cell layers. These cell layers are continuous with the epithelial layer of the epidermis. The **internal root sheath (13)** is composed of a thin, pale epithelial stratum (Henle's layer) and a thin, granular epithelial stratum (Huxley's layer). These two cell layers become indistinguishable as their cells merge with those in the expanded part of the hair follicle, called the **hair bulb (21)**. Internal to the cell layers of the internal root sheath (13) are cells that produce the **cuticle (12)** of the hair and the keratinized **cortex (11)** of the hair follicle, which appears as a pale-yellow layer. The **hair root (16)** and the **dermal papilla (18)** form the hair bulb (21), in which the external root sheath (14) and internal root sheath (13) merge into a undifferentiated group of cells, called the **hair matrix (17)**, situated above the dermal papilla (18). Cell mitoses and **melanin pigment (19)** can be seen in the matrix cells (17). Numerous **capillaries (20)** in the connective tissue supply blood to the dermal papilla (18).

In the connective tissue of the dermis (7) and adjacent to the hair follicle are visible transverse sections of the basal portion of a coiled **sweat gland (8, 9)**. The **secretory cells (9)** of the sweat gland are tall and stain light. Along the bases of the secretory cells (9) are flattened nuclei of the contractile **myoepithelial cells (10)**. Compared to the taller and lighter secretory cells (9), the **excretory ducts (8)** of the sweat gland are smaller in diameter, are lined with a stratified cuboidal epithelium, and are darker staining.

In this figure, a **sebaceous gland (4)** connected to the hair follicle is sectioned through the middle. The sebaceous gland (4) is lined with a stratified epithelium that has continuity with the external root sheath (14) of the hair follicle. The epithelium of the sebaceous gland is modified, and along its base is a row of columnar or cuboidal cells, called the **basal cells (3)**, the nuclei of which may be flattened. These cells rest on a basement membrane, which is surrounded by the connective tissue of the dermis (7). The basal cells (3) of the sebaaceous gland divide and fill the acinus of the gland with larger, polyhedral **secretory cells (5)** that enlarge, accumulate secretory material, and become round. The secretory cells (5) in the interior of the acinus then undergo **degeneration (2)**, a process in which the cells become the oily secretory product, called sebum, of the gland. Sebum passes through the short **duct of the sebaceous gland (1)** into the lumen of the hair follicle.

Each hair follicle is surrounded by numerous sebaceous glands (4), which lie in the connective tissue of the dermis (7) and in the angle between the hair follicle and the smooth muscle strip, called the **arrector pili muscle (6)**. When the arrector pili muscle contracts, the hair stands up, forming a dimple or "goose bump" on the skin and forcing the sebum out of the sebaceous gland into the lumen of the hair follicle.

FUNCTIONAL CORRELATIONS

Skin

Skin comes in direct contact with the external environment. As a result, skin performs numerous important functions, most of which are protective.

Protection

The **keratinized stratified epithelium** of the epidermis protects the body surfaces from mechanical abrasion and forms a physical barrier to pathogens and foreign microorganisms. Because the **glycolipid layer** is present between the cells of the stratum granulosum, the epidermis is **impermeable** to water as well. This layer also prevents the loss of body fluids through dehydration. Increased synthesis of the pigment melanin protects skin against ultraviolet radiation.

Temperature Regulation

Physical exercise or a warm environment increases **sweating**, which reduces body temperature following the **evaporation** of sweat from skin surfaces. In addition to sweating, temperature regulation involves increased **dilation** of blood vessels for maximum flow of blood to skin. This function also increases heat loss. Conversely, in cold temperatures, body heat is conserved by **constriction** of blood vessels and decreased flow of blood to skin.

Sensory Perception

The skin is a large **sense organ** of the external environment. Numerous encapsulated and free **sensory nerve endings** within the skin respond to stimuli for temperature (heat and cold), touch, pain, and pressure.

Excretion

Water, sodium salts, urea, and nitrogenous wastes are excreted to the surface of skin through the production of sweat by **sweat glands.**

Formation of Vitamin D

Vitamin D is formed from precursors that are synthesized in the epidermis during exposure of skin to **ultraviolet** rays from the sun. Vitamin D is essential for **calcium absorption** from intestinal mucosa and for proper mineral metabolism.

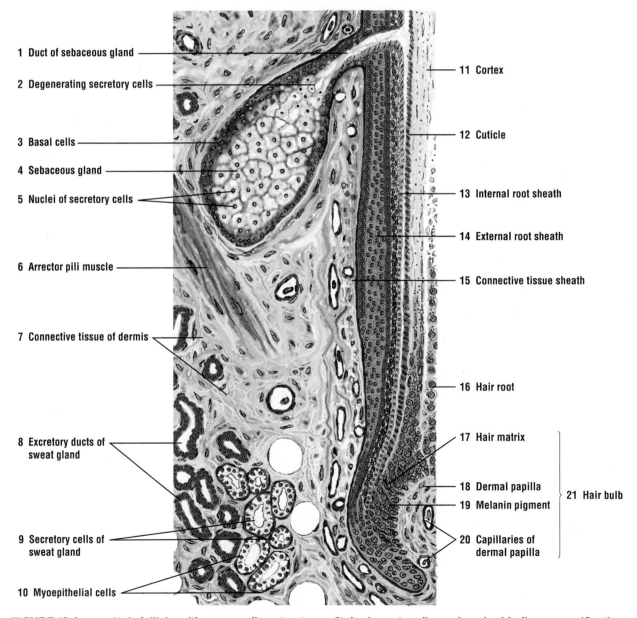

1 Duct of sebaceous gland

2 Degenerating secretory cells

3 Basal cells

4 Sebaceous gland

5 Nuclei of secretory cells

6 Arrector pili muscle

7 Connective tissue of dermis

8 Excretory ducts of sweat gland

9 Secretory cells of sweat gland

10 Myoepithelial cells

11 Cortex

12 Cuticle

13 Internal root sheath

14 External root sheath

15 Connective tissue sheath

16 Hair root

17 Hair matrix

18 Dermal papilla

19 Melanin pigment

20 Capillaries of dermal papilla

21 Hair bulb

FIGURE 10.4 ■ Hair follicle with surrounding structures. Stain: hematoxylin and eosin. Medium magnification.

FIGURE 10.5 ■ Thick Skin of the Palm, Superficial Cell Layers, and Melanin Pigment

Thick skin is best illustrated by examining a section from the palm. The epidermis of the thick skin exhibits five distinct cell layers and is much thicker than that of the thin skin (Figs. 10-1 to 10-3). Here, the different cells layers of the epidermis are illustrated in greater detail and at higher magnification on the right.

The outermost layer of the thick skin is the **stratum corneum (1, 9),** which is a wide layer of flattened, dead, or keratinized cells that are constantly being shed or **desquamated (8)** from the skin surface. Inferior to the stratum corneum (1, 9) is a narrow, lightly stained **stratum lucidum (2).** This thin layer is difficult to see in most slide preparations. At higher magnification, however, the outlines of flattened cells and eleidin droplets in this layer occasionally are seen.

Located below the stratum lucidum (2) is the **stratum granulosum (3, 11),** the cells of which are filled with dark-staining **keratohyalin granules (3).** Directly under the stratum granulosum (3, 11) is the thick **stratum spinosum (4, 12),** which is composed of several layers of polyhedral-shaped cells. These cells are connected to each other by spinous processes, or intercellular bridges, that represent the attachment sites of desmosomes (macula adherens).

The deepest cell layer in skin is the columnar **stratum basale (5, 13)** that rests on the connective tissue **basement membrane (6, 15).** Mitotic activity and the brown melanin pigment (5, 13) are normally seen in the deeper layers of stratum spinosum (4, 12) and stratum basale (5, 13).

The **excretory duct** of a **sweat gland (10)** located deep in the dermis penetrates the epidermis, loses its epithelial wall, and spirals through the epidermal cell layers (1 to 5) to the skin surface as small channels with a thin lining.

Dermal papillae (7) are prominent in thick skin. Some dermal papillae may contain tactile or sensory **Meissner's corpuscles (14)** and **capillary loops (16).**

FIGURE 10.6 ■ Thick Skin: Epidermis and Superficial Cell Layers

A higher-magnification photomicrograph shows a clear distinction between the different cell layers in the **epidermis (1)** of the thick skin of the palm. The outermost and thickest layer is the **stratum corneum (1a).** Inferior to the stratum corneum (1a) are from two to three layers of dark cells filled with granules; this is the **stratum granulosum (1b).** Below the stratum granulosum (1b) is the **stratum spinosum (1c),** a thicker layer of polyhedral cells. The deepest cell layer in the epidermis (1) is the **stratum basale (1d),** the cells of which contain brown **melanin granules (6).** The stratum basale (1d) is attached to a thin connective tissue **basement membrane (4)** that separates the epidermis (1) from the **dermis (2).** The connective tissue of the dermis (2) indents the epidermis (1) to form **dermal papillae (5).** The **excretory duct (3)** of a sweat gland deep in the dermis can be seen here passing through the dermis (2) and the cell layers of the epidermis (1).

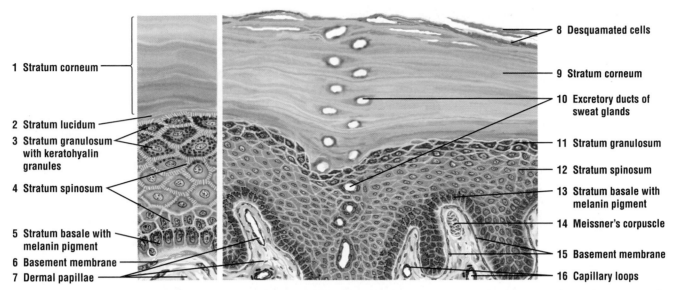

1 **Stratum corneum**

2 **Stratum lucidum**

3 **Stratum granulosum with keratohyalin granules**

4 **Stratum spinosum**

5 **Stratum basale with melanin pigment**

6 **Basement membrane**

7 **Dermal papillae**

8 **Desquamated cells**

9 **Stratum corneum**

10 **Excretory ducts of sweat glands**

11 **Stratum granulosum**

12 **Stratum spinosum**

13 **Stratum basale with melanin pigment**

14 **Meissner's corpuscle**

15 **Basement membrane**

16 **Capillary loops**

FIGURE 10.5 ■ Thick skin of the palm, superficial cell layers, and melanin pigment. Stain: hematoxylin and eosin. Medium magnification.

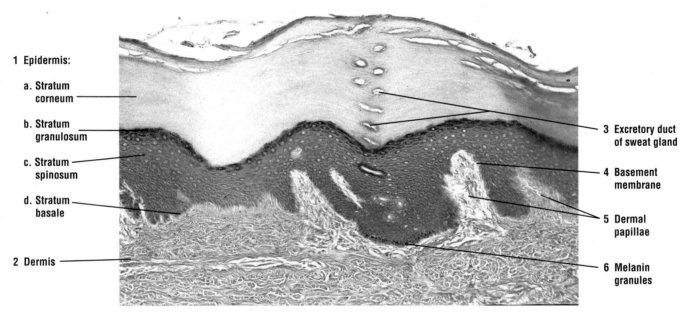

1 **Epidermis:**

   a. **Stratum corneum**

   b. **Stratum granulosum**

   c. **Stratum spinosum**

   d. **Stratum basale**

2 **Dermis**

3 **Excretory duct of sweat gland**

4 **Basement membrane**

5 **Dermal papillae**

6 **Melanin granules**

FIGURE 10.6 ■ Thick skin: epidermis and superficial cell layers. Stain: hematoxylin and eosin. 40×

FIGURE 10.7 ■ Thick Skin: Epidermis, Dermis, and Hypodermis of the Palm

A low-power photomicrograph illustrates the superficial and deep structures in the thick skin of the palm. The following cell layers are recognized in the **epidermis (6):** the **stratum corneum (7),** the **stratum granulosum (8),** and the **stratum basale (9).** Inferior to the epidermis (6) is the dense irregular connective tissue **dermis (5). Dermal papillae (11)** from the dermis indent the base of the epidermis (6). Deep in the dermis (5) and the **hypodermis (4)** are cross-sections of the coiled simple tubular **sweat glands (3)** and the **excretory ducts** of the **sweat glands (10).** A thick layer of **adipose tissue (1)** deep to the dermis (5) is called the **hypodermis (4)** or superficial fascia. The hypodermis (4) is not part of the integument. Two sensory receptors called the **Pacinian corpuscles (2)** are seen inferior to the adipose tissue (1) of the hypodermis (4).

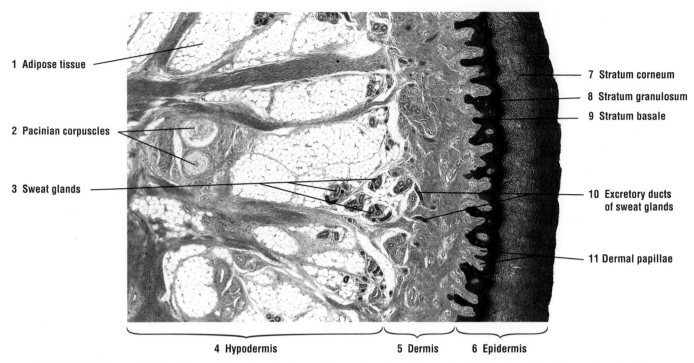

1 Adipose tissue

2 Pacinian corpuscles

3 Sweat glands

7 Stratum corneum

8 Stratum granulosum

9 Stratum basale

10 Excretory ducts
    of sweat glands

11 Dermal papillae

4 Hypodermis   5 Dermis   6 Epidermis

FIGURE 10.7 ■ Thick skin: epidermis, dermis, and hypodermis of the palm. Stain: hematoxylin and eosin. 17×

FIGURE 10.8 ■ Sweat Glands

The sweat gland is a simple, highly coiled, tubular gland that extends deep into the dermis or the upper hypodermis. To illustrate this extension, the sweat gland is shown in both cross-sectional (left) and three-dimensional views (side).

The coiled region of the sweat gland in the dermis is the **secretory portion (8)** region. The **secretory cells (3, 4)** are large, columnar, and stain light eosinophilic. Surrounding the secretory cells (3, 4) are thin, spindle-shaped **myoepithelial cells (5)** that are located between the base of the secretory cells (3, 4) and the basement membrane (not illustrated) that surrounds the cells.

A thinner, darker-staining **excretory duct (2, 7)** leaves the secretory region of the sweat gland. The cells of the excretory duct are smaller than the secretory cells (3, 4). Also, the excretory duct (2, 7) is smaller in diameter and is lined by deep-staining, stratified cuboidal cells. No myoepithelial cells are found around the excretory duct. As the excretory duct ascends, it straightens out and penetrates the cell layers of the **epidermis (1, 6),** where the duct loses its epithelial wall. In the epidermis (1, 6), the duct follows a spiral course through the cells to the skin surface.

FUNCTIONAL CORRELATIONS

Skin Derivatives or Appendages

Nails, hairs, and **sweat glands** are derivatives of skin that develop directly from the surface epithelium of the epidermis. During development, these appendages grow into and reside deep within the connective tissue of the **dermis.** Sweat glands may also extend deeper into the **subcutaneous layer,** or the **hypodermis.**

Hairs are the hard, cornified, cylindrical structures that arise from **hair follicles** in skin. One portion of the hair projects through the epithelium to the exterior surface; the other portion remains embedded in the dermis. Hair grows in the expanded portion at the base of the hair follicle, called the **hair bulb.** The base of the hair bulb is indented by a **connective tissue papilla,** which is a highly vascularized region that brings essential nutrients to hair follicle cells. Here, the hair cells divide, grow, cornify, and form the hair.

Associated with each hair follicle are one or more **sebaceous glands** that produce an oily secretion, called **sebum.** Also, extending from the connective tissue around the hair follicle to the **papillary layer** of the **dermis** are bundles of smooth muscle, called **arrector pili.** The sebaceous glands are between the arrector pili muscle and the hair follicle. Arrector pili muscles are controlled by the **autonomic nervous system** and contract during strong emotions, fear, and cold temperatures. Contraction of the arrector pili muscle erects the hair shaft, depresses the skin where it inserts, and produces a small bump on the skin surface (often called a "goose bump"). In addition, this contraction forces the sebum from sebaceous glands onto the hair follicle and skin. Sebum oils and keeps the skin smooth, waterproofs it, prevents it from drying, and gives it some antibacterial protection.

Sweat glands are widely distributed in skin and are divided into two types, eccrine and apocrine. **Eccrine** sweat glands are simple, coiled, tubular glands. Their **secretory portion** is found deep in the dermis, from which a coiled **excretory duct** leads to the skin surface. The eccrine sweat glands contain two cell types: **clear cells,** which have no secretory granules, and **dark cells,** which have secretory granules. Secretion from the dark cells is primarily mucous, whereas secretion from the clear cells is watery. Surrounding the basal region of the secretory portion of each sweat gland are **myoepithelial cells,** the contraction of which expels the secretion (sweat) from sweat glands. Eccrine sweat glands are most numerous in skin of the palms and soles. The eccrine sweat glands assist in temperature regulation. Sweat glands also excrete water, sodium salts, ammonia, uric acid, and urea.

Apocrine sweat glands are primarily limited to the axillary, anus, and areolar regions of the breast. These sweat glands are larger than eccrine sweat glands, and their ducts open into the hair follicle. Apocrine sweat glands produce a viscous secretion that acquires a distinct odor following bacterial decomposition.

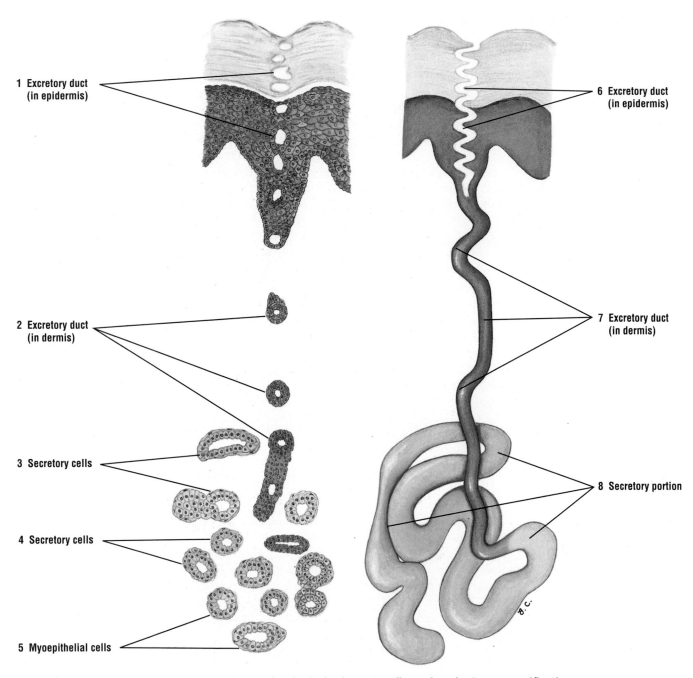

1 **Excretory duct**
   (in epidermis)

2 **Excretory duct**
   (in dermis)

3 **Secretory cells**

4 **Secretory cells**

5 **Myoepithelial cells**

6 **Excretory duct**
   (in epidermis)

7 **Excretory duct**
   (in dermis)

8 **Secretory portion**

FIGURE 10.8 ■ Sweat glands. Stain: hematoxylin and eosin. Low magnification.

FIGURE 10.9 ■ Glomus in the Dermis of Thick Skin

Arteriovenous anastomoses are numerous in the thick skin of the fingers and toes. In some arteriovenous anastomoses, direct connections exist between the arteries and veins; in others, the arterial portion of the anastomosis forms a specialized, thick-walled structure, called the **glomus (2).** The blood vessel in the glomus (2) is highly coiled or convoluted. As a result, more than one lumen of the coiled vessel may be seen in a transverse section of the glomus (2).

The smooth muscle cells in the tunica media of the glomus artery (2) enlarge and become **epithelioid cells (6).** The tunica media of the glomus artery (2) becomes thin again before it empties into a venule at the **arteriovenous junction (5).**

All arteriovenous anastomoses are richly innervated and supplied by blood vessels. A **connective tissue sheath (7)** encloses the glomus (2). The **dermis (4)** that surrounds the glomus (2) contains numerous **venules (8),** peripheral **nerves (1),** and excretory **ducts** of **sweat glands (3).**

FUNCTIONAL CORRELATIONS

Arteriovenous Anastomoses and Glomus

In numerous tissues, direct communications between arteries and veins, called **arteriovenous anastomoses,** bypass the capillaries. Their main functions are regulation of blood pressure, blood flow, and temperature as well as conservation of body heat. A more complex structure that also forms shunts is called a **glomus.** A glomus consists of a highly coiled arteriovenous shunt that is surrounded by collageneous connective tissue. The functions of the glomus are also to regulate blood flow and to conserve body heat. These structures are found in the fingertips, external ear, and other peripheral areas that are exposed to excessive cold temperatures and where arteriovenous shunts are neeeded.

FIGURE 10.10 ■ Pacinian Corpuscles in the Dermis of Thick Skin (Transverse and Longitudinal Sections)

Located deep in the **dermis (3)** of the thick skin and subcutaneous tissue are the **Pacinian corpuscles (2, 9).** Here, one Pacinian corpuscle is illustrated in longitudinal section (2) and one in transverse section (9).

Each Pacinian corpuscle (2, 9) is an ovoid structure with an elongated, central, myelinated **axon (2b, 9b).** The axon (2b, 9b) in the corpuscle is surrounded by **concentric lamellae (2a, 9a)** of compact collagenous fibers that become denser in the periphery to form the **connective tissue capsule (2c, 9c).** Between the connective tissue lamellae (2c, 9c) is a small amount of lymph-like fluid. In a transverse section, the layers of connective tissue lamellae (9a) surrounding the central axon (9c) of the Pacinian corpuscle (9) resemble a sliced onion.

In the connective tissue of the dermis (3) and surrounding the Pacinian corpuscles (2, 9) are numerous **adipose cells (5),** blood vessels such as a **venule (10),** peripheral **nerves (4, 6),** and cross-sections of the **excretory ducts (1)** and **secretory portions (8)** of sweat glands. The contractile **myoepithelial cells (7)** surround the secretory portion of the sweat gland (8).

The Pacinian corpuscles (2, 9) are important sensory receptors for pressure, vibration, and touch.

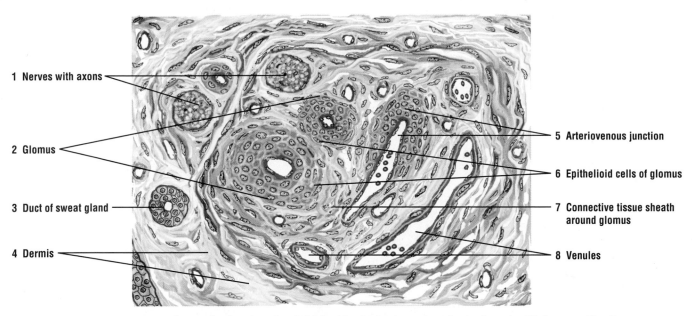

1 Nerves with axons

2 Glomus

3 Duct of sweat gland

4 Dermis

5 Arteriovenous junction

6 Epithelioid cells of glomus

7 Connective tissue sheath around glomus

8 Venules

FIGURE 10.9   ■   Glomus in the dermis of thick skin. Stain: hematoxylin and eosin. High magnification.

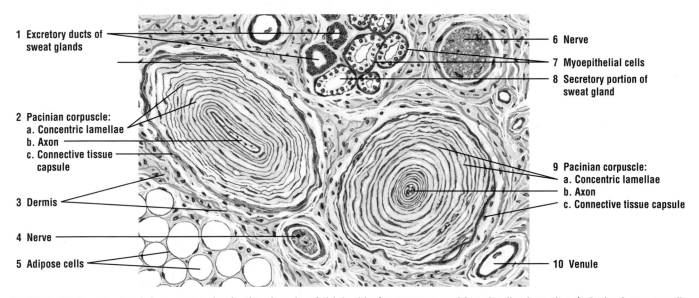

1 Excretory ducts of sweat glands

2 Pacinian corpuscle:
   a. Concentric lamellae
   b. Axon
   c. Connective tissue capsule

3 Dermis

4 Nerve

5 Adipose cells

6 Nerve

7 Myoepithelial cells

8 Secretory portion of sweat gland

9 Pacinian corpuscle:
   a. Concentric lamellae
   b. Axon
   c. Connective tissue capsule

10 Venule

FIGURE 10.10   ■   Pacinian corpuscles in the dermis of thick skin (transverse and longitudinal sections). Stain: hematoxylin and eosin. High magnification.

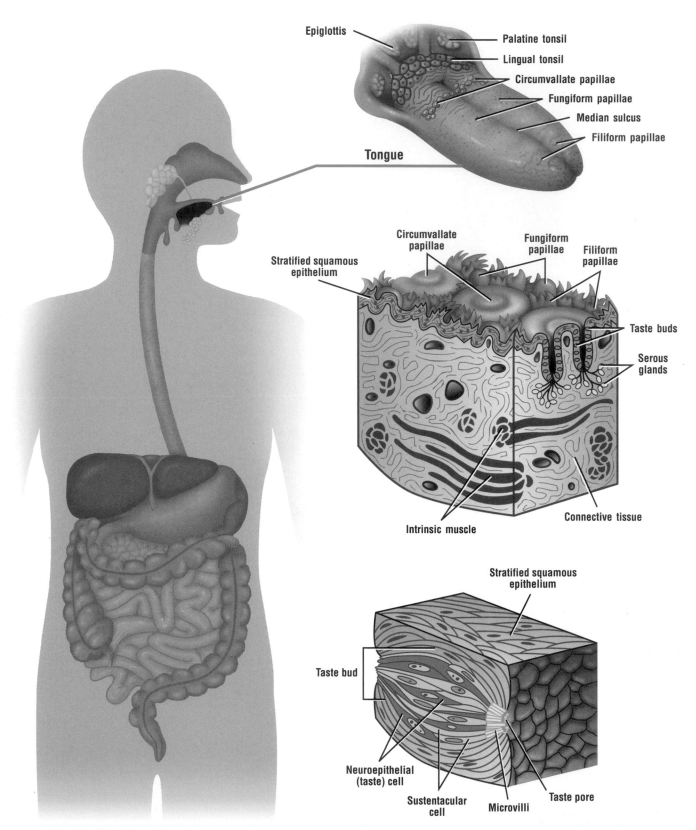

Epiglottis

Palatine tonsil

Lingual tonsil

Circumvallate papillae

Fungiform papillae

Median sulcus

Filiform papillae

Tongue

Circumvallate papillae

Fungiform papillae

Filiform papillae

Stratified squamous epithelium

Taste buds

Serous glands

Intrinsic muscle

Connective tissue

Stratified squamous epithelium

Taste bud

Neuroepithelial (taste) cell

Sustentacular cell

Microvilli

Taste pore

OVERVIEW FIGURE–ORAL CAVITY ■ Salivary glands and their connections to the oral cavity, morphology of the tongue in cross-section, and added detail of a taste bud.

CHAPTER 11

Digestive System: Oral Cavity and Salivary Glands

The digestive system is a long, hollow tube or tract that starts at the oral cavity and terminates at the anus. The system consists of the **oral cavity, esophagus, stomach, small intestine, large intestine, rectum,** and **anal canal.** Associated with the digestive tract are the accessory digestive organs: the **salivary glands,** the **liver,** and the **pancreas.** The accessory organs are located outside the digestive tract. Their secretory products are delivered to the digestive tract through excretory ducts that penetrate the digestive tract wall (Overview Figure—Oral Cavity).

The Oral Cavity

In the oral cavity, food is ingested, masticated (chewed), and lubricated by saliva for swallowing. Because food is physically broken down in the oral cavity, this region is lined by a protective, nonkeratinized, **stratified squamous epithelium,** which also lines the inner or labial surface of the lips.

The Lip

The oral cavity is formed, in part, by the lips and the cheeks. The lips are lined by a very thin skin that is covered by a stratified squamous keratinized epithelium. Blood vessels are close to the lip surface and impart a red color to the lips. The outer surface of the lip contains hair follicles, sebaceous glands, and sweat glands. The lips also contain skeletal muscle called **orbicularis oris.** Inside the free margin of the lip, the outer lining changes to a thicker, stratified squamous nonkeratinized oral epithelium. Beneath the oral epithelium are mucus-secreting **labial glands.**

The Tongue

The **tongue** is a muscular organ in the oral cavity. The core of the tongue consists of **connective tissue** and interlacing bundles of **skeletal muscle fibers.** The distribution and random orientation of individual skeletal muscle fibers in the tongue allows increased movement during chewing, swallowing, and speaking.

Papillae

The epithelium on the ventral surface of the tongue is smooth. In contrast, the epithelium on the dorsal surface of the tongue is irregular or rough because of numerous elevations or projections, called **papillae,** that are indented by the underlying connective tissue, called the **lamina propria.** All papillae on the tongue are covered by **stratified squamous epithelium** that shows partial or incomplete **keratinization.**

Four types of papillae are found on the tongue: filiform, fungiform, circumvallate, and foliate.

Filiform Papillae. The most numerous and smallest papillae on the surface of the tongue are the narrow, conical-shaped **filiform papillae.** They cover the entire dorsal surface of the tongue.

Fungiform Papillae. Less numerous but larger and broader then the filiform papillae are the **fungiform papillae.** These papillae exhibit a mushroom-like shape, are more prevalent in the anterior region of the tongue, and are interspersed among the filiform papillae. Fungiform papillae are also taller then the filliform papillae.

Circumvallate Papillae. **Circumvallate papillae** are much larger than fungiform or filiform papillae. Eight to 12 large circumvallatae papillae are located in the posterior region of the tongue. These papillae are characterized by deep moats, or **furrows,** that completely encircle them. Numerous excretory ducts from underlying **serous (von Ebner's) glands,** located in the connective tissue, empty into the base of the furrows.

Foliate Papillae. **Foliate papillae** are well developed in some animals but are rudimentary or poorly developed in humans.

Taste Buds

Located in the epithelium of the foliate and fungiform papillae and on the lateral sides of the circumvallate papillae are barrel-shaped structures called **taste buds.** The free surface of each taste bud contains an opening called the **taste pore.**

Located within each taste bud are elongated **neuroepithelial (taste) cells** that extend from the base of the taste bud to the taste pore. The apical region of each taste cell exhibits numerous **microvilli** that protrude through the taste pore. The taste cells are closely associated with afferent nerve fibers. Also present in the taste buds are elongated, supporting **sustentacular cells,** which are not sensory. At the base of each taste bud are **basal cells,** which are undifferentiated and are believed to serve as **stem cells** for the specialized cells in taste buds (Overview Figure—Oral Cavity).

Lymphoid Aggregations—Palatine Tonsils and Lingual Tonsils

The posterior third of the dorsal surface of the tongue is smooth, and it is lined by stratified squamous epithelium. Here, the surface shows numerous small bulges composed of masses of lymphoid aggregations, called the **palatine tonsils** and the **lingual tonsils.** Each tonsil is invaginated by the covering epithelium to form numerous crypts, around which are aggregations of lymphatic nodules.

FIGURE 11.1 ■ Lip (Longitudinal Section)

Thin skin, or thin **epidermis (11),** lines the external surface of the lip. The epidermis (11) is composed of stratified squamous keratinized epithelium with **desquamating surface cells (10).** Beneath the epidermis (11) is the **dermis (14)** with **sebaceous glands (2, 12),** that are associated with **hair follicles (4, 15),** and the simple tubular **sweat glands (16),** which are located deeper in the dermis (14). The dermis (14) also contains the **arrector pili muscles (3, 13),** which are smooth muscles that attach to the hair follicles (4, 15). Also visible in the lip periphery are **blood vessels (6),** such as an **artery (6a)** and a **venule (6b).** The core of the lip contains a layer of striated muscles, the **orbicularis oris (5, 17).**

The **transition zone (1)** of the skin epidermis (11) to the oral epithelium illustrates a mucocutaneous junction. The internal or oral surface of the lip is lined with a moist, stratified, squamous nonkeratinized **oral epithelium (8)** that is thicker than the epithelium of the epidermis (11). The surface cells of the oral epithelium (8), without becoming cornified, are sloughed off (desquamated) into the fluids of the mouth. In the deeper connective tissue of the lip are tubuloacinar, **mucus-secreting labial glands (9, 18).** The secretions from these glands moisten the oral mucosa. The small excretory ducts of the labial glands (9, 18) open into the oral cavity.

In the underlying connective tissue of the lip are also numerous **adipose cells (7),** blood vessels (6), and capillaries. Because the blood vessels (6) are very close to the surface, the color of the blood shows through the overlying thin epithelium, giving the lips their characteristic red color.

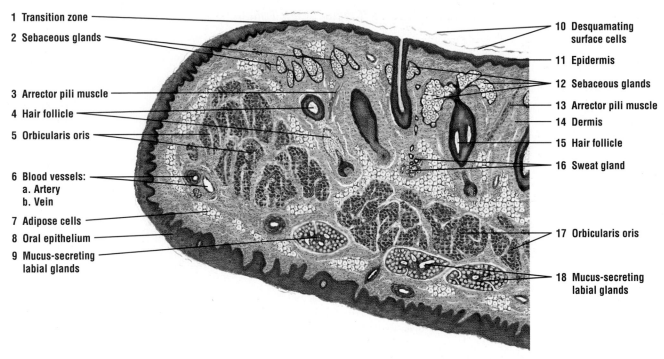

1 Transition zone
2 Sebaceous glands
3 Arrector pili muscle
4 Hair follicle
5 Orbicularis oris
6 Blood vessels:
   a. Artery
   b. Vein
7 Adipose cells
8 Oral epithelium
9 Mucus-secreting
   labial glands

10 Desquamating
   surface cells
11 Epidermis
12 Sebaceous glands
13 Arrector pili muscle
14 Dermis
15 Hair follicle
16 Sweat gland
17 Orbicularis oris
18 Mucus-secreting
   labial glands

FIGURE 11.1 ■ Lip (longitudinal section). Stain: hematoxylin and eosin. Low magnification.

FIGURE 11.2 ■ Anterior Region of the Tongue: Apex (Longitudinal Section)

This illustration shows a longitudinal section of an anterior portion of the tongue. The oral cavity is lined by a protective **mucosa (5)** that consists of an outer layer of **epithelium (5a)** and an underlying connective tissue layer, called the **lamina propria (5b)**.

The dorsal surface of the tongue is rough, and it is characterized by numerous mucosal projections, called **papillae (1, 2, 6)**. In contrast, the mucosa (5) of the ventral surface of the tongue is smooth. The slender, conical-shaped **filiform papillae (2, 6)** are the most numerous papillae, and they cover the entire dorsal surface of the tongue. The tips of the filiform papillae (2, 6) show partial keratinization.

Less numerous are the **fungiform papillae (1)**, which have a broad, round surface of non-cornified epithelium and a prominent core of **lamina propria (5b)**.

The core of the tongue consists of criss-crossing bundles of **skeletal muscle (3, 7)**. As a result, the skeletal muscles of the tongue are typically seen in longitudinal, transverse, or oblique planes of section. In the **connective tissue (9)** around the muscle bundles may be seen **blood vessels (8)**, such as an **artery (8a)**, a **vein (8b)**, and **nerve fibers (11)**.

In the lower half of the tongue and surrounded by skeletal muscle fibers (3, 7) is a portion of the **anterior lingual gland (10)**. This gland is of a mixed type, and it contains both **mucous acini (10b)** and **serous acini (10c)** as well as mixed acini. The **interlobular ducts (10a)** from the anterior lingual gland (10) pass into the larger **excretory duct** of the **lingual gland (12)** that opens into the oral cavity on the ventral surface of the tongue.

FIGURE 11.3 ■ Tongue: Circumvallate Papilla (Cross-Section)

A cross-section of a circumvallate papilla of the tongue is illustrated. The **lingual epithelium (2)** of the tongue that covers the circumvallate papilla is **stratified squamous epithelium (1)**. The underlying connective tissue, called the **lamina propria (3)**, exhibits numerous **secondary papillae (7)** that project into the overlying stratified squamous epithelium (2) of the papilla. A deep trench or **furrow (5, 10)** surrounds the base of each circumvallate papilla.

The oval **taste buds (4, 9)** are in the epithelium of the lateral surfaces of the circumvallate papilla and in the epithelium on the outer wall of the furrow (5, 10). Figure 11-5 illustrates the taste buds (4, 9) in greater detail with higher magnification.

Located deep in the lamina propria (3) and core of the tongue are numerous tubuloacinar **serous (von Ebner's) glands (6, 11)**, the **excretory ducts (6a, 11a)** of which open at the base of the circular furrows (5, 10) in the circumvallate papilla. The secretory product from the serous glands (6, 11) acts as a solvent for taste-inducing substances.

Most of the core of the tongue consists of interlacing bundles of **skeletal muscles (12)**. Examples of skeletal muscle fibers sectioned in the **longitudinal (12a)** and **transverse (12b)** planes are abundant. This interlacing arrangement of skeletal muscles (12) gives the tongue the mobility necessary for phonating, chewing, and swallowing. The lamina propria (3) surrounding the serous glands (6, 11) and muscles also contains an abundance of **blood vessels (8)**.

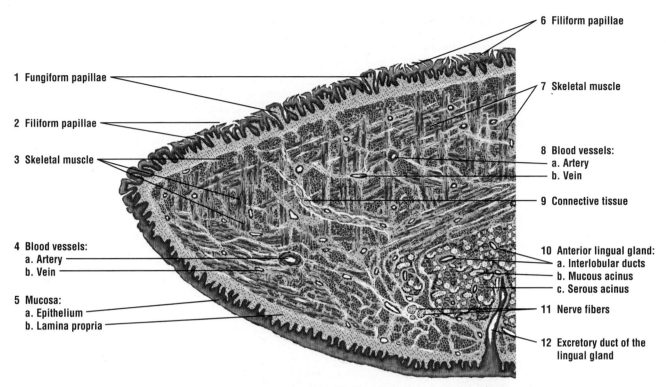

1 Fungiform papillae

2 Filiform papillae

3 Skeletal muscle

4 Blood vessels:
   a. Artery
   b. Vein

5 Mucosa:
   a. Epithelium
   b. Lamina propria

6 Filiform papillae

7 Skeletal muscle

8 Blood vessels:
   a. Artery
   b. Vein

9 Connective tissue

10 Anterior lingual gland:
   a. Interlobular ducts
   b. Mucous acinus
   c. Serous acinus

11 Nerve fibers

12 Excretory duct of the lingual gland

FIGURE 11.2 ■ Anterior region of the tongue: apex (longitudinal section). Stain: hematoxylin and eosin. Low magnification.

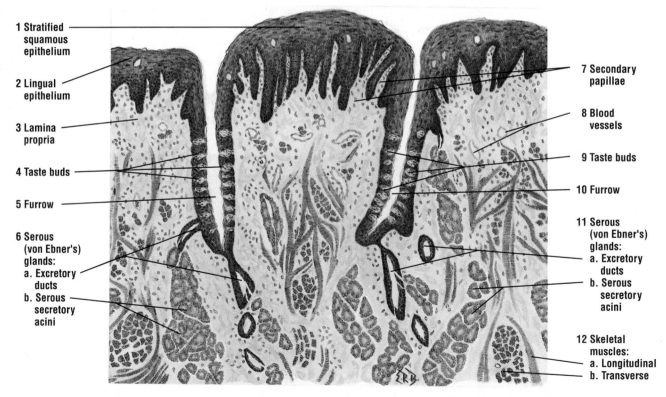

1 Stratified squamous epithelium

2 Lingual epithelium

3 Lamina propria

4 Taste buds

5 Furrow

6 Serous (von Ebner's) glands:
   a. Excretory ducts
   b. Serous secretory acini

7 Secondary papillae

8 Blood vessels

9 Taste buds

10 Furrow

11 Serous (von Ebner's) glands:
   a. Excretory ducts
   b. Serous secretory acini

12 Skeletal muscles:
   a. Longitudinal
   b. Transverse

FIGURE 11.3 ■ Tongue: circumvallate papilla (cross-section). Stain: hematoxylin and eosin. Medium magnification.

FIGURE 11.4 ◼ Tongue: Filiform and Fungiform Papillae

A low-power photomicrograph shows a section of the dorsal surface of the tongue. In the center is a large fungiform papilla (2). The surface of the fungiform papilla (2) is covered by stratified squamous epithelium (3) that is not cornified or keratinized. The fungiform papilla (2) also exhibits numerous taste buds (4) in the epithelium on the apical surface of the papilla, which is in contrast to the circumvallate papillae, in which the taste buds are located in the peripheral epithelium (see Fig. 11-3).

The underlying connective tissue core, called the **lamina propria (5)**, projects into the surface epithelium of the fungiform papilla (2) to form numerous indentations. Surrounding the fungiform papilla (2) are the slender **filiform papillae (1)**, the conical tips of which are covered by stratified squamous epithelium that exhibits partial keratinization.

FIGURE 11.5 ◼ Tongue: Taste Buds

The **taste buds (5, 12)** at the bottom of a **furrow (14)** of the circumvallate papilla are illustrated in greater detail. The taste buds (5, 12) are embedded within and extend the full thickness of the stratified **lingual epithelium (1)** of the circumvallate papilla. The taste buds (5, 12) are distinguished from the surrounding stratified epithelium (1) by their oval shapes and elongated (modified columnar) cells, which are arranged perpendicular to the epithelium (1).

Several types of cells are found in the taste buds (5, 12). Three types can be identified in this illustration. The supporting or **sustentacular cells (3, 8)** are elongated and exhibit a darker cytoplasm and a slender, dark nucleus. The taste or **gustatory cells (7, 11)** exhibit a lighter cytoplasm and a more oval, lighter nucleus. The **basal cells (13)** are located at the periphery of the taste bud (5, 12) near the basement membrane.

Because unmyelinated nerve fibers are associated with both sustentacular cells (3, 8) and gustatory cells (7, 11), both types may be responsible for taste functions. The basal cells (13) give rise to both sustentacular cells (3, 8) and gustatory cells (7, 11).

Each taste bud (5, 12) exhibits a small opening onto the epithelial surface called the **taste pore (9)**. The apical surfaces of both the sustentacular cells (3, 8) and the gustatory cells (7, 11) exhibit long **microvilli (taste hairs) (4)** that extend into and protrude through the taste pore (9) into the furrow (14) that surrounds the circumvallate papilla.

The underlying **lamina propria (2)** adjacent to the epithelium and the taste buds (5, 12) consists of loose connective tissue with numerous **blood vessels (6, 10)** and nerve fibers.

FUNCTIONAL CORRELATIONS

Tongue and Taste Buds

The main functions of the tongue during food processing are to perceive **taste** and to assist in mastication (chewing) and swallowing of the food mass, called a **bolus.** In the oral cavity, taste sensations are detected by receptor taste cells in the **taste buds** of the **fungiform** and **circumvallate papillae** of the tongue. In addition to the tongue, where they are most numerous, taste buds are also found in the mucous membrane of the **soft palate, pharynx,** and **epiglottis.**

Substances to be tasted are first dissolved in the **saliva** present in the oral cavity during food intake. In addition to saliva, taste buds in the epithelium of circumvallate papillae are continuously washed by watery secretions that are produced by the underlying **serous (von Ebner's) glands.** This secretion enters the **furrow** at the base of the papillae and dissolves different substances, which then enter the **taste pores** in the taste buds. The taste cells are stimulated by coming in direct contact with the dissolved substances.

There are four basic taste sensations: **sour, salt, bitter,** and **sweet.** All remaining taste sensations are various combinations of these four basic tastes. The tip of the tongue is most sensitive to sweet and salt, the posterior portion of the tongue to bitter, and the lateral edges of the tongue to sour taste sensations.

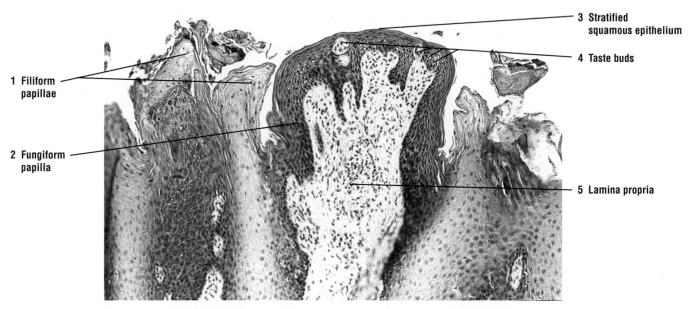

3 Stratified
   squamous epithelium

4 Taste buds

1 Filiform
  papillae

2 Fungiform
  papilla

5 Lamina propria

FIGURE 11.4 ■ Tongue: filiform and fungiform papillae. Stain: hematoxylin and eosin. 25×

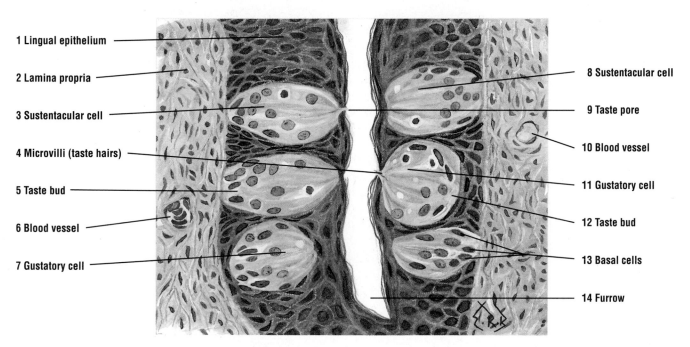

1 Lingual epithelium

2 Lamina propria

3 Sustentacular cell

4 Microvilli (taste hairs)

5 Taste bud

6 Blood vessel

7 Gustatory cell

8 Sustentacular cell

9 Taste pore

10 Blood vessel

11 Gustatory cell

12 Taste bud

13 Basal cells

14 Furrow

FIGURE 11.5 ■ Tongue: taste buds. Stain: hematoxylin and eosin. High magnification.

FIGURE 11.6 ■ Posterior Tongue: Behind Circumvallate Papilla and Near the Lingual Tonsil (Longitudinal Section)

The anterior two-thirds of the tongue are separated from the posterior third by a depression, or a sulcus terminalis. The posterior region of the tongue is located behind the circumvallate papillae and near the lingual tonsils. The dorsal surface of the posterior region typically exhibits large **mucosal ridges (1)** and elevations or **folds (7)** that resemble the large fungiform papillae of the anterior tongue. A **stratified squamous epithelium (6)** without keratinization covers the mucosal ridges (1) and folds (7). The filiform and fungiform papillae normally seen in the anterior region of the tongue are absent from the posterior tongue. Instead, lymphatic nodules of the lingual tonsils can be seen in these folds (7).

The **lamina propria (7)** of the mucosa is wider but similar to that in the anterior two-thirds of the tongue. Under the stratified squamous epithelium (6) are aggregations of **diffuse lymphatic tissue (2)**, accumulations of **adipose tissue (4)**, **nerve fibers (3)** (in longitudinal section), and blood vessels, such as an **artery (8)** and a **vein (9)**.

Deep in the connective tissue of the lamina propria (7) and between the interlacing **skeletal muscle fibers (5)** are the **mucous acini** of the **posterior lingual glands (11).** The **excretory ducts (10)** of the posterior lingual glands (11) open onto the dorsal surface of the tongue, usually between the bases of the mucosal ridges and folds (1, 7). The posterior lingual glands (11) come in contact with the serous (von Ebner's) glands of the circumvallate papilla in the anterior region of the tongue. In the posterior region, the posterior lingual glands (11) extend through the root of the tongue.

FIGURE 11.7 ■ Lingual Tonsils (Transverse Section)

The lingual tonsils are aggregations of small, individual tonsils, each with its own **tonsillar crypt (2, 8).** Lingual tonsils are situated on the dorsal surface of the posterior region or the root of the tongue. A nonkeratinized **stratified squamous epithelium (1)** lines the tonsils and their crypts (2, 8). The tonsillar crypts (2, 8) form deep invaginations on the surface of the tongue and may extend deep into the **lamina propria (5).**

Numerous **lymphatic nodules (3, 9),** some of which exhibit **germinal centers (3, 9),** are located in the lamina propria (5) below the stratified squamous surface epithelium (1). Dense **lymphatic infiltration (4, 10)** surrounds the individual lymphatic nodules (3, 9) of the tonsils.

Deep in the lamina propria (5) are fat cells of the **adipose tissue (7)** and the secretory **mucous acini** of the **posterior lingual glands (11).** Small excretory ducts from the lingual glands (11) unite to form larger **excretory ducts (6).** Most of the excretory ducts (6) open into the tonsillar crypts (2, 8), although some may open directly onto the lingual surface. Interspersed among the connective tissue of the lamina propria (5), the adipose tissue (7), and the secretory mucous acini of the posterior ingual glands (11) are fibers of the **skeletal muscles (12)** of the tongue.

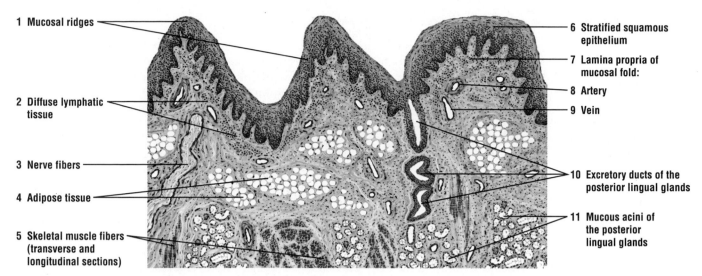

1 Mucosal ridges

2 Diffuse lymphatic tissue

3 Nerve fibers

4 Adipose tissue

5 Skeletal muscle fibers (transverse and longitudinal sections)

6 Stratified squamous epithelium

7 Lamina propria of mucosal fold:

8 Artery

9 Vein

10 Excretory ducts of the posterior lingual glands

11 Mucous acini of the posterior lingual glands

FIGURE 11.6 ■ Posterior tongue: behind circumvallate papillae and near the lingual tonsil (longitudinal section). Stain: hematoxylin and eosin. Low magnification.

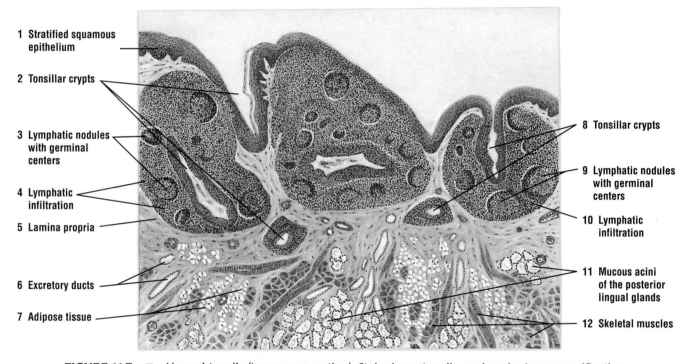

1 Stratified squamous epithelium

2 Tonsillar crypts

3 Lymphatic nodules with germinal centers

4 Lymphatic infiltration

5 Lamina propria

6 Excretory ducts

7 Adipose tissue

8 Tonsillar crypts

9 Lymphatic nodules with germinal centers

10 Lymphatic infiltration

11 Mucous acini of the posterior lingual glands

12 Skeletal muscles

FIGURE 11.7 ■ Lingual tonsils (transverse section). Stain: hematoxylin and eosin. Low magnification.

FIGURE 11.8 ◼ Longitudinal Section of a Dried Tooth

This illustration shows a longitudinal section of a dried, nondecalcified, and unstained tooth. The mineralized parts of a tooth are the enamel, the dentin, and the cementum. **Dentin (3)** is covered by **enamel (1)** in the region that projects above the gum. Enamel is not present at the root of the tooth, and here, the dentin is covered by **cementum (6).** Cementum (6) contains lacunae with the cementum-producing cells, called cementocytes, and their connecting canaliculi. Dentin (3) surrounds both the **pulp cavity (5)** and its extension into the root of the tooth, called the **root canal (11).** In living persons, the pulp cavity and root canal are filled with fine connective tissue, fibroblasts, histiocytes, and dentin-forming cells, called odontoblasts. Blood capillaries and nerves enter the pulp cavity (5) through an **apical foramen (13)** at the tip of each root.

Dentin (3) exhibits wavy, parallel dentinal tubules. The earlier, or primary, dentin is located at the periphery of the tooth. The later, or secondary, dentin lies along the pulp cavity, where it is formed throughout life by odontoblasts. In the crown of a dried tooth at the **dentinoenamel junction (2)** are numerous irregular, air-filled spaces that appear black in this section. In living persons, these **interglobular spaces (4, 10)** are filled with incompletely calcified dentin (interglobular dentin). In the root, similar areas, although smaller and spaced more closely together, are present close to the dentinal-cementum junction, where they form the **granular layer (of Tomes) (12).**

The dentin in the crown of the tooth is covered with a thicker layer of enamel (1) that is composed of enamel rods or prisms held together by an interprismatic cementing substance. The **lines of Retzius (7)** represent variations in the rate of enamel deposition. Light rays passing through a dried section of the tooth are refracted by twists that occur in the enamel rods as they course toward the surface of the tooth. These are the light **lines of Schreger (8).** Poor calcification of enamel rods during enamel formation can produce **enamel tufts (9)** that extend from the dentinoenamel junction into the enamel (see Fig. 11-9).

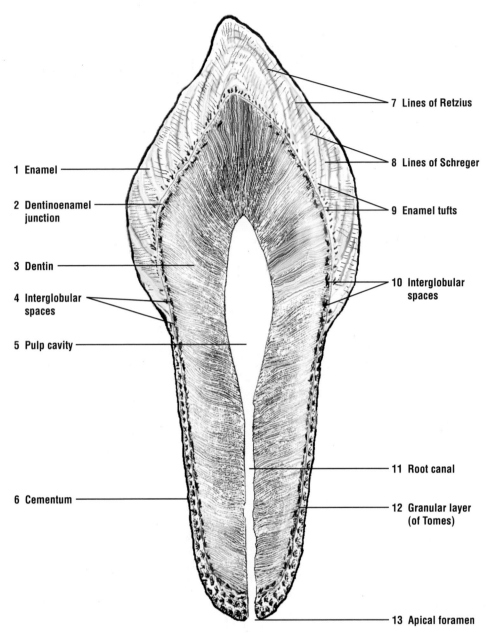

1 Enamel

2 Dentinoenamel
junction

3 Dentin

4 Interglobular
spaces

5 Pulp cavity

6 Cementum

7 Lines of Retzius

8 Lines of Schreger

9 Enamel tufts

10 Interglobular
spaces

11 Root canal

12 Granular layer
(of Tomes)

13 Apical foramen

FIGURE 11.8 ■ Longitudinal section of a dried tooth. Ground and unstained. Low magnification.

FIGURE 11.9 ■ Dried Tooth: Dentinoenamel Junction

A section of the **dentin matrix (4)** and **enamel (5)** at the **dentinoenamel junction (1)** are illustrated at a higher magnification. Cells called ameloblasts produce the enamel as successive segments that form elongated **enamel rods (7)** or prisms. The **enamel tufts (6),** which are the poorly calcified, twisted enamel rods or prisms, extend from the dentinoenamel junction (1) into the enamel (5). Dentin matrix (4) is produced by cells called odontoblasts. The odontoblastic processes of the odontoblasts occupy tunnel-like spaces in the dentin, forming the clearly visible **dentin tubules (3)** and the black, air-filled **interglobular spaces (2).**

FIGURE 11.10 ■ Dried Tooth: Cementum and Dentin Junction

The junction between the **dentin matrix (5)** and the **cementum (2)** is illustrated with higher magnification at the root of the tooth. At this junction is a layer of small interglobular spaces, called the **granular layer (of Tomes) (7).** Internal to this layer in the dentin matrix (5) are the large, irregular **interglobular spaces (4, 8)** that are commonly seen in the crown of the tooth but may also be present in the root of the tooth.

Cementum (2) is a thin layer of bony material that is secreted by cells called cementoblasts (mature forms are called cementocytes). The bone-like cementum exhibits **lacunae (1)** that house the cementocytes and numerous **canaliculi (3)** for the cytoplasmic processes of cementocytes.

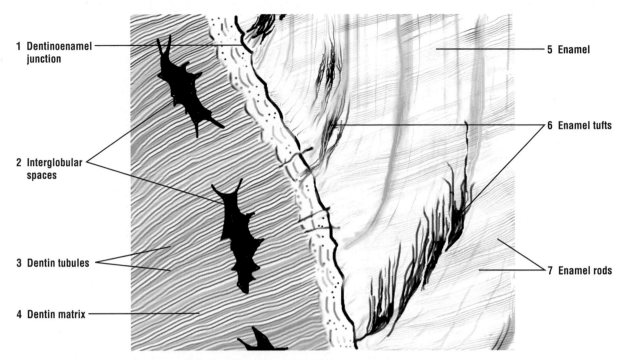

1 Dentinoenamel junction

2 Interglobular spaces

3 Dentin tubules

4 Dentin matrix

5 Enamel

6 Enamel tufts

7 Enamel rods

FIGURE 11.9 ■ Dried tooth. Dentinoenamel junction. Ground and unstained. Medium magnification.

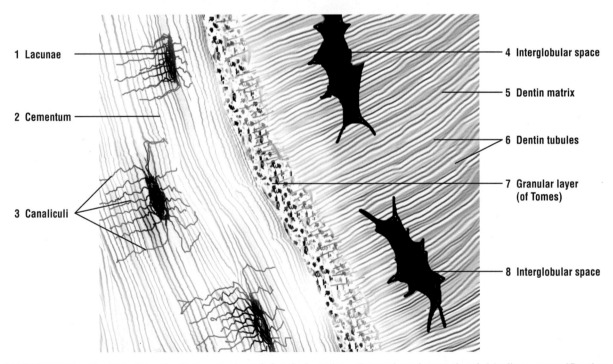

1 Lacunae

2 Cementum

3 Canaliculi

4 Interglobular space

5 Dentin matrix

6 Dentin tubules

7 Granular layer (of Tomes)

8 Interglobular space

FIGURE 11.10 ■ Dried tooth. Cementum and dentin junction. Ground and unstained. Medium magnification.

FIGURE 11.11 ▤ Developing Tooth (Longitudinal Section)

A developing tooth is shown embedded in a socket, the **dental alveolus (23)** in the **bone (9)** of the jaw. The stratified squamous nonkeratinized **oral epithelium (1, 11)** covers the developing tooth. The underlying connective tissue in the digestive tube is called the **lamina propria (2, 12)**. A downgrowth from the oral epithelium (1, 11) invades the lamina propria (2, 12) and the primitive connective tissue as the **dental lamina (3).** A layer of primitive **connective tissue (8, 17)** surrounds the developing tooth and forms a compact layer around the tooth, called the **dental sac (8, 17).**

The dental lamina (3) from the oral epithelium (1, 11) proliferates and gives rise to a cap-shaped enamel organ that consists of the **external enamel epithelium (4),** the extracellular **stellate reticulum (5, 14),** and the enamel-forming **ameloblasts** of the **inner enamel epithelium (6).** The ameloblasts of the inner enamel epithelium (6) secrete the hard **enamel (7, 13)** around the **dentin (16).** The enamel (7, 13) appears as a narrow band of dark-red colored material.

At the concave or the opposite end of the enamel organ, the **dental papilla (21)** originates from the primitive connective tissue **mesenchyme (21)** and forms the dental pulp, or core, of the developing tooth. **Blood vessels (20)** and nerves extend into and innervate the dental papilla (21) from below. The mesenchymal cells in the dental papilla (21) differentiate into **odontoblasts (15, 19)** and form the outer margin of the dental papilla (21). The odontoblasts (15, 19) secrete an uncalcified dentin, called **predentin (18).** As predentin (18) calcifies, it forms a layer of pink-staining **dentin (16)** that lies adjacent to the dark-staining enamel (7, 13).

At the base of the tooth, the external enamel epithelium (4) and the ameloblasts of the inner enamel epithelium (6) continue to grow downward and form the bilayered **epithelial root sheath (of Hertwig) (10, 22).** The cells of the epithelial root sheath (10, 22) induce the adjacent mesenchymal cells (21) to differentiate into odontoblasts (15, 19) and to form dentin (16).

FIGURE 11.12 ▤ Developing Tooth: Dentinoenamel Junction in Detail

A section of the dentinoenamel junction from a developing tooth is illustrated at high magnification. On the left is a small area of **stellate reticulum (1)** of enamel adjacent to the tall, columnar **ameloblasts (2)** that secrete the **enamel (3).** During enamel (3) formation, the apical extensions of ameloblasts become transformed into terminal processes (of Tomes). The mature enamel (3) consists of calcified, elongated **enamel rods (4)** or prisms that are barely visible in the dark-stained enamel (3). The enamel rods (4) extend through the thickness of the enamel (3).

On the right are the nuclei of **mesenchymal cells** in the **dental papilla (5).** The **odontoblasts (6)** are located adjacent to the dental papilla (5). The odontoblasts (6) secrete the uncalcified organic matrix of **predentin (8),** which later calcifies into **dentin (9).** The odontoblasts (6) exhibit slender, apical extensions, called **odontoblast processes (of Tomes) (7),** that penetrate both the predentin (8) and the dentin (9).

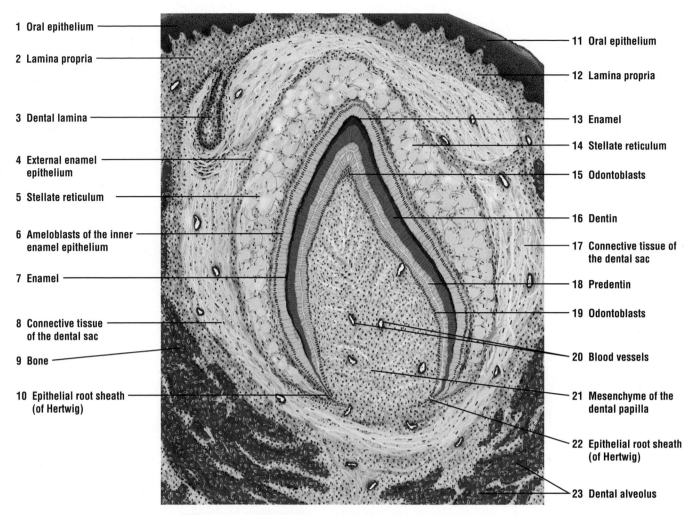

1 Oral epithelium

2 Lamina propria

3 Dental lamina

4 External enamel epithelium

5 Stellate reticulum

6 Ameloblasts of the inner enamel epithelium

7 Enamel

8 Connective tissue of the dental sac

9 Bone

10 Epithelial root sheath (of Hertwig)

11 Oral epithelium

12 Lamina propria

13 Enamel

14 Stellate reticulum

15 Odontoblasts

16 Dentin

17 Connective tissue of the dental sac

18 Predentin

19 Odontoblasts

20 Blood vessels

21 Mesenchyme of the dental papilla

22 Epithelial root sheath (of Hertwig)

23 Dental alveolus

FIGURE 11.11 ■ Developing tooth (longitudinal section). Stain: hematoxylin and eosin. Low magnification.

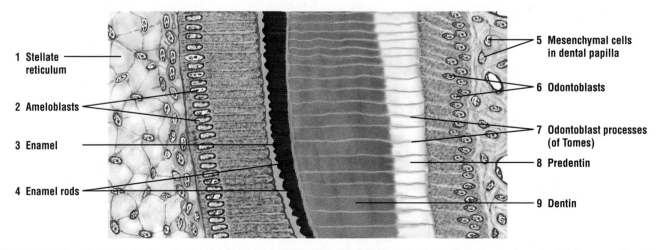

1 Stellate reticulum

2 Ameloblasts

3 Enamel

4 Enamel rods

5 Mesenchymal cells in dental papilla

6 Odontoblasts

7 Odontoblast processes (of Tomes)

8 Predentin

9 Dentin

FIGURE 11.12 ■ Developing tooth: dentinoenamel junction in detail. Stain: hematoxylin and eosin. High magnification.

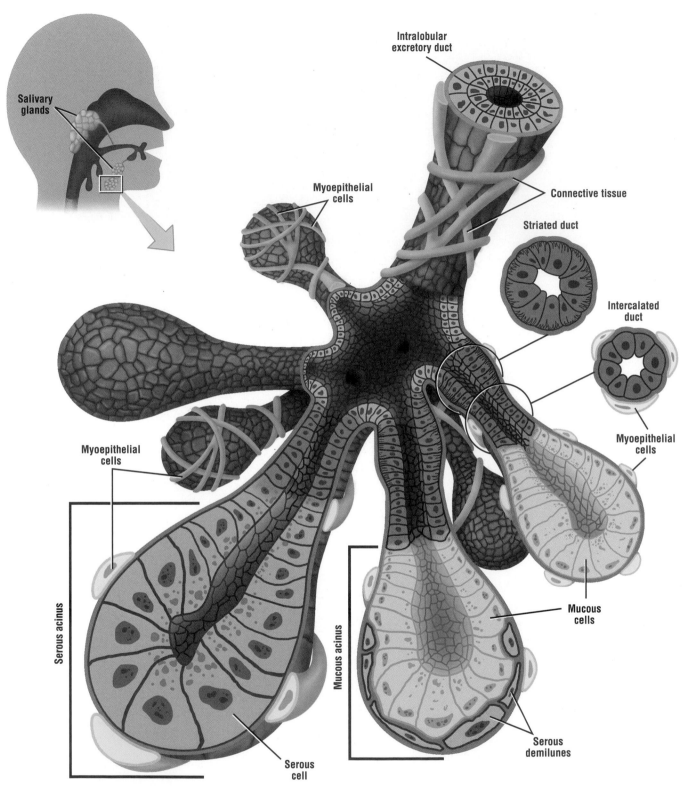

Intralobular
excretory duct

Myoepithelial
cells

Connective tissue

Striated duct

Intercalated
duct

Myoepithelial
cells

Mucous
cells

Serous
demilunes

Salivary
glands

Myoepithelial
cells

Serous acinus

Mucous acinus

Serous
cell

OVERVIEW FIGURE–SALIVARY GLANDS ■ Different types of acini (serous acini, mucous acini, and serous demilunes), different duct types (intercalated, striated, and interlobular), and myoepithelial cells of a salivary gland.

The Major Salivary Glands

There are three major **salivary glands:** the parotid, the submandibular, and the sublingual. Salivary glands are located outside of the oral cavity, and they convey their secretions into the mouth via large **excretory ducts.** The paired **parotid glands,** which are located anterior and inferior to the external ear, are the largest of the salivary glands. The smaller, paired **submandibular (submaxillary) glands** are located inferior to the mandible in the floor of the mouth. The smallest salivary glands are the **sublingual glands,** which are aggregates of smaller glands located inferior to the tongue.

Salivary glands are composed of cellular **secretory units,** called **acini** (singular, acinus), and numerous **excretory ducts.** The secretory units are small, sac-like dilations located at the end of the first segment of the excretory duct system called the **intercalated ducts.**

Cells of the Salivary Gland Acini

Two types of cells comprise the secretory acini of salivary glands: serous and mucous (Overview Figure 11—Salivary Glands).

Serous cells in the acini are pyramidal in shape. Their spherical or round nuclei are displaced basally by secretory granules that accumulate in the upper or apical regions of the cytoplasm.

Mucous cells are similar in shape to serous cells, but their cytoplasm is completely filled with a light-staining, secretory product, called **mucus.** As a result, the accumulated secretory granules flatten the nucleus and displace it to the base of the cytoplasm.

In some salivary glands, both mucous and serous cells are present in the same secretory acinus. In these mixed acini, where mucous cells predominate, serous cells form a crescent or moon-shaped cap over the mucous cells, called **serous demilune.** The secretions from serous cells in the demilunes enter the lumen of the acinus through tiny intercellular canaliculi between mucous cells.

Myoepithelial cells are flattened cells that surround both serous and mucous acini. Myoepithelial cells are also highly branched and **contractile.** They are sometimes called basket cells, because they surround the acini with their branches like a basket. Myoepithelial cells are located between the cell membrane of the secretory cells in acini and the surrounding basement menbrane.

Salivary Gland Ducts

Connective tissue fibers subdivide the salivary glands into numerous **lobules,** in which the secretory units and their excretory ducts are found.

Intercalated Ducts. Both serous, mucous, and mixed secretory acini initially empty their secretions into the **intercalated ducts.** These are the smallest ducts in the salivary glands, with small lumina that are lined by low cuboidal epithelium. Contractile myoepithelial cells surround some portions of intercalated ducts.

Striated Ducts. Several intercalated ducts merge to form the larger **striated ducts.** These ducts are lined by columnar epithelium and, with proper staining, exhibit tiny basal striations. These striations correspond to the basal infoldings of the cell membrane and the cellular interdigitations. Located in these basal infoldings are numerous and elongated mitochondria.

Excretory Intralobular Ducts. Striated ducts, in turn, join to form larger **intralobular ducts** of gradually increasing size that are surrounded by increased layers of connective tissue fibers.

Interlobular and Interlobar Ducts. Intralobular ducts join to form the larger **interlobular ducts** and **interlobar ducts.** The terminal portion of these large ducts conveys saliva from the salivary glands to the oral cavity. Larger interlobular ducts may be lined with stratified epithelium, either low cuboidal or columnar (Overview Figure—Salivary Glands).

FIGURE 11.13 ■ Salivary Gland: Parotid

The parotid salivary gland is a large serous gland that is classified as a compound tubuloacinar gland (see Fig. 2-15). The upper portion of this illustration depicts a section of the parotid gland at lower magnification, with details of specific features represented at higher magnification in separate boxes below.

The parotid gland is surrounded by a connective tissue capsule, from which arise numerous **septa (2, 8)** that subdivide the gland into lobes and lobules. Located in the connective tissue septa (2, 8) between the lobules are an **arteriole (12)**, a **venule (13)**, **interlobular excretory ducts (1, 4, 9, IV)**, and **adipose cells (intralobular) (3)**.

Each salivary gland lobule consists of secretory cells that form the **serous acini (5, 10, 16, I)** and whose pyramid-shaped cells are arranged around a lumen. The spherical nuclei of the serous cells are located at the base of the slightly basophilic cytoplasm. In certain sections, the lumen in all serous acini (5, 10, 16, I) is not always visible. At higher magnification, small **secretory granules (15, I)** are visible in the cell apices of the serous acini (15, I). The number of secretory granules in these cells varies with the functional activity of the gland. The serous acini (5, 10, 16, I) are also surrounded by thin, contractile **myoepithelial cells (14, I)** that are located between the basement membrane and the serous cells. Because of their small size, only the nuclei are visible in the myoepithelial cells (14, I).

The secretory acini empty their product into narrow channels, called the **intercalated ducts (6, 11, II)**. These ducts have small lumina, are lined by a simple squamous or low cuboidal epithelium, and are often surrounded by myoepithelial cells (see labels 23 and III in Fig. 11-14). The secretory product from the intercalated ducts (6, 11, II) drains into larger **striated ducts (7, III)**. These ducts have larger lumina and are lined by simple columnar cells that exhibit **basal striations (17, III)**. The striations in the striated ducts (7, III) are formed by deep infoldings of the basal cell membrane.

The striated ducts (7, III) empty their product into the **interlobular excretory ducts (1, 4, 9, IV)** that are located in the **interlobular connective tissue septa (2, 8)** that surround the salivary gland lobules. The lumina of interlobular excretory ducts (1, 4, 9, IV) become progressively wider, and the epithelium taller, as the ducts increase in size. The ductal epithelium (IV) increases from columnar to pseudostratified or stratified columnar in large excretory (lobar) ducts that drain the lobes of the parotid gland.

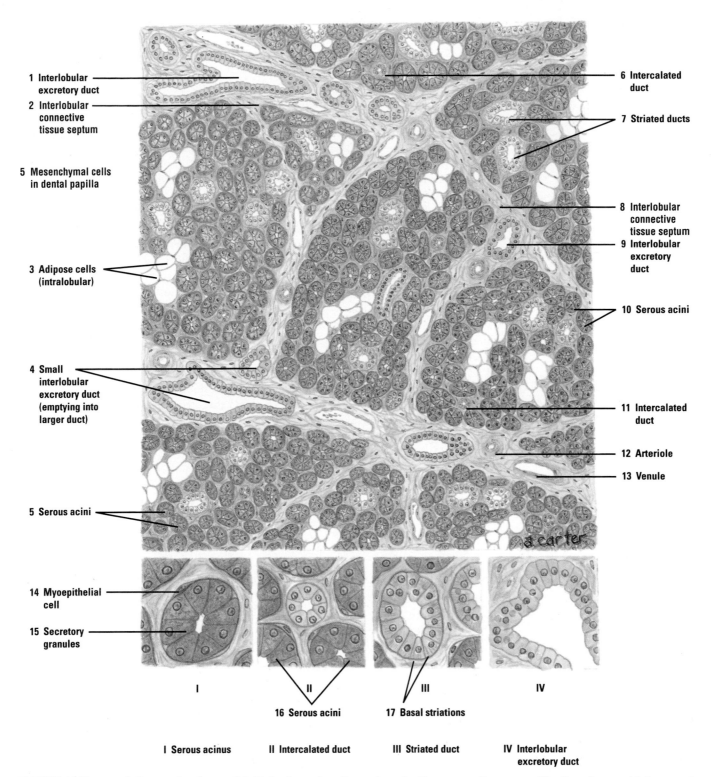

1 Interlobular excretory duct
2 Interlobular connective tissue septum
5 Mesenchymal cells in dental papilla
3 Adipose cells (intralobular)
4 Small interlobular excretory duct (emptying into larger duct)
5 Serous acini

6 Intercalated duct
7 Striated ducts
8 Interlobular connective tissue septum
9 Interlobular excretory duct
10 Serous acini
11 Intercalated duct
12 Arteriole
13 Venule

14 Myoepithelial cell
15 Secretory granules

16 Serous acini
17 Basal striations

I   II   III   IV

I Serous acinus   II Intercalated duct   III Striated duct   IV Interlobular excretory duct

FIGURE 11.13 ■ Salivary gland: parotid. Stain: hematoxylin and eosin. Upper: medium magnification. Lower: high magnification.

FIGURE 11.14   ■   Salivary Gland: Submandibular

The submandibular is also a compound tubuloacinar gland. However, the submandibular gland is a mixed gland, containing both serous and mucous acini, with serous acini predominating. The presence of both serous and mucous acini distinguishes the submandibular gland from the parotid gland, which is a purely serous gland.

This illustration depicts several lobules of the submandibular gland in which a **few mucous acini (6, 11, 14, II)** are intermixed with **serous acini (7, 18, I)**. The detailed features of the acini and ducts of the gland are illustrated at higher magnification in separate boxes at the bottom.

The serous acini (7, 18, I) are similar to those in the parotid gland (see Fig. 11-13). These acini are characterized by smaller and darker-staining pyramidal cells, a spherical basal nucleus, and apical **secretory granules (20, I).** The mucous acini (6, 11, 14, II) are larger than the serous acini (7, 18, I), have larger lumina, and exhibit more variation in size and shape. The mucous cells (6, 11, 14, II) are columnar, with pale or almost colorless cytoplasm after staining. The nuclei of mucous cells (6, 11, 14, II) are flattened and pressed against the base of the cell membrane.

The mixed acini (serous and mucous) are normally the mucous acini that are surrounded or capped by one or more serous cells, forming a crescent-shaped **serous demilune (8, 12).** The thin, contractile **myoepithelial cells (21, 22, 23)** surround the serous (I) and mucous (II) acini, and the **intercalated duct (III).**

The duct system of the submandibular gland is similar to that of the parotid gland. The intralobular **intercalated ducts (9, 13, 15, 19, III)** have small lumina and are shorter, whereas the **striated ducts (5, 16, IV)**, with distinct **basal striations (24)** in the cells, are longer than in the parotid gland. This figure also illustrates a mucous acinus (14) that opens into an intercalated duct (15), which then joins a larger striated duct (16). **Interlobular excretory ducts (3, 17)** are located in the **interlobular connective tissue septa (4)** that divide the gland into lobules and lobes. Also located in the connective tissue septa (4) are nerves, an **arteriole (1)**, a **venule (2)**, and **adipose cells (10).**

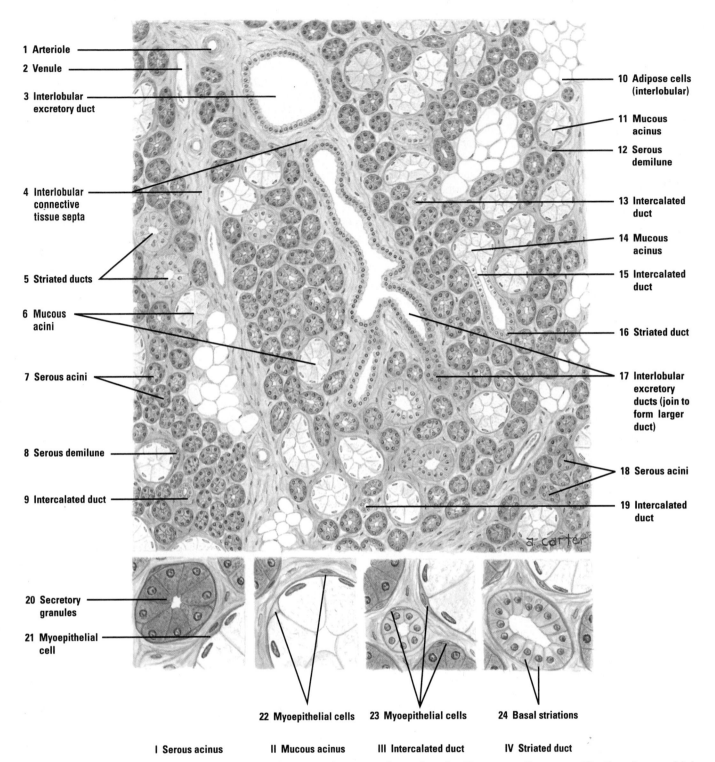

1 Arteriole

2 Venule

3 Interlobular excretory duct

4 Interlobular connective tissue septa

5 Striated ducts

6 Mucous acini

7 Serous acini

8 Serous demilune

9 Intercalated duct

10 Adipose cells (interlobular)

11 Mucous acinus

12 Serous demilune

13 Intercalated duct

14 Mucous acinus

15 Intercalated duct

16 Striated duct

17 Interlobular excretory ducts (join to form larger duct)

18 Serous acini

19 Intercalated duct

20 Secretory granules

21 Myoepithelial cell

22 Myoepithelial cells

23 Myoepithelial cells

24 Basal striations

I Serous acinus

II Mucous acinus

III Intercalated duct

IV Striated duct

a. carter

FIGURE 11.14 ■ Salivary gland: submandibular. Stain: hematoxylin and eosin. Upper: medium magnification. Lower: high magnification.

FIGURE 11.15 ■ Salivary Gland: Sublingual

The sublingual gland is also a compound, mixed tubuloacinar gland that resembles the submandibular gland, because it contains both serous and mucous acini. Most, however, are **mucous acini (5, 15, I)** and mucous acini capped **with serous demilunes (9, 14, 18, 19, II)**. The light-stained mucous acini (5, 15, I) are conspicuous in this section. Purely serous acini are scarce in the sublingual gland; however, the composition of the gland varies. In this medium-magnification illustration, **serous acini (3, 16)** appear frequently, whereas in other sections, serous acini may be absent. At higher magnification, **myoepithelial cells (17, I)** are seen around individual acini.

In comparison to other salivary glands, the duct system of the sublingual gland is different. The **intercalated ducts (2, 10, III)** are short or absent, and they are not readily observed in a given section. In contrast, the nonstriated **intralobular excretory ducts (4, 6, IV)** are more prevalent in the sublingual glands. The intralobular excretory ducts (4, 6, IV) are equivalent to the striated ducts of the submandibular and parotid glands, but they lack the extensive membrane infolding and basal striations.

The **interlobular connective tissue septa (13)** are also more abundant in the sublingual than in the parotid and submandibular glands. An **arteriole (12)**, a **venule (8),** nerve fibers, and **interlobular excretory ducts (1, 11)** are seen in the septa. The epithelial lining of the interlobular excretory ducts (1, 11) varies from low columnar in the smaller ducts to pseudostratified or stratified columnar in the larger ducts.

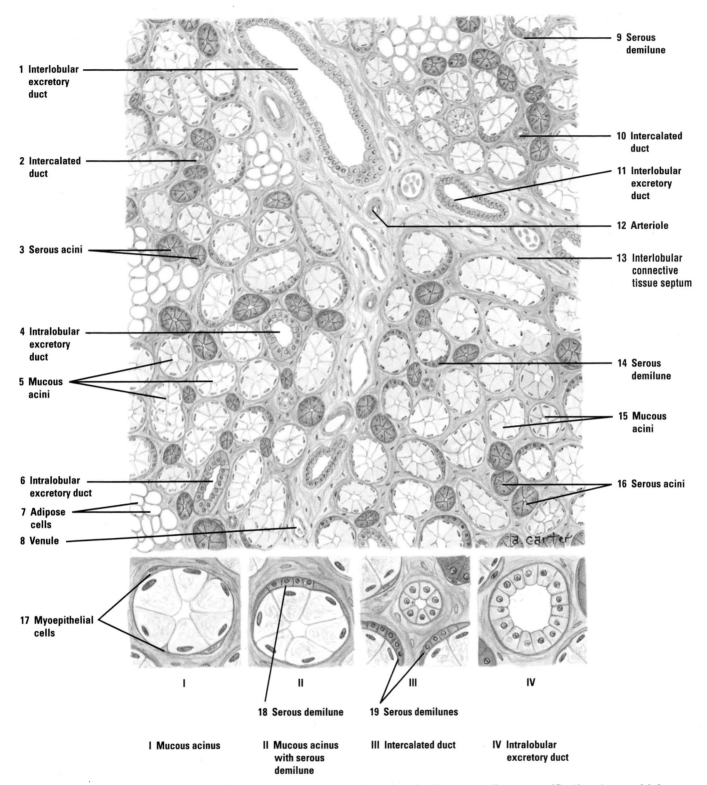

1 Interlobular excretory duct

2 Intercalated duct

3 Serous acini

4 Intralobular excretory duct

5 Mucous acini

6 Intralobular excretory duct

7 Adipose cells

8 Venule

9 Serous demilune

10 Intercalated duct

11 Interlobular excretory duct

12 Arteriole

13 Interlobular connective tissue septum

14 Serous demilune

15 Mucous acini

16 Serous acini

17 Myoepithelial cells

18 Serous demilune

19 Serous demilunes

I   II   III   IV

I Mucous acinus

II Mucous acinus with serous demilune

III Intercalated duct

IV Intralobular excretory duct

FIGURE 11.15 ■ Salivary gland: sublingual. Stain: hematoxylin and eosin. Upper: medium magnification. Lower: high magnification.

FIGURE 11.16 ■ Serous Salivary Gland: Parotid

This photomicrograph illustrates a section of the parotid salivary gland. In humans, the parotid gland is entirely composed of **serous acini (1)** and excretory ducts. In this illustration, the cytoplasm of serous cells in the serous acini (1) is filled with tiny secretory granules. A small **intercalated duct (2),** with its cuboidal epithelium, is surrounded by the serous acini (1). Also visible on the right is a larger, lighter-staining excretory duct, called the **striated duct (3).**

FIGURE 11.17 ■ Mixed Salivary Gland: Sublingual

The sublingual salivary gland exhibits both **mucous acini (2)** and **serous acini (3).** The mucous acini (2), with their cytoplasm filled with **mucus (1),** are larger and lighter staining than the serous acini (3), which are darker staining and have tiny secretory granules in the apical cytoplasm. The serous acini (3) that surround the mucous acini (2) form crescent-shaped structures, called **serous demilunes (4).** A tiny excretory **intercalated duct (5),** lined by cuboidal epithelium, and a larger **striated duct (6),** with columnar epithelium, are also visible.

FUNCTIONAL CORRELATIONS

Salivary Glands and Saliva

Salivary glands produce approximately 1 L/day of a watery secretion, called **saliva,** that enters the oral cavity via different large excretory ducts. **Myoepithelial cells** surround the secretory acini and the intercalated ducts in the salivary glands. On contraction, these cells expel the secretory products from the different acini.

Saliva is a mixture of secretions that are produced by cells in different salivary glands. Although the major component is **water,** saliva also contains ions, mucus, enzymes, and antibodies (immunoglobulins). The sight, smell, thought, taste, or actual presence of food in the mouth causes an **autonomic stimulation** of the salivary glands that increases production of saliva and stimulates its release into the oral cavity.

Saliva performs numerous important functions. It moistens the chewed food, and it provides solvents that allow the food to be tasted. Saliva also lubricates the bolus of chewed food for easier swallowing and passage through the esophagus to the stomach. In addition, saliva contains numerous **electrolytes** (calcium, potassium, sodium, chloride, bicarbonate ions, and others). A digestive enzyme, **salivary amylase,** is present in saliva as well. This enzyme is mainly produced by the **serous acini** in the salivary glands, and it initiates the breakdown of starch into smaller carbohydrates during the short time that food is present in the oral cavity. Once in the stomach, food is acidified by gastric juices, an action that decreases amylase activity and carbohydrate digestion.

Saliva also functions in controlling **bacterial flora** in the mouth and protecting the oral cavity against pathogens. Another salivary enzyme, **lysozyme,** which is also secreted by serous cells, hydrolyzes the cell walls of bacteria and inhibits their growth in the oral cavity. In addition, saliva contains salivary **antibodies.** The antibodies (primarily immunoglobulin A) are produced by the **plasma cells** in the connective tissue of salivary glands. The antibodies form complexes with antigens, and they assist with immunological defense against oral bacteria. Salivary acinar cells secrete a component that binds to and transports the immunoglobulins from plasma cells in the connective tissue into saliva.

As saliva flows through the duct system of salivary glands, the striated ducts modify its ionic content by selective transport, resorption, or secretions of ions. Sodium and chloride ions are actively reabsorbed from saliva, whereas potassium and bicarbonate ions are added to salivary secretions. The numerous infoldings of the basal cell membrane or the striations seen in the striated ducts contain elongated mitochondria. These structures are characteristic features of cells that transport fluids and electrolytes across cell membranes.

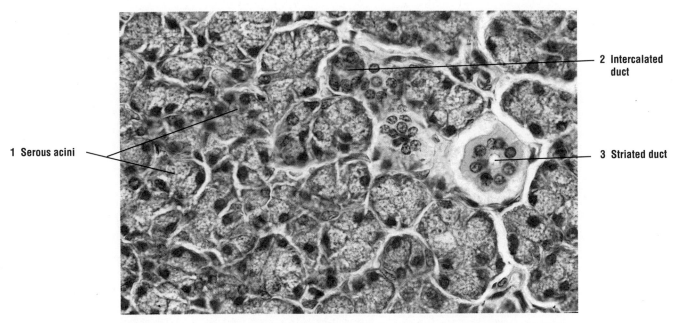

1 Serous acini

2 Intercalated duct

3 Striated duct

FIGURE 11.16 ■ Serous salivary gland: parotid. Stain: hematoxylin and eosin. 165×

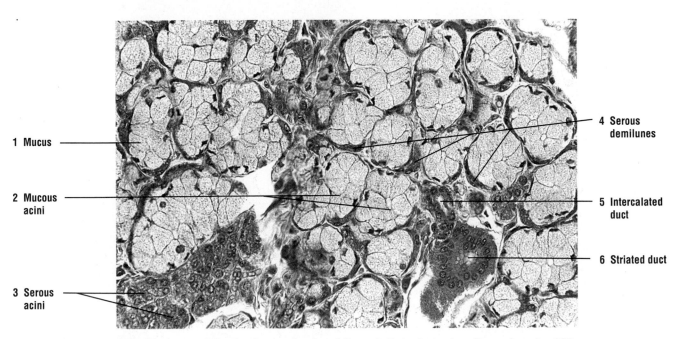

1 Mucus

2 Mucous acini

3 Serous acini

4 Serous demilunes

5 Intercalated duct

6 Striated duct

FIGURE 11.17 ■ Mixed salivary gland: sublingual. Stain: hematoxylin and eosin. 165×

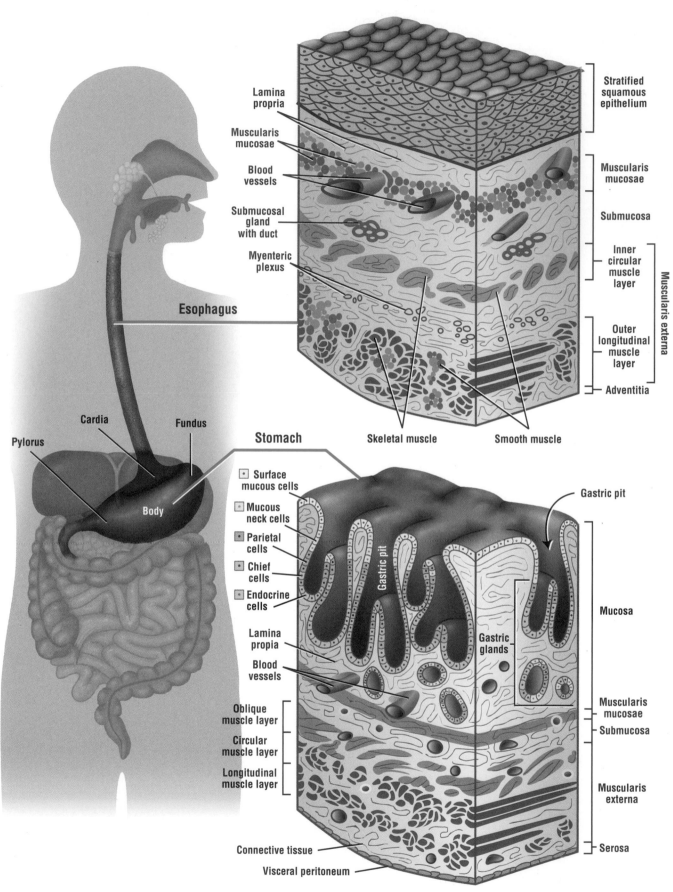

Lamina propria

Muscularis mucosae

Blood vessels

Submucosal gland with duct

Myenteric plexus

Stratified squamous epithelium

Muscularis mucosae

Submucosa

Inner circular muscle layer

Outer longitudinal muscle layer

Muscularis externa

Adventitia

Esophagus

Skeletal muscle

Smooth muscle

Cardia

Fundus

Pylorus

Body

Stomach

· **Surface mucous cells**

· **Mucous neck cells**

· **Parietal cells**

· **Chief cells**

· **Endocrine cells**

Gastric pit

Gastric pit

Lamina propia

Blood vessels

Gastric glands

Mucosa

Muscularis mucosae

Submucosa

Oblique muscle layer

Circular muscle layer

Longitudinal muscle layer

Muscularis externa

Connective tissue

Serosa

Visceral peritoneum

OVERVIEW FIGURE ■ Detailed illustration comparing the structural differences of the four layers (mucosa, submucosa, muscularis externa, and adventitia/serosa) in the wall of the esophagus and stomach.

Digestive System:
Esophagus and Stomach

General Plan of the Digestive System

The digestive (gastrointestinal) tract is a long, hollow tube that extends from the esophagus to the rectum. It includes the esophagus, stomach, small intestine (duodenum, jejunum, and ileum), large intestine (colon), and rectum. The wall of the digestive tube exhibits four layers that show a basic histologic organization. These layers are the mucosa, submucosa, muscularis externa, and serosa or adventitia. Because of the different functions of the digestive organs in the digestive process, the morphology of these layers exhibits variations.

The **mucosa** is the innermost layer of the digestive tube. It consists of a covering **epithelium** and glands that extend into the underlying layer of loose connective tissue, called the **lamina propria.** An inner circular and outer longitudinal layers of smooth muscle, called the **muscularis mucosae,** form the outer boundary of the mucosa.

The **submucosa** is located below the mucosa. It consists of dense irregular connective tissue, with numerous blood and lymph vessels, and a **submucosal (Meissner's) nerve plexus.** This nerve plexus contains postganglionic parasympathetic neurons. The neurons and axons of the submucosal nerve plexus control the motility of the mucosa and the secretory activities of associated mucosal glands. In the initial portion of the small intestine, called the **duodenum,** the submucosa contains numerous branched mucous glands.

The **muscularis externa** is a thick, smooth muscle layer that is located inferior to the submucosa. Except for the large intestine, this layer is composed of an inner layer of circular smooth muscle and outer layer of longitudinal smooth muscle. Situated between the two smooth muscle layers of the muscularis externa is connective tissue and another nerve plexus, called the **myenteric (Auerbach's) nerve plexus.** This plexus also contains some postganglionic parasympathetic neurons and controls the motility of smooth muscles in the muscularis externa.

The **serosa** is a thin layer of loose connective tissue that surrounds the visceral organs. It may or may not be covered by a thin, outer layer of squamous epithelium, called the **mesothelium.** If the mesothelium covers the visceral organs, then the organs are within the abdominal or pelvic cavities (**intraperitoneal**), and the outer layer is called serosa. The serosa covers the outer surface of the abdominal portion of the esophagus, stomach, and small intestine. It also covers parts of the colon (ascending and descending colon), but only on the anterior and lateral surfaces, because their posterior surfaces are bound to the posterior abdominal body wall and are not covered by the mesothelium (see overview figure).

When the wall of the digestive tube is not covered by mesothelium, it lies outside the peritoneal cavity and is called **retroperitoneal.** In this case, the outermost layer adheres to the body wall and consists only of a connective tissue layer, called the **adventitia.**

The characteristic features and functions of each layer in the digestive tube are discussed in detail with each illustration of the different organs.

Esophagus

The **esophagus** is a soft tube approximately 10 inches in length that extends from the **pharynx** to the **stomach.** It is located posterior to the trachea and in the mediastinum of the **thoracic cavity.**

After descending in the thoracic cavity, the esophagus penetrates the muscular **diaphragm.** A short section of the esophagus is present in the abdominal cavity before it terminates at the stomach.

In the thoracic cavity, the esophagus is surrounded only by a connective tissue layer. As a result, the outermost layer in the esophagus is called the **adventitia.** In the abdominal cavity, a simple squamous mesothelium lines the outermost wall of the short segment of the esophagus to form the serosa.

Internally, the esophageal lumen is lined with moist, **nonkeratinized stratified squamous epithelium.** When the esophagus is empty, the lumen exhibits numerous, but temporary, **longitudinal folds** of mucosa. The outer wall of the esophagus, the **muscularis externa,** contains a mixture of different types of muscle fibers. In the upper third of the esophagus, the muscularis externa contains striated **skeletal muscle fibers.** In the middle third, the muscularis externa contains both **skeletal** and **smooth muscle fibers.** In the lower third, the esophagus is comprised entirely of **smooth muscle fibers** (see overview figure).

Stomach

The stomach is an expanded, hollow organ that is situated between the esophagus and the small intestine. At the esophageal-stomach junction is an abrupt transition from the stratified squamous epithelium of the esophagus to the **simple columnar epithelium** of the stomach. The luminal surface of the stomach is pitted with numerous tiny openings, called **gastric pits.** These are formed by the luminal epithelium that invaginates the underlying connective tissue **lamina propria** of the **mucosa.** The tubular **gastric glands** are located below the luminal epithelium, and they open directly into the gastric pits to deliver their secretions into the stomach lumen. The gastric glands descend through the lamina propria to the **muscularis mucosae.**

Below the mucosa of the stomach is the dense connective tissue **submucosa,** which contains large blood vessels and nerves. The thick, muscular wall of the stomach, the **muscularis externa,** exhibits three muscle layers instead of the two that are normally seen in the esophagus and small intestine. The outer layer of the stomach is covered by the **serosa** or visceral peritoneum.

Anatomically, the stomach is divided into the narrow **cardia,** where the esophagus terminates; an upper, dome-shaped **fundus;** a lower **body** or **corpus;** and a funnel-shaped, terminal region, called the **pylorus.**

The fundus and the body comprise about two-thirds of the stomach, and they have identical histologies. As a result, the stomach has only three distinct histologic regions. The fundus and the body form the major portions of stomach. Their mucosae consist of deep **gastric glands** that produce most of the **gastric secretions** or juices for digestion. Also, all stomach regions exhibit **rugae,** which are the longitudinal folds of the mucosa and submucosa. These folds are temporary and dissapear when the stomach is distended with fluid or solid material (Overview Figure 12).

FIGURE 12.1 ■ Wall of the Upper Esophagus (Transverse Section)

The esophagus is a long, hollow tube, the wall of which consists of the mucosa, submucosa, muscularis externa, and adventitia. In this illustration, the upper portion of the esophagus has been sectioned in a transverse plane.

The **mucosa (1)** of the esophagus consists of three parts: an inner lining of nonkeratinized **stratified squamous epithelium (1a);** an underlying, thin layer of fine connective tissue, called the **lamina propria (1b);** and a layer of longitudinal smooth muscle fibers, called the **muscularis mucosae (1c).** All three layers are shown here in the transverse plane. The **connective tissue papillae (9)** of the lamina propria (1b) indent the epithelium (1a). Found in the lamina propria (1b) are small **blood vessels (8),** diffuse lymphatic tissue, and a small **lymphatic nodule (8).**

The **submucosa (3)** in the esophagus is a wide layer of moderately dense irregular connective tissue that often contains **adipose tissue (12).** The **mucous acini** of the **esophageal glands proper (2)** are present in the submucosa (3) at intervals throughout the length of the esophagus. The **excretory ducts** of the **esophageal glands (10)** pass through the muscularis mucosae (1c) and the lamina propria (1b) to open into the esophageal lumen. The dark-staining ductal epithelium of the glands merges with the stratified squamous surface epithelium (1a) of the esophagus (see Fig. 12-2). Numerous blood vessels, such as a **vein** and an **artery (11),** are found in the connective tissue of the submucosa (4).

Located inferior to the submucosa (3) is the **muscularis externa (4),** which is composed of two well-defined muscle layers: an **inner circular muscle layer (4a)** and the **outer longitudinal muscle layer (4b),** the muscle fibers of which are shown here sectioned in a transverse plane. A thin layer of **connective tissue (12)** lies between the inner circular muscle layer (4a) and the outer longitudinal muscle layer (4b).

The muscularis externa (4) of the esophagus is highly variable in different species. In humans, the muscularis externa (4) in the upper third of the esophagus consists primarily of striated skeletal muscles. In the middle third, the inner circular muscle layer (4a) and the outer longidutinal muscle layer (4b) exhibit a mixture of both smooth muscle and skeletal muscle fibers. In the lower third, only smooth muscle is present.

The **adventitia (5)** of the esophagus consists of a loose connective tissue layer that blends with the adventitia of the trachea and the surrounding structures. **Adipose tissue (14),** large blood vessels (**artery** and **vein [15]**), and **nerve fibers (6)** are numerous in the connective tissue of the adventitia (5).

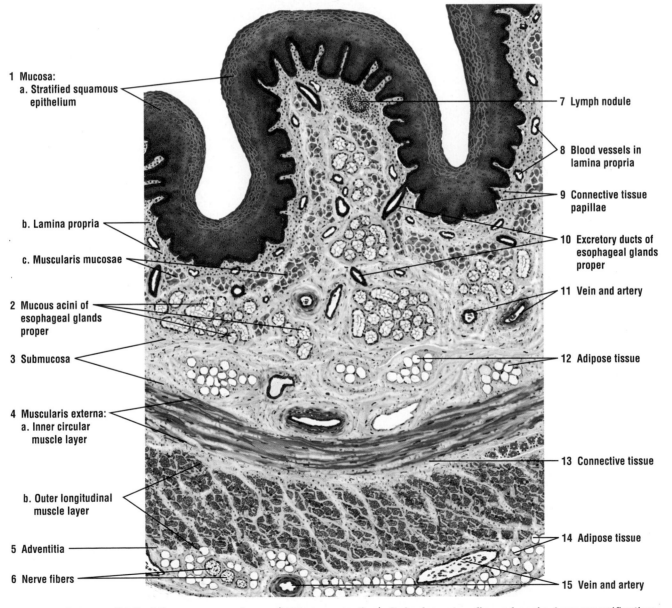

1 Mucosa:
  a. Stratified squamous epithelium

7 Lymph nodule

8 Blood vessels in lamina propria

9 Connective tissue papillae

b. Lamina propria

c. Muscularis mucosae

10 Excretory ducts of esophageal glands proper

2 Mucous acini of esophageal glands proper

11 Vein and artery

3 Submucosa

12 Adipose tissue

4 Muscularis externa:
  a. Inner circular muscle layer

13 Connective tissue

b. Outer longitudinal muscle layer

14 Adipose tissue

5 Adventitia

6 Nerve fibers

15 Vein and artery

FIGURE 12.1 ■ Wall of the upper esophagus (transverse section). Stain: hematoxylin and eosin. Low magnification.

FIGURE 12.2 ■ Upper Esophagus (Transverse Section)

The following two sections illustrate the difference between the upper and lower esophageal wall.

The different layers of the esophagus are easily distinguishable. The mucosa of the upper esophagus (as in Fig.12-1) consists of a stratified squamous nonkeratinized **epithelium (1)**, a connective tissue **lamina propria (2)**, and a layer of smooth muscle **musclaris mucosae (3)** (transverse plane). A small **lymphatic nodule (4)** is visible in the lamina propria (2). In the **submucosa (7)** are cells of adipose tissue and **mucous acini** of the **esophageal glands proper (6)**, with their **excretory ducts (5)**. The muscularis externa of the uppper esophagus consists of an **inner circular layer (10)** and an **outer longitudinal layer (14)** of skeletal muscles, separated by a layer of **connective tissue (11)**. The outermost layer around the esophagus is the connective tissue **adventitia (8)**, with adipose tissue, **nerves (13)**, a **vein (9)**, and an **artery (12)**.

FIGURE 12.3 ■ Lower Esophagus (Transverse Section)

This illustration shows the terminal portion of the esophagus after it has penetrated the diaphragm and entered the peritoneal cavity near the stomach.

The layers in the wall of the lower esophagus are similar to those in the upper region, except for regional modifications (see Fig. 12-2). As in the upper esophagus, the **mucosa (1)** of the lower esophagus consists of stratified squamous nonkeratinized **epithelium (1a)**, the connective tissue **lamina propria (1b)**, and a smooth muscle layer **musclaris mucosae (1c)** (transverse section). Also visible are the **connective tissue papillae (2)** of the lamina propria (1b) that indent the lining epithelium (1a) and a **lymphatic nodule (3)**.

The connective tissue **submucosa (6)** also contains mucous acini of the **esophageal glands proper (5)**, their **excretory ducts (4)**, and **adipose tissue (7)**. In some regions of the esophagus, these glands may be absent.

The major differences between the upper and lower esophagus are seen in the next two layers. The **muscularis externa (10)** in the lower esophagus consists entirely of smooth muscle layers: an **inner circular muscle layer (10a)** and an **outer longitudinal muscle layer (10b)**. The outermost layer of the lower esophagus is the **serosa (8)**, or visceral peritoneum. Serosa (8) consists of a connective tissue layer that is lined by a simple squamous layer mesothelium. In contrast, the adventitia that surrounds the esophagus in the thoracic region consists only of a connective tissue layer.

In the upper esophagus, less connective tissue is present in the lamina propria (1b), around the smooth muscle fibers of the muscularis externa (10), and in the serosa (8).

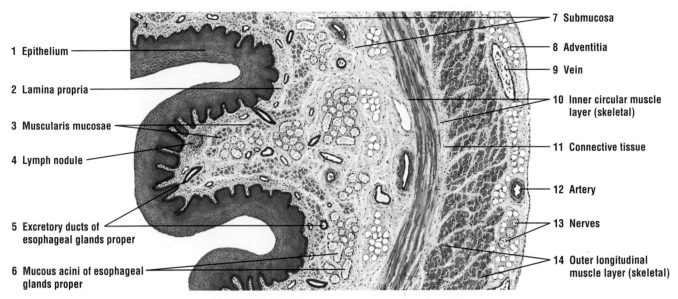

1 Epithelium

2 Lamina propria

3 Muscularis mucosae

4 Lymph nodule

5 Excretory ducts of esophageal glands proper

6 Mucous acini of esophageal glands proper

7 Submucosa

8 Adventitia

9 Vein

10 Inner circular muscle layer (skeletal)

11 Connective tissue

12 Artery

13 Nerves

14 Outer longitudinal muscle layer (skeletal)

FIGURE 12.2 ■ Upper esophagus (transverse section). Stain: hematoxylin and eosin. Low magnification.

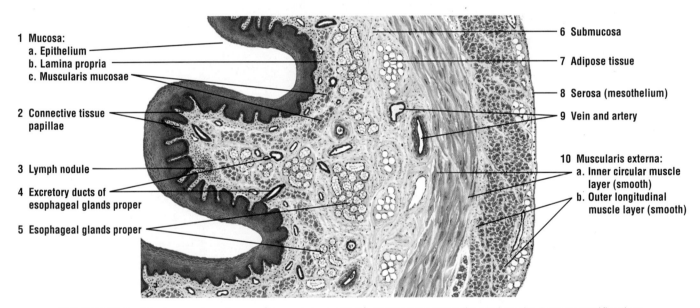

1 Mucosa:
  a. Epithelium
  b. Lamina propria
  c. Muscularis mucosae

2 Connective tissue papillae

3 Lymph nodule

4 Excretory ducts of esophageal glands proper

5 Esophageal glands proper

6 Submucosa

7 Adipose tissue

8 Serosa (mesothelium)

9 Vein and artery

10 Muscularis externa:
  a. Inner circular muscle layer (smooth)
  b. Outer longitudinal muscle layer (smooth)

FIGURE 12.3 ■ Lower esophagus (transverse section). Stain: hematoxylin and eosin. Low magnification.

FIGURE 12.4 ■ Upper Esophagus: Mucosa and Submucosa (Longitudinal Section)

This higher-magnification illustration of the upper esophagus has been sectioned longitudinally. The smooth muscle fibers of the **muscularis mucosae (9)** exhibit a longitudinal orientation, and the fibers of the inner circular mucle layer are cut in a transverse section.

The esophagus is lined with stratified squamous **epithelium (7).** Squamous cells form the outermost layers of the epithelium, the numerous polyhedral cells form the intermediate layers, and low columnar cells form the basal layer. Mitotic activity can be seen in the deeper layers of the epithelium. The connective tissue **lamina propria (8)** contains numerous blood vessels, aggregates of lymphocytes, and a small **lymphatic nodule (2). Connective tissue papillae (1)** from the lamina propria (8) indent the surface epithelium (7). The muscularis mucosae (9) is illustrated here as bundles of smooth muscle fibers sectioned in a longitudinal plane.

The underlying **submucosa (3, 10)** contains **mucous acini** of the **esophageal glands proper (4).** Small **excretory ducts (11)** from these glands, lined with simple epithelium, join the larger excretory ducts that are lined with stratified epithelium. One of the excretory ducts joins the stratified squamous epithelium (7) of the esophageal lumen. Also in the submucosa (3, 10) are blood vessels, such as a **vein** and **artery (12), nerves (5),** and **adipose tissue (6).**

In the upper esophagus, the **inner circular muscle layer (13)** of the muscularis externa consists of skeletal muscle. A portion of this layer is illustrated in a transverse plane at the bottom of the figure.

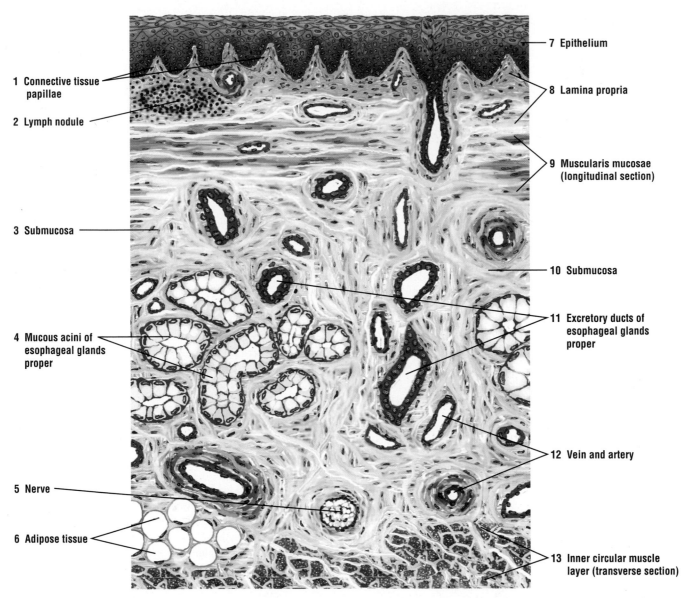

1 Connective tissue
  papillae

2 Lymph nodule

3 Submucosa

4 Mucous acini of
  esophageal glands
  proper

5 Nerve

6 Adipose tissue

7 Epithelium

8 Lamina propria

9 Muscularis mucosae
  (longitudinal section)

10 Submucosa

11 Excretory ducts of
   esophageal glands
   proper

12 Vein and artery

13 Inner circular muscle
   layer (transverse section)

FIGURE 12.4 ■ Upper esophagus: mucosa and submucosa (longitudinal section). Stain: hematoxylin and eosin. Medium magnification.

FIGURE 12.5 ■ Lower Esophageal Wall (Transverse Section)

A low-magnification photomicrograph illustrates the lower portion of the esophagus and all layers of the mucosa. The mucosa consists of a thick, but nonkeratinized, **stratified squamous epithelium (1)**, a connective tissue **lamina propria (2)**, and a thin strip of smooth muscle **muscularis mucosae (3)**.

FUNCTIONAL CORRELATIONS

Esophagus

The major function of the esophagus is to convey liquids and/or a mass of chewed food (**bolus**) from the oral cavity to the stomach. For this function, the lumen of the esophagus is lined by a protective **nonkeratinized stratified squamous epithelium.** Aiding in this function are esophageal glands in the connective tissue of the wall. Two types of glands are found in the wall of the esophagus. The **esophageal cardiac glands** are present in the **lamina propria** of the upper and lower regions of the esophagus. These glands have a morphology similar to those found in the cardia of the stomach, where the esophagus terminates. The **esophageal glands proper** are located in the connective tissue of the submucosa. Both types of glands produce the secretory product **mucus,** which is conducted in **excretory ducts** through the epithelium to lubricate the esophageal lumen. The swallowed material is moved from one end of the esophagus to the other by strong muscular contractions, called **peristalsis.** At the lower end of the esophagus, a muscular **gastroesophageal sphincter** constricts the lumen and prevents regurgitation of swallowed material back into the esophagus.

FIGURE 12.6 ■ Esophageal-Stomach Junction

At its terminal end, the esophagus joins the stomach and forms the esophageal-stomach junction. The nonkeratinized **stratified squamous epithelium (1)** of the **esophagus** abruptly changes to the simple columnar, mucus-secreting **gastric epithelium (10)** of the cardia region of the **stomach.**

At the esophageal-stomach junction, the **esophageal glands proper (7)** may be seen in the **submucosa (8).** Excretory ducts (4, 6) from these glands course through the **muscularis mucosae (5)** and the **lamina propria (2)** of the esophagus and into its lumen. In the lamina propria (2) of the esophagus near the stomach region are the **esophageal cardiac glands (3).** Both the esophageal glands proper (7) and the esophageal cardiac glands (3) secrete mucus.

The lamina propria of the esophagus (2) continues into the **lamina propria** of the **stomach (12),** where it becomes filled with **gastric** and **cardiac glands (16, 17)** and with diffuse lymphatic tissue. The lamina propria of the stomach (12) is penetrated by shallow **gastric pits (11),** into which the gastric glands (16, 17) empty.

The upper region of the stomach contains two types of glands. The simple tubular cardiac glands (17) are limited to the transition region, the cardia of the stomach. These glands are lined with pale-staining, mucus-secreting columnar cells. Below the cardiac region of the stomach are the simple tubular gastric glands (16), some of which exhibit basal branching.

In contrast to the cardiac glands (17), the gastric glands (16) contain four types of cells: the pale-staining **mucous neck cells (13);** the large, eosinophilic **parietal cells (14);** the basophilic **zymogenic (chief) cells (15);** and several different types of endocrine cells (not illustrated), which are collectively called the enteroendocrine cells.

The **muscularis mucosae** of the **stomach (18)** also continues with the muscularis mucosae of the esophagus (5). In the esophagus, the muscularis mucosae (5) is usually a single layer of longitudinal smooth muscle fibers, whereas in the stomach, a second layer of smooth muscle, called the inner circular layer, is added.

The **submucosa (8, 19)** and the **muscularis externa (9, 21)** of the esophagus are continuous with those of the stomach. **Blood vessels (20)** are found in the submucosa (8, 19), from which smaller blood vessels are distributed to other regions of the stomach.

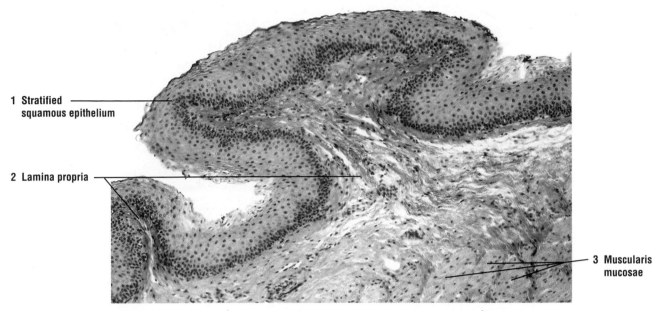

1 Stratified
  squamous epithelium

2 Lamina propria

3 Muscularis
  mucosae

FIGURE 12.5 ■ Lower esophageal wall (transverse section). Stain: mallory-azan. 30×

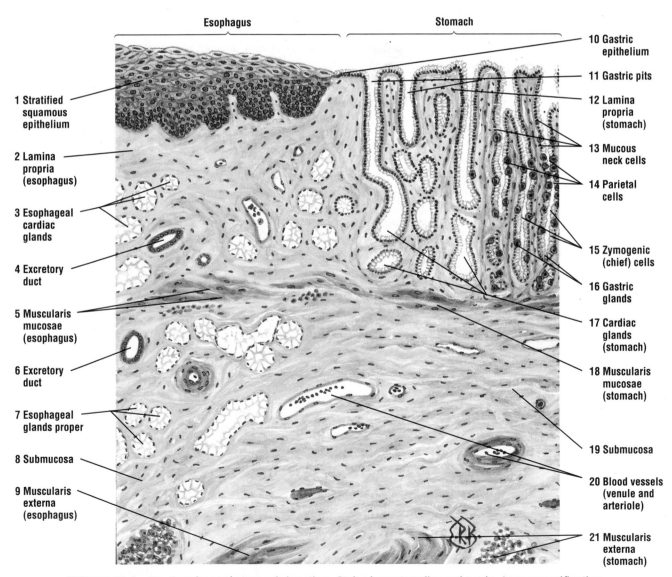

Esophagus   Stomach

1 Stratified
  squamous
  epithelium

2 Lamina
  propria
  (esophagus)

3 Esophageal
  cardiac
  glands

4 Excretory
  duct

5 Muscularis
  mucosae
  (esophagus)

6 Excretory
  duct

7 Esophageal
  glands proper

8 Submucosa

9 Muscularis
  externa
  (esophagus)

10 Gastric
   epithelium

11 Gastric pits

12 Lamina
   propria
   (stomach)

13 Mucous
   neck cells

14 Parietal
   cells

15 Zymogenic
   (chief) cells

16 Gastric
   glands

17 Cardiac
   glands
   (stomach)

18 Muscularis
   mucosae
   (stomach)

19 Submucosa

20 Blood vessels
   (venule and
   arteriole)

21 Muscularis
   externa
   (stomach)

FIGURE 12.6 ■ Esophageal-stomach junction. Stain: hematoxylin and eosin. Low magnification.

FIGURE 12.7 ■ Esophageal-Stomach Junction

A low-magnification photomicrograph illustrates the esophageal-stomach junction. The esophagus is characterized by a thick, protective, nonkeratinized **stratified squamous epithelium (1)**. Inferior to the epithelium (1) is the **lamina propria (2)**, below which is the smooth muscle **muscularis mucosae (3)**. The lamina propria (2) indents the undersurface of the esophageal epithelium to form the connective tissue papillae. The esophageal-stomach junction is characterized by an abrupt transition from the stratified epithelium (1) of the esophagus to the **simple columnar epithelium (4)** of the stomach. The surface of the stomach also exhibits numerous **gastric pits (5)**, into which the **gastric glands (6)** open. The **lamina propria (7)** of the stomach, in contrast to that of the esophagus, is seen as thin strips of connective tissue between the tightly packed gastric glands (6).

FIGURE 12.8 ■ Stomach: Fundus and Body Regions (Transverse Section)

The three histologic regions of the stomach are the cardia, the fundus and body, and the pylorus. The fundus and body constitute the most extensive region in the stomach. The stomach wall exhibits four general regions: the **mucosa (1, 2, 3)**, the **submucosa (4)**, the **muscularis externa (5, 6, 7)**, and the **serosa (8)**.

The mucosa consists of the **surface epithelium (1)**, **lamina propria (2)**, and **muscularis mucosae (3)**. The surface of the stomach is lined by simple columnar **epithelium (1, 11)** that extends into and lines the **gastric pits (10)**, which are tubular infoldings of the surface epithelium (11). In the fundus, the gastric pits (10) are not deep, and they extend into the mucosa about one-fourth of its thickness. Beneath the epithelium is the loose connective tissue **lamina propria (2, 12)** that fills the spaces between the gastric glands. A thin, smooth muscle **muscularis mucosae (3, 15)**, consisting of an inner circular and an outer longitudinal layers, forms the outer boudary of the mucosa. Thin strands of smooth muscle from the muscularis mucosae (3, 15) extend into the lamina propria (2, 12) between the **gastric glands (13, 14)** and toward the surface epithelium (1, 11); these smooth muscle strands are illustrated at higher magnification in Figure 12-9 (label 8).

The gastric glands (13, 14) are packed in the lamina propria (2, 12) and occupy the entire mucosa (1, 2, 3). The gastric glands open into the bottom of the gastric pits (10). The surface epithelium of the gastric mucosa, from the cardiac to the pyloric region, consists of the same cell type. The cells that comprise the gastric glands, however, distinguish the regional differences of the stomach. Two distinct cell types can be identified in the gastric glands. The acidophilic **parietal cells (13)** are located in the upper portions of the glands, whereas the basophilic **chief** (zymogenic) **cells (14)** occupy the lower regions. The subglandular regions of the lamina propria (2, 12) may contain either lymphatic tissue or small **lympha nodules (16)**.

The mucosa of the empty stomach exhibits temporary folds, called **rugae (9)**. Rugae (9) are formed during the contractions of the smooth muscle layer, the muscularis mucosae (3, 15). As the stomach fills, the rugae disappear and form a smooth mucosa.

The submucosa (4) lies below the muscularis mucosae (3, 15). In the empty stomach, submucosa (4) can extend into the rugae (9). The submucosa (4) contains denser irregular connective tissue and more **collagen fibers (17)** than the lamina propria (2, 12). In addition, the submucosa (4) contains lymph vessels, **capillaries (22)**, large **arterioles (18)**, and **venules (19)**. Isolated or clusters of parasympathetic ganglia of the **submucosal (Meissner's) nerve plexus (21)** can be seen deeper in the submucosa.

The muscularis externa (5, 6, 7) consists of three layers of smooth muscle, each of which is oriented in a different plane: an inner **oblique muscle layer (5)**, a middle **circular muscle layer (6)**, and an outer **longitudinal muscle layer (7)**. The oblique layer is not complete, and it is not always seen in sections of the stomach wall. In this illustration, the circular layer has been sectioned longitudinally, and the longitudinal layer has been sectioned transversely. Located between the circular and longitudinal smooth muscle layers is a **myenteric (Auerbach's) nerve plexus (23)** of parasympathetic ganglia and nerve fibers.

The serosa (8) consists of a thin, outer layer of connective tissue that overlies the muscularis externa (5, 6, 7) and is covered by a simple squamous mesothelium of the **visceral peritoneum (8)**. The serosa can contain **adipose cells (24)**.

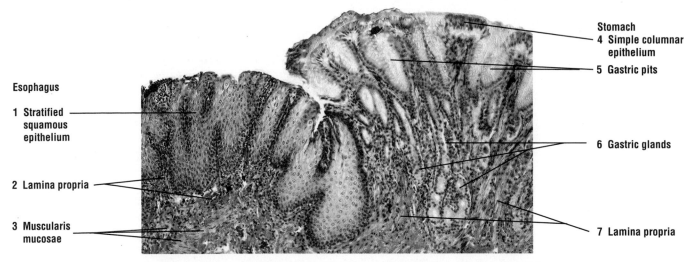

Esophagus

1 Stratified squamous epithelium

2 Lamina propria

3 Muscularis mucosae

Stomach
4 Simple columnar epithelium

5 Gastric pits

6 Gastric glands

7 Lamina propria

FIGURE 12.7 ■ Esophageal-stomach junction. Stain: mallory-azan. 30×

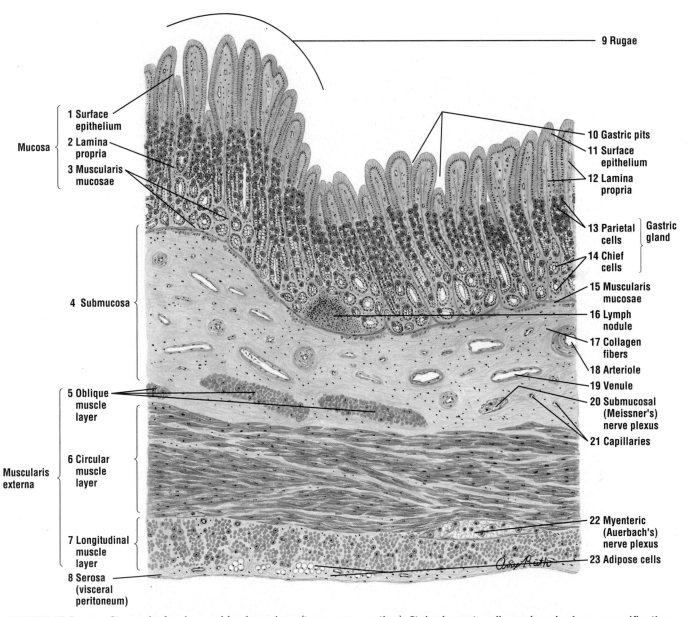

Mucosa

1 Surface epithelium

2 Lamina propria

3 Muscularis mucosae

4 Submucosa

Muscularis externa

5 Oblique muscle layer

6 Circular muscle layer

7 Longitudinal muscle layer

8 Serosa (visceral peritoneum)

9 Rugae

10 Gastric pits

11 Surface epithelium

12 Lamina propria

13 Parietal cells ⎤ Gastric
14 Chief cells ⎦ gland

15 Muscularis mucosae

16 Lymph nodule

17 Collagen fibers

18 Arteriole

19 Venule

20 Submucosal (Meissner's) nerve plexus

21 Capillaries

22 Myenteric (Auerbach's) nerve plexus

23 Adipose cells

FIGURE 12.8 ■ Stomach: fundus and body regions (transverse section). Stain: hematoxylin and eosin. Low magnification.

FIGURE 12.9 ■ Stomach: Mucosa of the Fundus and Body (Transverse Section)

The mucosa and submucosa of the fundic region of the stomach are illustrated at a higher magnification. The simple columnar **surface epithelium (1, 13)** extends into the **gastric pits (11),** into which the tubular **gastric glands (5)** open. The **lamina propria (6)** fills the spaces between the packed gastric glands (5) and extends from the surface epithelium (1) to the **muscularis mucosae (9).**

The lamina propria (6), which consists of fine reticular and collagen fibers, is better seen in the **mucosal ridges (2).** Scattered throughout the lamina propria (6) are the fibroblast nuclei, accumulations of lymphoid tissue in the form of a **lymphatic nodule (17),** lymphocytes, and other loose connective tissue cells.

The gastric glands (5) extend the length of the mucosa. In the deeper regions of the mucosa, the gastric glands may branch. As a result, the gastric glands appear as transverse and oblique sections. Each gastric gland consists of three regions. At the junction of the gastric pit with the gastric gland is the **isthmus (14),** which is lined by surface epithelial cells (1, 13) and **parietal cells (4).** Lower in the gland is the **neck (15),** which contains mainly **mucous neck cells (3)** and some parietal cells (4). The base, or **fundus (16),** is the deep portion of the gland, which is composed predominantly of **chief (zymogenic) cells (7)** and a few parietal cells (4). The fundic glands also contain undifferentiated cells and enteroendocrine cells (not illustrated) that secrete different hormones to regulate the digestive system.

Three types of cells can be identified in the fundic gastric glands. The mucous neck cells (3) are located just below the gastric pits (11) and are interspersed between the parietal cells (4) in the neck region of the glands. The parietal cells (4) stain uniformly acidophilic (pink), which distinguishes them from other cells in the fundic glands. In contrast, the chief (zymogenic) cells (7) are basophilic and, thus, are distinguishable from the acidophilic parietal cells (4).

The muscularis mucosae (9) in the stomach is composed of two thin strips of smooth muscle, the **inner circular layer (9a)** and **outer longitudinal layer (9b).** In this illustration, the inner circular layer (9a) is sectioned longitudinally, and the outer layer (9b) is sectioned transversely. Extending upward from the muscularis mucosae (9b) to the surface epithelium (1, 13) are **smooth muscle strands (8, 12).**

Below the muscularis mucosae (9) is the **submucosa (10)** with denser connective tissue. **Collagen fibers (18)** and the nuclei of **fibroblasts (19)** are seen in the submucosa (10). The submucosa (10) also contains **arterioles (20), venules (21),** lymphatics, capillaries, and adipose tissue.

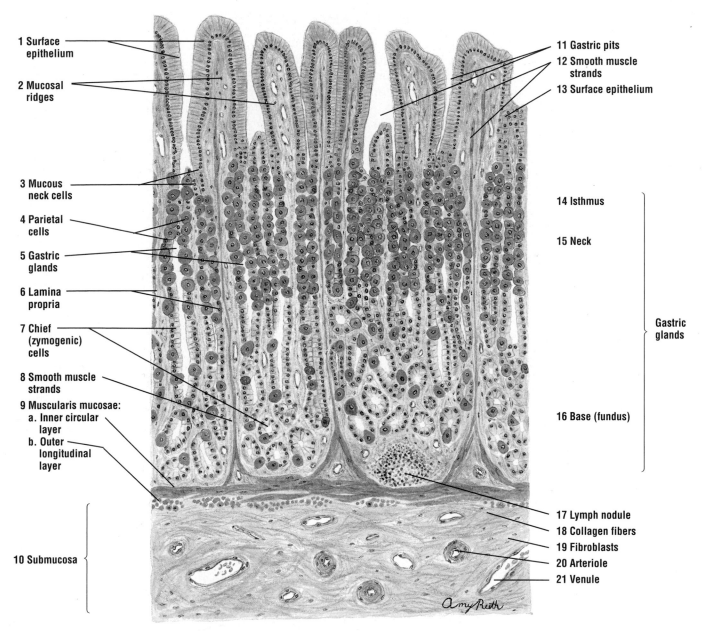

1 Surface epithelium

2 Mucosal ridges

3 Mucous neck cells

4 Parietal cells

5 Gastric glands

6 Lamina propria

7 Chief (zymogenic) cells

8 Smooth muscle strands

9 Muscularis mucosae:
   a. Inner circular layer
   b. Outer longitudinal layer

10 Submucosa

11 Gastric pits

12 Smooth muscle strands

13 Surface epithelium

14 Isthmus

15 Neck

16 Base (fundus)

17 Lymph nodule

18 Collagen fibers

19 Fibroblasts

20 Arteriole

21 Venule

Gastric glands

FIGURE 12.9 ■ Stomach: mucosa of the fundus and body (transverse section). Stain: hematoxylin and eosin. Medium magnification.

FIGURE 12.10 ■ Stomach: Fundus and Body Regions (Plastic Section)

This low-magnification photomicrograph illustrates the mucosa of the stomach wall. The fundus and body regions of the stomach have identical histologies. The stomach surface is lined by mucus-secreting **simple columnar epithelium (1)** that extends down into the **gastric pits (2).** In the fundus and body, the gastric pits (2) are shallow. Draining into the gastric pits (2) are the **gastric glands (5),** with different cell types. The cells of the gastric glands (5) are packed, and their lumina are not clearly visible. The large, pale-staining cells in the gastric glands (5) are the acid-secreting **parietal cells (3),** which are more numerous in the upper regions of the gastric glands (5). The darker-staining cells are the **chief (zymogenic) cells (6),** which are mostly located in the basal regions of the gastric glands (5). Between the gastric glands (5) are strips of the connective tissue **lamina propria (7).** A thin strip of the smooth muscle, the **muscularis mucosae (8),** separates the mucosa from the **submucosa (4)** of the stomach.

FUNCTIONAL CORRELATIONS

Gastric Glands and Cell Types

The **cardia** and **pylorus** are located at opposite ends of the stomach. The cardia surrounds the entrance of the esophagus into the stomach, and at the esophageal-stomach junction are the **cardiac glands.** The pylorus is the most inferior region of the stomach. It terminates at the border of the initial portion of the small intestine, called the **duodenum.** In the cardia, the **gastric pits** are shallow, whereas in the pylorus, the gastric pits are deep. Gastric glands in these two regions have similar histologies, however, and their cells are predominantly **mucus-secreting.**

In contrast, the gastric glands in the fundus and body of the stomach contain three major cell types. Located in the upper region of the gastric glands, near the gastric pits, are the **mucous neck cells.** The **parietal cells** are large, polygonal cells with a distinctive eosinophilic cytoplasm. They are located primarily in the upper half of the gastric glands and are squeezed between other gastric gland cells. Located predominantly in the lower region of the gastric glands are the basophilic-staining, cuboidal **chief (zymogenic) cells.**

In addition to the cells in the gastric glands, the mucosa of the digestive tract also contains a wide distribution of **enteroendocrine,** or gastrointestinal endocrine, **cells.** These cells are widely distributed in different digestive organs and are located both among and between existing exocrine cells. Unless histologic sections of digestive organs are prepared with special stains, these cells are poorly seen.

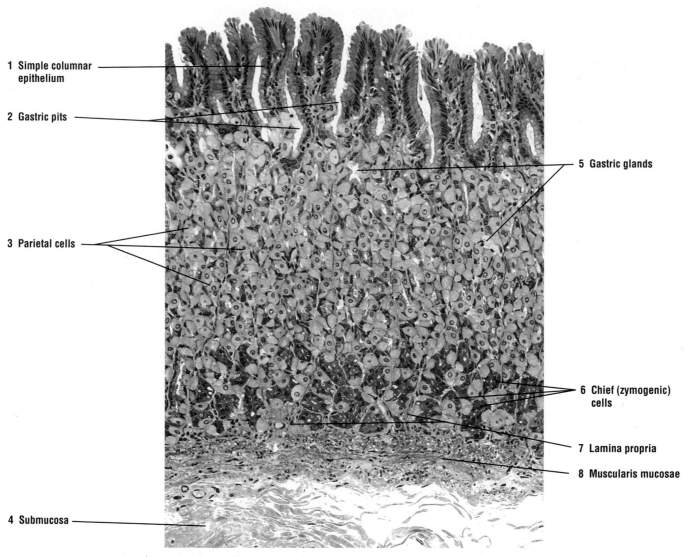

1 Simple columnar
  epithelium

2 Gastric pits

3 Parietal cells

4 Submucosa

5 Gastric glands

6 Chief (zymogenic)
  cells

7 Lamina propria

8 Muscularis mucosae

FIGURE 12.10 ■ Stomach: fundus and body regions (plastic section). Stain: hematoxylin and eosin. 50×

FIGURE 12.11 ■ Stomach: Superficial Region of the Gastric (Fundic) Mucosa

Higher magnification of the superficial region of the stomach shows the cells that comprise the mucosa of the fundus and body.

The columnar **surface epithelium** (1) exhibits basal, oval nuclei and a lightly stained cytoplasm because of the presence of mucigen droplets. The surface epithelium (1) is separated from the **lamina propria (3, 7, 8)** by a thin **basement membrane (2).** The lamina propria (3, 7, 8) is vascular and contains **blood vessels (9).** The surface epithelium (1) also extends downward into the **gastric pits (4).**

The **gastric glands (5)** lie in the lamina propria (3, 7, 8) below the gastric pits (4). The **neck region** of the gastric glands (5) is lined with **mucous neck cells (10)** that have round, basal nuclei. The constricted necks of the gastric glands (5) open through a short transition region into the bottom of the gastric pits (4).

The **parietal cells (6, 11)** are large cells with a pyramidal shape, round nuclei, and highly acidophilic cytoplasm, and they are interspersed among the mucous neck cells (10). Some pyramidal cells (6, 11) may be binucleate (two nuclei). The free surfaces of parietal cells (6, 11) open into the lumen of the gastric glands (5). The parietal cells (6, 11) are the most conspicuous cells in the gastric mucosa, and they are found predominantly in the upper third to upper half of the gastric glands (5).

Deeper in the lower half of the gastric glands (5) are found the basophilic **chief (zymogenic) cells (12),** which also border on the lumen of the gland. Parietal cells (6, 11) are also seen here.

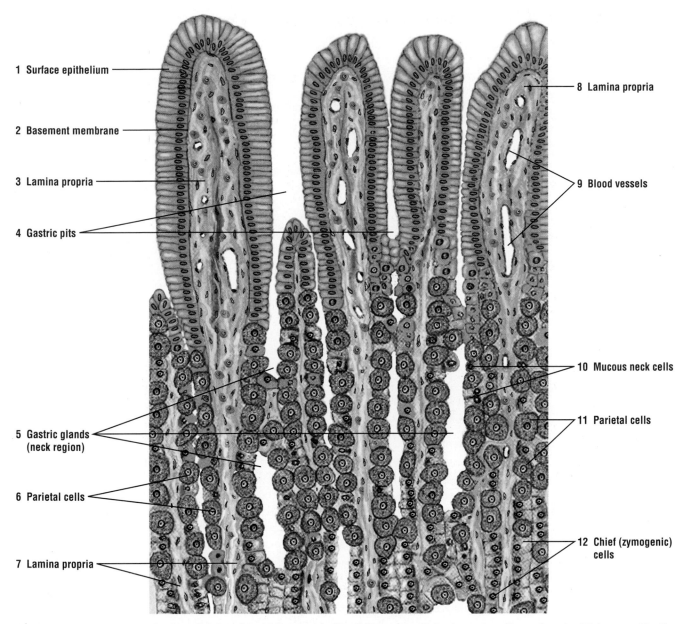

1 Surface epithelium

2 Basement membrane

3 Lamina propria

4 Gastric pits

5 Gastric glands
   (neck region)

6 Parietal cells

7 Lamina propria

8 Lamina propria

9 Blood vessels

10 Mucous neck cells

11 Parietal cells

12 Chief (zymogenic)
   cells

FIGURE 12.11   ■   Stomach: superficial region of the gastric (fundic) mucosa. Stain: hematoxylin and eosin. High magnification.

FIGURE 12.12 ■ Stomach: Basal Region of the Gastric (Fundic) Mucosa

The **gastric glands (1, 9)** in the body and fundus of the stomach show **basal branching (9).** In the upper regions of the gastric glands, the **chief (zymogenic) cells (6, 10)** border the lumen of the gastric glands (1, 9). In the basal region of the gastric mucosa, the **parietal cells (2)** are wedged against the basement membrane and are not always in direct contact with the lumen.

The connective tissue **lamina propria (3, 7)** surrounds the gastric glands (1). A small **lymphatic nodule (4)** is located in the lamina propria (3) adjacent to the the gastric glands (1, 9). The two layers of the **muscularis mucosae (5),** the inner circular layer and the outer longitudinal layer, are seen below the gastric glands (1, 9). **Smooth muscle strands (8)** extend upward from the muscularis mucosae (5) into the lamina propria (3, 7) between the gastric glands (1, 9).

Adjacent to the muscularis mucosae (5) is the connective tissue **submucosa (11).**

FUNCTIONAL CORRELATIONS

Stomach

The stomach performs numerous functions. It **receives, stores, mixes,** and **digests** ingested food products, and it secretes different hormones that regulate digestive functions. Some functions are **mechanical** and **chemical** and are specifically designed to reduce the mass of ingested food material, or **bolus,** to a semiliquid mass, called **chyme.** The mechanical reduction of the bolus is performed by strong, muscular peristaltic contractions of the stomach wall when the food enters the stomach. With the pylorus closed, the muscular contractions churn and mix the stomach contents with **gastric juices** that are produced by the **gastric glands. Neurons** and **axons** in the **submucosal nerve plexus** and **myenteric nerve plexus** of the stomach wall regulate the peristaltic activity. The stomach also performs some absorptive functions; however, these functions are primarily limited to the absorption of water, alcohol, salts, and certain drugs.

Gastric Gland Cells in the Body and Fundus of the Stomach

Chemical reduction of food in the stomach is the main function of the gastric secretions that are produced by the different cells in the gastric glands, especially those cells located in the fundus and body regions of the stomach. The main components of the gastric secretions are **pepsin, hydrochloric acid, mucus, intrinsic factor, water, lysozyme,** and different **electrolytes.**

Luminal cells line the stomach and secrete thick layers of **mucus,** the main function of which is to cover, lubricate, and protect the stomach surface from the corrosive actions of chemicals secreted by different cells in the gastric glands.

Parietal cells are located in the upper regions of the gastric glands. They secrete the major component of gastric juice, **hydrochloric acid.** In humans, parietal cells also produce **gastric intrinsic factor,** a glycoprotein that is necessary for the absorption of **vitamin B_{12}** from the small intestine. Vitamin B_{12} is necessary for **erythrocyte** (red blood cell) production (**erythropoiesis**) in the red bone marrow. Deficiency of this vitamin leads to the development of **pernicious anemia,** a disorder of erythrocyte formation.

Chief (zymogenic) cells are filled with secretory granules that contain the proenzyme **pepsinogen,** which is an inactive precursor of **pepsin.** Release of pepsinogen during gastric secretion into the acidic environment of the stomach converts the inactive pepsinogen into the highly active, proteolytic enzyme pepsin.

Enteroendocrine cells secrete a variety of **polypeptides** and **proteins** with hormonal activity that influence different functions of the digestive tract. They are called enteroendocrine cells because they produce gastric hormones and are located in the digestive organs. The enteroendocrine cells are also called **APUD cells** because they can take up the precursors of amines and decarboxylate them. These cells are not confined to the gastrointestinal tract; they are also found in the respiratory and other organs of the body, where they are also known by different names. Additional details, description, and illustration of known enteroendocrine (APUD) cells are found in Chapter 13.

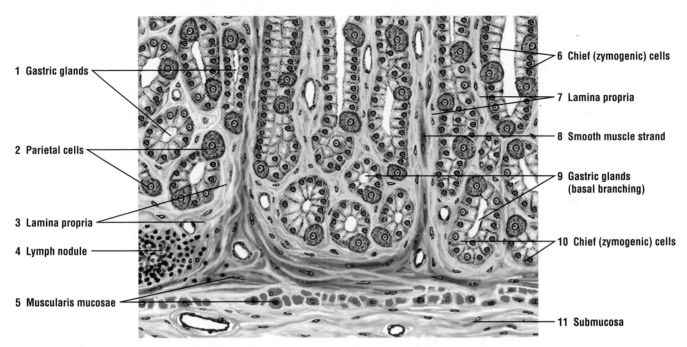

1 Gastric glands

2 Parietal cells

3 Lamina propria

4 Lymph nodule

5 Muscularis mucosae

6 Chief (zymogenic) cells

7 Lamina propria

8 Smooth muscle strand

9 Gastric glands (basal branching)

10 Chief (zymogenic) cells

11 Submucosa

FIGURE 12.12 ■ Stomach: basal region of the gastric (fundic) mucosa. Stain: hematoxylin and eosin. High magnification.

FIGURE 12.13 ■ Stomach: Mucosa of the Pyloric Region

In the pyloric region of the stomach, the **gastric pits (4, 12)** are deeper than those in the body or fundic regions. The gastric pits (4, 12) extend into the mucosa to about half or more of its thickness. The simple **columnar mucous epithelium (10)** that lines the surface of the stomach also extends into and lines the gastric pits (4, 12).

The **pyloric glands (5, 6, 14)** are either branched or coiled, tubular mucous glands. Similar to the cardia region of the stomach, only one type of cell is found in the epithelium of these glands. This tall columnar cell with a granular cytoplasm stains lightly because of its mucigen content, and it has a flattened or oval nucleus at its base. The pyloric glands (5, 6, 14) open into the bottom of the gastric pits (4, lower leader). Enteroendocrine cells are also present in this region and can be demonstrated using a special stain.

The remaining structures in this region of the stomach are similar to those in other regions. The **lamina propria (13)** contains diffuse lymphatic tissue and an occasional **lymphatic nodule (16)** adjacent to a **capillary (17)**. The lymphatic nodule (16) may increase in size and penetrate the **muscularis mucosae (18)** and reach the **submucosa (20),** in which are found blood vessels, such as **arterioles (8)** and **venules (9, 19),** of different size. Smooth **muscle fibers (7, 15)** from the circular layer of the **muscularis mucosae (18)** pass upward into the lamina propria (13) between the pyloric glands (6) and into the **mucosal ridges (3).**

FUNCTIONAL CORRELATIONS

Cells in Pyloric Gastric Glands

Pyloric glands contain the same cell types as those found in cardiac glands of the stomach. Mucus-secreting cells predominate in these glands. In addition to producing **mucus,** these cells also secrete an enzyme, called **lysozyme,** that destroys bacteria in the stomach.

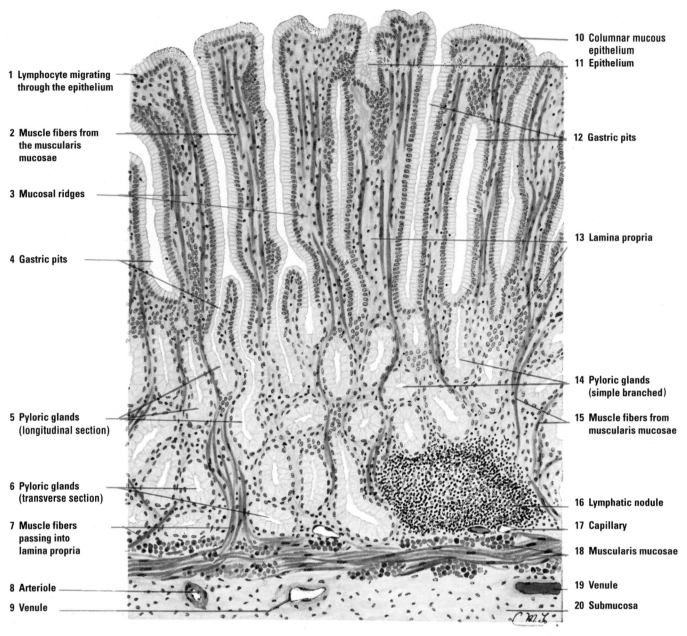

1 Lymphocyte migrating through the epithelium

2 Muscle fibers from the muscularis mucosae

3 Mucosal ridges

4 Gastric pits

5 Pyloric glands (longitudinal section)

6 Pyloric glands (transverse section)

7 Muscle fibers passing into lamina propria

8 Arteriole

9 Venule

10 Columnar mucous epithelium

11 Epithelium

12 Gastric pits

13 Lamina propria

14 Pyloric glands (simple branched)

15 Muscle fibers from muscularis mucosae

16 Lymphatic nodule

17 Capillary

18 Muscularis mucosae

19 Venule

20 Submucosa

FIGURE 12.13 ■ Stomach: mucosa of the pyloric region. Stain: hematoxylin and eosin. Medium magnification.

FIGURE 12.14 ■ Pyloric-Duodenal Junction

The **pylorus (1)** of the stomach is separated from the **duodenum (11)** of the small intestine by a thick, smooth muscle layer, called the **pyloric sphincter (8),** that is formed by the thickened circular layer of the **muscularis externa** of the **stomach (9).**

At the junction with the duodenum, the **mucosal ridges (4)** of the stomach around the **gastric pits (3)** become broader, more irregular, and their shape more variable. Coiled tubular **pyloric (mucous) glands (6),** located in the **lamina propria (5),** open at the bottom of the gastric pits (3). **Lymphatic nodules (16)** are seen between the pylorus (1) and the duodenum (11).

The mucus-secreting **stomach epithelium (2)** changes to **intestinal epithelium (12)** in the duodenum. The intestinal epithelium (12) consists of goblet cells and columnar cells with striated borders (microvilli) that are present throughout the length of the small intestine. The duodenum (11) contains **villi (13),** a specialized surface modification (singular, villus). Each villus (13) is a leaf-shaped surface projection. Between individual villi are the **intervillous spaces (14)** of the intestinal lumen.

Short, simple, tubular **intestinal glands** (crypts of Lieberkühn) **(15)** are present in the lamina propria of the duodenum (11). These glands consist primarily of goblet cells and cells with striated borders (microvilli) of the surface epithelium.

Duodenal (Brunner's) **glands (18)** occupy most of the **submucosa (19)** in the upper duodenum (11), and they are the characteristic features of the duodenum. The ducts of the duodenal glands (18) penetrate the **muscularis mucosae (17)** of the duodenum and enter the base of the intestinal glands (15), disrupting the muscularis mucosae (17) in this region. Except for the esophageal (submucosal) glands proper, the duodenal glands (18) are the only submucosal glands in the digestive tract. In the **muscularis externa** of the **stomach (9)** and of the **duodenum (20)** are neurons and axons of the **myenteric nerve plexus (10, 21).**

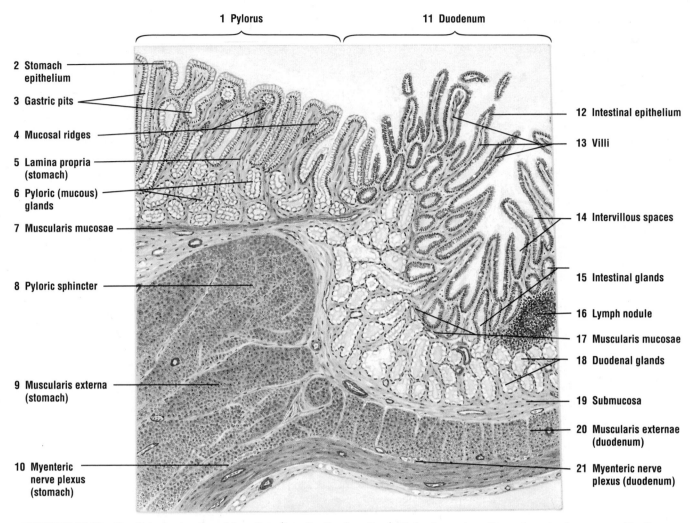

1 Pylorus

11 Duodenum

2 Stomach epithelium

3 Gastric pits

4 Mucosal ridges

5 Lamina propria (stomach)

6 Pyloric (mucous) glands

7 Muscularis mucosae

8 Pyloric sphincter

9 Muscularis externa (stomach)

10 Myenteric nerve plexus (stomach)

12 Intestinal epithelium

13 Villi

14 Intervillous spaces

15 Intestinal glands

16 Lymph nodule

17 Muscularis mucosae

18 Duodenal glands

19 Submucosa

20 Muscularis externae (duodenum)

21 Myenteric nerve plexus (duodenum)

FIGURE 12.14 ■ Pyloric-duodenal junction (longitudinal section). Stain: hematoxylin and eosin. Low magnification.

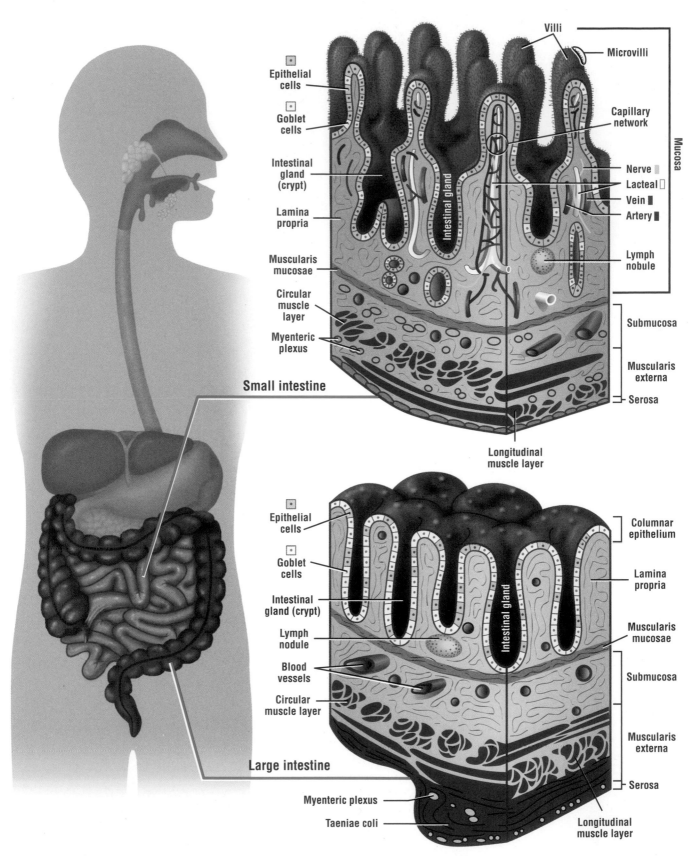

Villi

Microvilli

Epithelial cells

Goblet cells

Capillary network

Mucosa

Intestinal gland (crypt)

Intestinal gland

Nerve ▦

Lacteal ▢

Vein ▪

Artery ▪

Lamina propria

Muscularis mucosae

Lymph nobule

Circular muscle layer

Submucosa

Myenteric plexus

Small intestine

Muscularis externa

Serosa

Longitudinal muscle layer

Epithelial cells

Goblet cells

Columnar epithelium

Intestinal gland

Lamina propria

Intestinal gland (crypt)

Lymph nodule

Muscularis mucosae

Blood vessels

Submucosa

Circular muscle layer

Muscularis externa

Large intestine

Serosa

Myenteric plexus

Taeniae coli

Longitudinal muscle layer

OVERVIEW FIGURE ■ Structural differences between the wall of the small intestine and large intestine, with emphasis on different layers of the wall.

CHAPTER 13

Digestive System: Small and Large Intestines

Small Intestine

The **small intestine** is a long, convoluted tube approximately 5 to 7 m in length; it is the longest section of the digestive tract. The small intestine extends from the junction with the stomach to join with the **large intestine,** or **colon.** For descriptive purposes, the small intestine is divided into three parts: the duodenum, the jejunum, and the ileum. Although the microscopic differences among these three segments are minor, they allow identification of the individual segments.

The main function of the small intestine is the digestion of gastric contents and the absorption of nutrients into blood capillaries and/or lymphatic lacteals.

Surface Modifications for Absorption

The mucosa of the small intestine exhibits specialized structural modifications that increase the cellular surface area for the absorption of nutrients and fluids. These modifications include the plicae circulares, villi, and microvilli.

In contrast to the rugae of the stomach, the **plicae circulares** are permanent, spiral folds or elevations of the mucosa (with a submucosal core) that extend into the intestinal lumen. The plicae circulares are most prominent in the proximal portion of the small intestine, where most absorption takes place; they decrease in prominence toward the ileum.

Villi are permanent, finger-like projections of the **lamina propria** of the mucosa that extend into the intestinal lumen. They are covered by **simple columnar epithelium** and are also more prominent in the proximal portion of the small intestine. The height of the villi decreases toward the ileum. The connective tissue core of each villus contains a lymphatic capillary, called a **lacteal,** as well as blood capillaries and individual strands of smooth muscles (see overview figure).

Microvilli are cytoplasmic extensions that cover the apices of the intestinal absorptive cells. They are visible under a light microscope as a **striated (brush) border.**

Cells, Glands, and Lymphatic Nodules

The epithelium that lines the stomach surface contains only one cell type (mucus-secreting). In contrast, the surface of the small intestine contains numerous cell types.

Columnar absorptive cells are the most common cell types in the intestinal epithelium. These cells are tall columnar, with a prominent striated (brush) border or **microvilli.** A thick **glycocalyx** coat covers and protects the microvilli from the corrosive chemicals.

Goblet cells are interspersed among the columnar absorptive cells of the intestinal epithelium. They increase in number toward the distal region of the small intestine (ileum).

Enteroendocrine or **APUD** (amine precursor uptake and decarboxylation) cells are scattered throughout the epithelium of the villi and intestinal glands.

Intestinal glands (crypts of Lieberkühn) are located throughout the small intestinal mucosa. These glands open into the intestinal lumen at the base of the villi. The surface epithelium of the villi also extends into and lines the intestinal glands.

Duodenal (Brunner's) glands are primarily found in the submucosa of the initial portion of the duodenum, and they are highly characteristic of this region of the small intestine. These are branched, tubuloacinar glands, with light-staining mucous cells. The ducts of the duodenal glands penetrate the muscularis mucosae to discharge their secretory product at the base of intestinal glands.

Undifferentiated cells exhibit mitotic activity and are located in the base of intestinal glands. They function as stem cells and replace worn-out columnar absorptive cells, goblet cells, and intestinal gland cells.

Paneth cells are located at the base of intestinal glands. They are characterized by the presence of deep-staining eosinophilic granules in their cytoplasm.

Peyer's patches are numerous aggregations of closely packed, permanent **lymphatic nodules.** They are found primarily in the wall of the terminal portion of small intestine (ileum). These nodules occupy a large portion of the lamina propria and submucosa of the ileum.

M cells are highly specialized epithelial cells that cover the Peyer's patches and large lymphatic nodules; they are not found anywhere else in the intestine. M cells phagocytose luminal antigens and present them to the lymphocytes and macrophages in the lamina propria.

Regional Differences

The **duodenum** is the shortest segment of the small intestine. The villi in this region are broad, tall, and numerous, with fewer goblet cells in the epithelium. Duodenal (Brunner's) glands with mucus-secreting cells in the submucosa characterize this region.

The **jejunum** exhibits fewer villi than the duodenum, and the villi here are both shorter and narrower. More goblet cells are also found in the epithelium.

The **ileum** contains few villi, and these villi are narrower and shorter than those in jejunum. In addition, the epithelium contains more goblet cells than the duodenum or jejunum. The lymphatic nodules are particularly large and numerous in the ileum, where they aggregate in the lamina propria and submucosa to form the prominent Peyer's patches.

Large Intestine (Colon)

The large intestine is situated between the anus and the terminal end of the ileum. It is shorter and less convoluted than the small intestine. It is composed of an initial segment, called the **cecum;** the ascending, transverse, descending, and sigmoid colon; and the rectum and anus.

Chyme enters the large intestine from the ileum through the ileocecal valve. Unabsorbed and undigested food residues from the small intestine are forced into the large intestine by the strong peristaltic actions of smooth muscles in the muscularis externa. The residues that enter the large intestine are in a semifluid state; however, by the time they reach the terminal portion of the large intestine, these residues become semisolid **feces.**

Histologic Differences between the Small and Large Intestine (Colon)

The large intestine lacks the plicae circulares and villi of the small intestine. Intestinal glands are also present in the large intestine and are similar to those in the small intestine. Glands of the large intestine, however, are deeper (longer) and lack the Paneth cells in their bases. The epithelium of the large intestine also contains different enteroendocrine cells.

Although present in the small intestine, goblet cells are more numerous in the large intestinal epithelium. Also, the number of goblet cells increases from the cecum toward the terminal portion of the sigmoid colon. The lamina propria of the large intestine contains many solitary lymphatic nodules, lymphocyte accumulations, plasma cells, and macrophages.

The muscularis externa of the large intestine and cecum shows a unique arrangement. The inner circular smooth muscle layer is present. The outer longitudinal muscle layer, however, does not surround the large intestine. Instead, this layer is arranged into three longitudinal muscle strips, called **taeniae coli.** The contractions or tonus in the taeniae coli form sacculations in the large intestine, called **haustras** (see overview figure).

FIGURE 13.1 ■ Small Intestine: Duodenum (Longitudinal Section)

The wall of the duodenum consists of four layers: the mucosa, with the **lining epithelium (7a),** **lamina propria (7b),** and **muscularis mucosae (9, 12);** the underlying connective tissue **submucosa (13),** with the mucous **duodenal** (Brunner's) **glands (3, 13);** the two smooth muscle layers of the **muscularis externa (14);** and the visceral peritoneum, or **serosa (15).** These layers are continuous with those of the stomach, small intestine, and large intestine (colon).

The small intestine is characterized by finger-like extensions, called **villi (7)** (singular, villus); a lining epithelium (7a) of columnar cells lined with microvilli that form the striated borders; light-staining **goblet cells (2);** and short, tubular **intestinal glands** (crypts of Lieberkühn) **(4, 8)** in the lamina propria (7b). Duodenal glands (3, 13) in the submucosa (13) characterize the duodenum. These glands are absent in the rest of the small intestine (jejunum and ileum) and large intestine.

The villi (7) are mucosal surface modifications. Between the villi (7) are the **intervillous spaces (1).** The lining epithelium (7a) covers each villus and the intestinal glands (4, 8). Each villus (7) contains a core of lamina propria (7b), strands of **smooth muscle fibers (10)** that extend upward into the villi from the **muscularis mucosae (9, 12),** and a central lymphatic vessel, called the **lacteal (11)** (see Fig. 13-7).

The intestinal glands (4, 8) are located in the lamina propria (7b) and open into the intervillous spaces (1). In certain sections of the duodenum, the submucosal duodenal glands (13) extend into the lamina propria (3). The lamina propria (7b) also contains fine connective tissue fibers with reticular cells, diffuse lymphatic tissue, and/or **lymphatic nodules (5).**

The submucosa (13) in the duodenum is almost completely filled with branched, tubular duodenal glands (13). The duodenal glands (13) disrupt the muscularis mucosae (9, 12) when they penetrate into the lamina propria (3). The secretions from the duodenal glands (3) enter at the bottom of the intestinal glands (4, 8).

In a cross-section of the duodenum, the muscularis externa (14) consists of an **inner circular (14a)** and an **outer longitudinal (14b)** layer of smooth muscle. In this figure, however, the duodenum has been cut in a longitudinal plane, and the direction of the fibers in these two smooth muscle layers is reversed. Parasympathetic ganglion cells of the **myenteric** (Auerbach's) **nerve plexus (6),** found in the small and large intestine, are visible in the connective tissue between the two muscle layers of the muscularis externa (14). Similar, but smaller, plexuses of ganglion cells are also found in the submucosa (not illustrated) in the small and large intestine.

The **serosa (15),** or visceral peritoneum, contains the connective tissue cells, blood vessels, and adipose cells. The serosa forms the outermost layer of the first part of the duodenum.

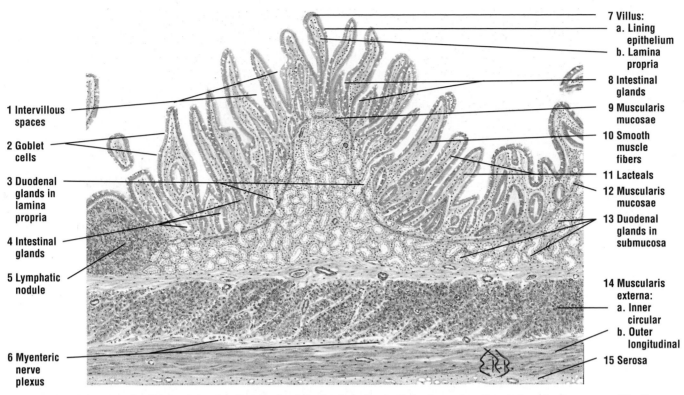

1 Intervillous spaces

2 Goblet cells

3 Duodenal glands in lamina propria

4 Intestinal glands

5 Lymphatic nodule

6 Myenteric nerve plexus

7 Villus:
a. Lining epithelium
b. Lamina propria

8 Intestinal glands

9 Muscularis mucosae

10 Smooth muscle fibers

11 Lacteals

12 Muscularis mucosae

13 Duodenal glands in submucosa

14 Muscularis externa:
a. Inner circular
b. Outer longitudinal

15 Serosa

FIGURE 13.1 ■ Small intestine: duodenum (longitudinal section). Stain: hematoxylin and eosin. Low magnification.

FIGURE 13.2 ■ Small Intestine: Duodenum (Transverse Section)

A low-magnification photomicrograph illustrates a transverse section of the duodenum. The luminal surface of the duodenum exhibits **villi (2)** that are covered by **simple columnar epithelium (1),** with a brush border. The core of each villus (2) contains **lamina propria (4, 6),** in which are found connective tissue cells, lymphoid cells, plasma cells, macrophages, smooth muscle cells, and others. In addition, the lamina propria (4, 6) contains blood vessels and the dilated, blind-ending lymphatic channels, called **lacteals (3).** Between the villi (2) are the **intestinal glands (7)** that extend to the **muscularis mucosae (8).** Inferior to the muscularis mucosae (8) is the dense irregular connective tissue of the **submucosa (9).** In the duodenum, the submucosa (9) is filled with light-staining, mucus-secreting **duodenal glands (5),** the ducts of which pierce the muscularis mucosae (8) to deliver their secretory product at the base of the intestinal glands (7). Surrounding the submucosa (9) and the duodenal glands (5) is the **muscularis externa (10).**

FUNCTIONAL CORRELATIONS

Duodenum

A characteristic feature of the duodenum is the branched, tubuloacinar **duodenal (Brunner's) glands** in the submucosa. Their excretory ducts penetrate the muscularis mucosae to deliver their secretions at the base of the intestinal glands. Duodenal glands secrete or release their product into the lumen in response to the entrance of acidic chyme from the stomach and to parasympathetic stimulation by the vagus nerve.

The main function of the duodenal glands is to protect the duodenal mucosa from the highly corrosive action of the gastric contents. Also, alkaline **mucus** and **bicarbonate ions** in the duodenal gland secretions buffer or neutralize the acidic chyme, which provides a more favorable environment for digestive enzymes that enter the duodenum from the pancreas.

Duodenal glands also produce a polypeptide hormone, called **urogastrone.** This hormone inhibits secretion of hydrochloric acid by the parietal cells in the stomach and increases epithelial proliferation in the small intestine.

FIGURE 13.3 ■ Small Intestine: Jejunum and Ileum (Transverse Section)

The histologies of the lower duodenum, jejunum, and ileum are similar to that of the upper duodenum (see Fig. 13-1). The only exceptions are the duodenal (Brunner's) glands, which usually are limited to the submucosa in the upper part of the duodenum and are not found in the jejunum and ileum.

This figure illustrates the **villi (2)** and a permanent fold of the small intestine, called the **plica circularis (10).** Both the mucosa and **submucosa (4, 16)** form the many plicae circulares (10).

In the lumen, each villus (2) exhibits a columnar **lining epithelium (1),** with a striated border and goblet cells; a core of **lamina propria (3),** with diffuse lymphatic tissue; and strands or strips of smooth muscle fibers that extend into the lamina propria (3) from the **muscularis mucosae (6).** Each villus also contains a central lacteal and capillaries (see Fig. 13-7).

The **intestinal glands** (crypts of Lieberkühn) **(5, 12)** are located in the lamina propria (3) and open into the **intervillous space (11).** A **lymphatic nodule (14)** extends from the lamina propria (3) of the mucosa into the submucosa (16), disrupting the **muscularis mucosae (13, 15)** that is adjacent to the intestinal glands (12).

In the small intestine, the **muscularis externa** contains an **inner circular smooth muscle (7)** layer and an **outer longitudinal smooth muscle (8)** layer. A visceral peritoneum, or **serosa (18),** surrounds the small intestine. Under the serosal lining are connective tissue fibers, blood vessels, and **adipose cells (9).**

Parasympathetic ganglion cells of the **myenteric plexus (17)** are present in the connective tissue between the muscle layers of the the muscularis externa. Similar submucosal plexus are pres-ent in the submucosa of the small intestine, but are not illustrated in this figure.

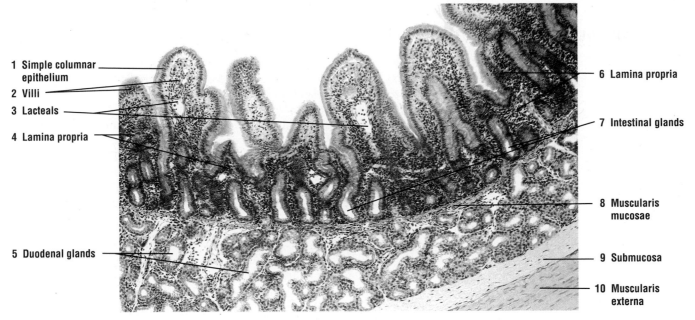

1 Simple columnar epithelium
2 Villi
3 Lacteals
4 Lamina propria
5 Duodenal glands
6 Lamina propria
7 Intestinal glands
8 Muscularis mucosae
9 Submucosa
10 Muscularis externa

FIGURE 13.2 ■ Small intestine: duodenum (transverse section). Stain: hematoxylin and eosin. 25×

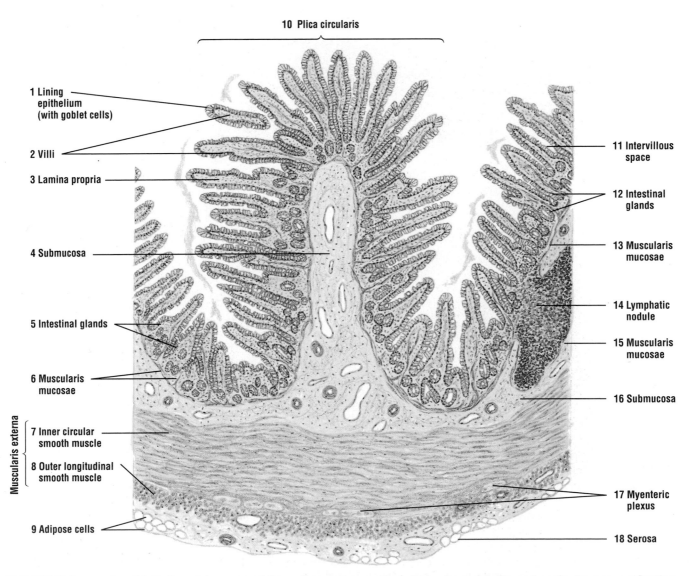

10 Plica circularis

1 Lining epithelium (with goblet cells)
2 Villi
3 Lamina propria
4 Submucosa
5 Intestinal glands
6 Muscularis mucosae
Muscularis externa
7 Inner circular smooth muscle
8 Outer longitudinal smooth muscle
9 Adipose cells

11 Intervillous space
12 Intestinal glands
13 Muscularis mucosae
14 Lymphatic nodule
15 Muscularis mucosae
16 Submucosa
17 Myenteric plexus
18 Serosa

FIGURE 13.3 ■ Small intestine: jejunum and ileum (transverse section). Stain: hematoxylin and eosin. Low magnification.

FIGURE 13.4 ■ Intestinal Glands with Paneth Cells and Enteroendocrine Cells

Adjacent to the **muscularis mucosae (5, 10)** are the **intestinal glands (7),** with **goblet cells (2)** and cells with striated borders. At the base of the intestinal glands (7) are pyramid-shaped cells with large, acidophilic granules that fill most of the cytoplasm and displace the nucleus toward the base of the cell. These are the **Paneth cells (4, 9),** which are found throughout the small intestine.

Enteroendocrine cells **(3, 8)** are interspersed among the intestinal gland (7) cells, the **mitotic cells (1, 6),** the goblet cells (2), and the Paneth cells (4, 9). Enteroendocrine cells (3, 8) contain fine granules in the basal cytoplasm. Most enteroendocrine cells (3, 8) take up and decarboxylate precursors of biogenic monoamines and, therefore, are designated as APUD (amine precursor uptake and decarboxylation) cells. The APUD cells are found in the epithelia of the gastrointestinal tract (stomach as well as small and large intestines), respiratory tract, pancreas, and thyroid glands.

FIGURE 13.5 ■ Small Intestine: Jejunum with Paneth Cells

A low-magnification photomicrograph illustrates the mucosa of the jejunum. The **villi (1)** are lined by **simple columnar epithelium (2),** with a brush border. Between the columnar cells are the mucus-filled **goblet cells (3).** In the **lamina propria (6)** of each villus are lymphoid cells, macrophages, smooth muscle cells, **blood vessels (7),** and lymphatic lacteals (not visible). Between the villi are the **intestinal glands (8),** the bases of which contain red-staining or eosinophilic secretory granules of **Paneth cells (9).** The intestinal glands (8) end near the **muscularis mucosae (4),** inferior to which is the **submucosa (5).**

FUNCTIONAL CORRELATIONS

Paneth Cells and Enteroendocrine Cells in the Small Intestine

Paneth cells, which are located in the bases of the intestinal glands, produce **lysozyme,** an antibacterial enzyme that digests bacterial cell walls and destroys bacteria. Paneth cells may also have some phagocytic functions. Thus, these cells have an important role in controlling the microbial flora of the small intestine.

Enteroendocrine cells in the small intestine secrete numerous **regulatory hormones,** including **gastric inhibitory peptide, secretin,** and **cholecystokinin (pancreozymin).** These intestinal hormones control the release of gastric and pancreatic secretions, induce intestinal motility, and stimulate contraction of the gallbladder to release bile.

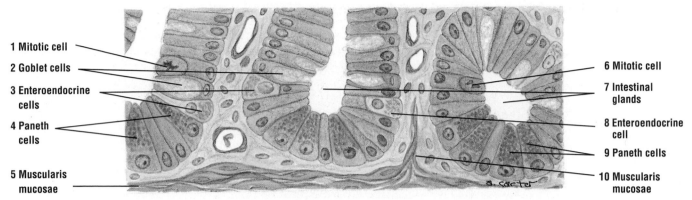

1 Mitotic cell
2 Goblet cells
3 Enteroendocrine cells
4 Paneth cells
5 Muscularis mucosae

6 Mitotic cell
7 Intestinal glands
8 Enteroendocrine cell
9 Paneth cells
10 Muscularis mucosae

FIGURE 13.4 ■ Intestinal glands with paneth cells and enteroendocrine cells. Stain: hematoxylin and eosin, plastic section. High magnification.

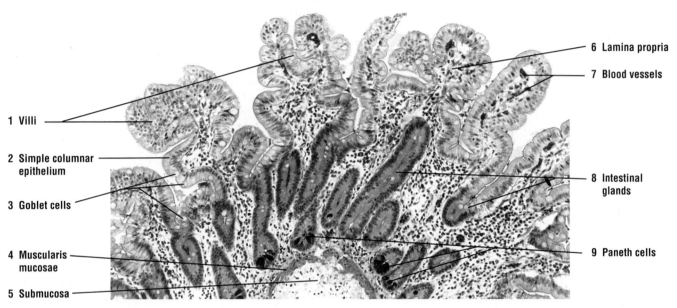

1 Villi
2 Simple columnar epithelium
3 Goblet cells
4 Muscularis mucosae
5 Submucosa

6 Lamina propria
7 Blood vessels
8 Intestinal glands
9 Paneth cells

FIGURE 13.5 ■ Small intestine: jejunum with paneth cells. Stain: mallory-azan. 40×

FIGURE 13.6 ◾ Small Intestine: Ileum with Lymphatic Nodules (Peyer's Patches) (Transverse Section)

A characteristic feature of the ileum is the aggregations of **lymphatic nodules (5, 12),** called **Peyer's patches (5, 12).** Each Peyer's patch is an aggregation of numerous lymphatic nodules that are located in the wall of the ileum, opposite the mesentery attachment. Most lymphatic nodules (5, 12) exhibit **germinal centers (5).** The lymphatic nodules (5, 12) usually coalesce, and the boundaries between them become indistinct.

The lymphatic nodules (5, 12) originate in the diffuse lymphatic tissue of the **lamina propria (10).** Villi are absent in the area of the intestinal lumen where the nodules reach the surface of the mucosa. Typically, the lymphatic nodules (5, 12) extend into the **submucosa (6),** disrupt the **muscularis mucosae (13),** and spread out in the loose connective tissue of the submucosa (6).

Also illustrated are the **surface epithelium (1)** that covers the **villi (2, 8)** as well as the **intestinal glands (4, 11), lacteals (3, 9)** in the villi, the **inner circular layer (14a)** and **outer longitudinal layer (14b)** of the **muscularis externa (14),** and the **serosa (visceral peritoneum) (7).**

FIGURE 13.7 ◾ Small Intestine: Villi

Several **villi (1)** are sectioned longitudinally and transversely and are illustrated at a higher magnification. The simple columnar **surface epithelium (2)** that covers the villi (1) contains mucus-secreting **goblet cells (7)** and absorptive cells with **striated borders (microvilli) (3).** To show mucus, this section was stained for carbohydrates. As a result, the goblet cells (7) are stained magenta red.

A thin **basement membrane (8)** is visible between the surface epithelium (2) and the **lamina propria (4).** In the core of the lamina propria (4) are connective tissue cells and collagen fibers, blood cells, and **smooth muscle fibers (5).** Also in each villus (but not always seen in sections) is a **central lacteal (6),** which is a lymphatic vessel lined with endothelium. Arterioles, one or more venules, and **capillaries (9)** are also visible in the villi.

FUNCTIONAL CORRELATIONS

Peyer's Patches in the Ileum

Overlying the large lymphoid nodules of Peyer's patches are specialized epithelial cells, called **M (membranous epithelial) cells.** The cell membranes of M cells show deep invaginations that contain macrophages and lymphocytes. The lymphatic nodules of Peyer's patches contain **B lymphocytes, T lymphocytes, macrophages,** and **plasma cells.** The M cells continually sample the **antigens** of the intestinal lumen, ingest the antigens, and present them to the underlying lymphocytes and macrophages in the lamina propria.

Small Intestine

The small intestine performs numerous digestive functions, including (1) continuation and completion of **digestion** (initiated in the oral cavity and stomach) of food products (chyme) by chemicals and enzymes produced in the liver and pancreas and by cells in its own mucosa, (2) selective **absorption** of nutrients into the blood and lymph capillaries, (3) **transportation** of chyme and digestive waste material to the large intestine, and (4) release of different **hormones** into the bloodstream to regulate the secretory functions and motility of digestive organs.

On the surface epithelium, **goblet cells** secrete **mucus** that lubricates, coats, and protects the intestinal surface from the corrosive actions of digestive chemicals and enzymes. The outer **glycocalyx** coat on absorptive cells not only protects the intestinal surface from digestion but also contains the enzymes that are required for terminal digestion of food products. These enzymes are produced by absorptive epithelial cells.

Absorption of nutrients into the cell interior occurs via diffusion, facilitated diffusion, osmosis, and active transport. Intestinal cells absorb **amino acids, glucose,** and **fatty acids**—the end products of protein, carbohydrate, and fat digestion, respectively. Amino acids, water, various ions, and glucose are transported through intestinal cells into the **capillaries** in the villi. Most of the long-chain fatty acids and monoglycerides, however, do not enter the capillaries; instead, they enter the tiny, blind-ending lymphatic vessels, called **lacteals,** in the lamina propria of each villus.

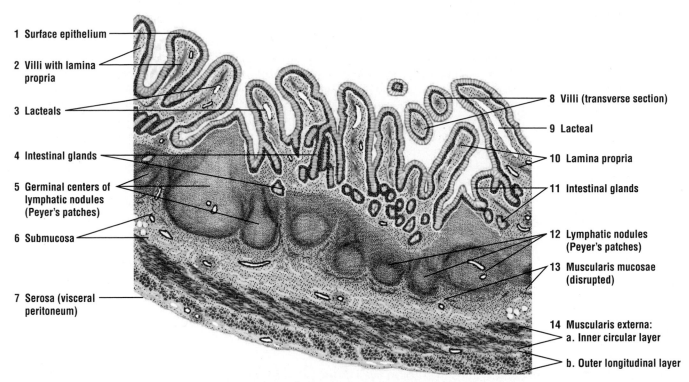

1 Surface epithelium

2 Villi with lamina propria

3 Lacteals

4 Intestinal glands

5 Germinal centers of lymphatic nodules (Peyer's patches)

6 Submucosa

7 Serosa (visceral peritoneum)

8 Villi (transverse section)

9 Lacteal

10 Lamina propria

11 Intestinal glands

12 Lymphatic nodules (Peyer's patches)

13 Muscularis mucosae (disrupted)

14 Muscularis externa:
a. Inner circular layer
b. Outer longitudinal layer

FIGURE 13.6 ■ Small intestine: ileum with lymphatic nodules (Peyer's patches) (transverse section). Stain: hematoxylin and eosin. Low magnification.

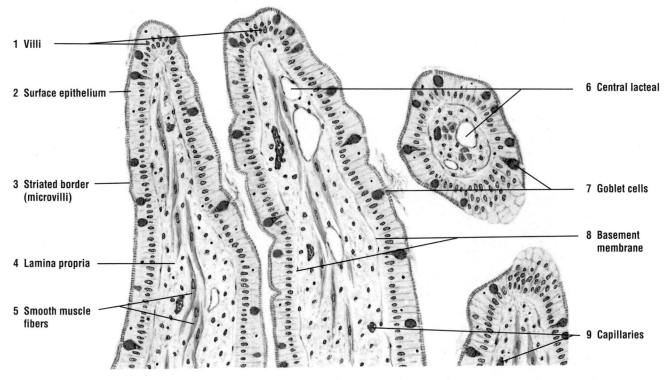

1 Villi

2 Surface epithelium

3 Striated border (microvilli)

4 Lamina propria

5 Smooth muscle fibers

6 Central lacteal

7 Goblet cells

8 Basement membrane

9 Capillaries

FIGURE 13.7 ■ Small intestine: villi. Stain: periodic acid-Schiff. Medium magnification.

FIGURE 13.8 ■ Large Intestine: Colon and Mesentery (Panoramic View, Transverse Section)

The wall of the colon has the same basic layers as the small intestine. The **mucosa (4, 5, 6, 7)** consists of simple columnar **epithelium (4), intestinal glands (5), lamina propria (6),** and **muscularis mucosae (7).** The underlying **submucosa (8)** contains connective tissue cells and fibers, various blood vessels, and nerves. Two smooth muscle layers form the **muscularis externa (13).** The **serosa** (visceral peritoneum) **(3)** and the **serosa** of the **mesentery (17)** cover the transverse colon and sigmoid colon. Several modifications in the colon wall distinguish it from other regions of the digestive tract (tube).

The colon does not have villi or plicae circulares, and the luminal surface of the mucosa is smooth. In the undistended colon, the mucosa (4, 5, 6, 7) and submucosa (8) exhibit **temporary folds (12).** In the lamina propria (6) and the submucosa (8) of the colon are **lymphatic nodules (9, 11).**

The smooth muscle layers in the muscularis externa (13) of the colon are modified. The **inner circular muscle layer (16)** is continuous in the colon wall, whereas the outer muscle layer is condensed into three broad, longitudinal bands, called **taeniae coli (1, 10).** A very thin **outer longitudinal muscle layer (15),** which is often discontinuous, is found between the taeniae coli (1, 10). The parasympathetic ganglion cells of the **myenteric (Auerbach's) nerve plexus (2, 14)** are found between the two smooth muscle layers of the muscularis externa (13).

The transverse and sigmoid colon are attached to the body wall by a **mesentery (18).** As a result, the serosa (3, 17) is the outermost layer.

FIGURE 13.9 ■ Large Intestine: Colon Wall (Transverse Section)

A low-magnification photomicrograph illustrates a portion of the colon wall. The simple columnar epithelium contains the **absorptive columnar cells (1)** and the mucus-filled **goblet cells (2, 6),** which increase in number toward the terminal end of the colon. The **intestinal glands (4)** in the colon are deep and straight, and they extend through the **lamina propria (3)** to the **muscularis mucosae (8).** The lamina propria (3) and **submucosa (9)** are filled with aggregations of lymphoid cells and **lymphatic nodules (5, 7).**

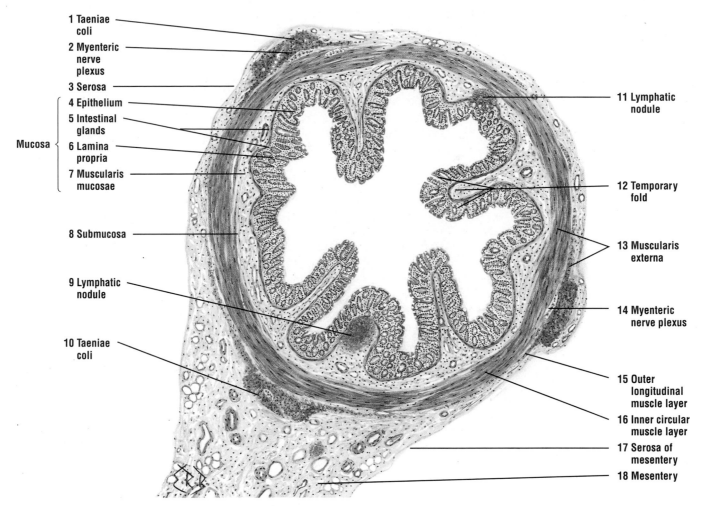

1 Taeniae coli
2 Myenteric nerve plexus
3 Serosa
4 Epithelium
5 Intestinal glands
6 Lamina propria
7 Muscularis mucosae

Mucosa

8 Submucosa
9 Lymphatic nodule
10 Taeniae coli

11 Lymphatic nodule
12 Temporary fold
13 Muscularis externa
14 Myenteric nerve plexus
15 Outer longitudinal muscle layer
16 Inner circular muscle layer
17 Serosa of mesentery
18 Mesentery

FIGURE 13.8 ■ Large intestine: colon and mesentery (panoramic view, transverse section). Stain: hematoxylin and eosin. Low magnification.

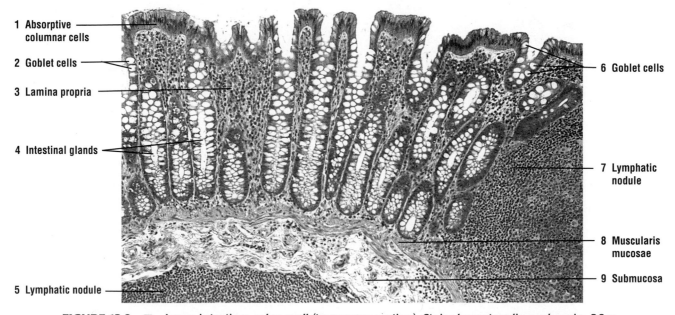

1 Absorptive columnar cells
2 Goblet cells
3 Lamina propria
4 Intestinal glands
5 Lymphatic nodule

6 Goblet cells
7 Lymphatic nodule
8 Muscularis mucosae
9 Submucosa

FIGURE 13.9 ■ Large intestine: colon wall (transverse section). Stain: hematoxylin and eosin. 30×

FIGURE 13.10 ■ Large Intestine: Colon Wall (Transverse Section)

A section of undistended colon wall shows the **temporary fold (9)** of the **mucosa (2, 3, 4)** and **submucosa (5, 12).** The four layers of the wall that are continuous with those of the small intestine are the mucosa (2, 3, 4), submucosa (5, 12), **muscularis externa (6),** and **serosa (7).**

Villi are absent in the colon, but the **lamina propria (3)** is indented by long **intestinal glands** (crypts of Lieberkühn) **(1, 10)** that extend through the lamina propria (3) to the **muscularis mucosae (4, 11).**

The **lining epithelium (2),** with numerous **goblet cells (2),** is simple columnar and continues into the intestinal glands (1, 10). Some of the intestinal glands (1, 10) are sectioned in longitudinal, transverse, and oblique planes.

The lamina propria (2), as in the small intestine, contains abundant diffuse lymphatic tissue. A distinct **lymphatic nodule (13)** can be seen deep in the lamina propria (3). Some of the larger lymphatic nodules may extend through the muscularis mucosae (4, 11) into the submucosa (5, 12).

The muscularis externa (6) is atypical. The longitudinal layer of the muscularis externa (6) is arranged into strips or bands of smooth muscle, called the **taeniae coli (15).** As in the circular layer, the taeniae coli (15) are supplied by **blood vessels (16).** The parasympathetic ganglia of the **myenteric plexus (8, 14)** are located between the muscle layers of the muscularis externa (6).

The serosa (7) covers the connective tissue and **adipose cells (17)** in the transverse and sigmoid colon. The ascending and descending colon are retroperitoneal, and their posterior surface is lined with adventitia.

FUNCTIONAL CORRELATIONS

Large Intestine

The principal functions of the large intestine are to absorb **water** and **minerals (electrolytes)** from the indigestible material that was transported from the ileum of the small intestine and to compact them into feces for elimination from the body. Consistent with these functions, the epithelium of the large intestine contains **columnar absorptive cells** (similar to those in the epithelium of the small intestine) and mucus-secreting **goblet cells,** which produce mucus for lubricating the lumen of the large intestine to facilitate passage of the feces. No digestive enzymes or chemicals are produced by the cells of the large intestine.

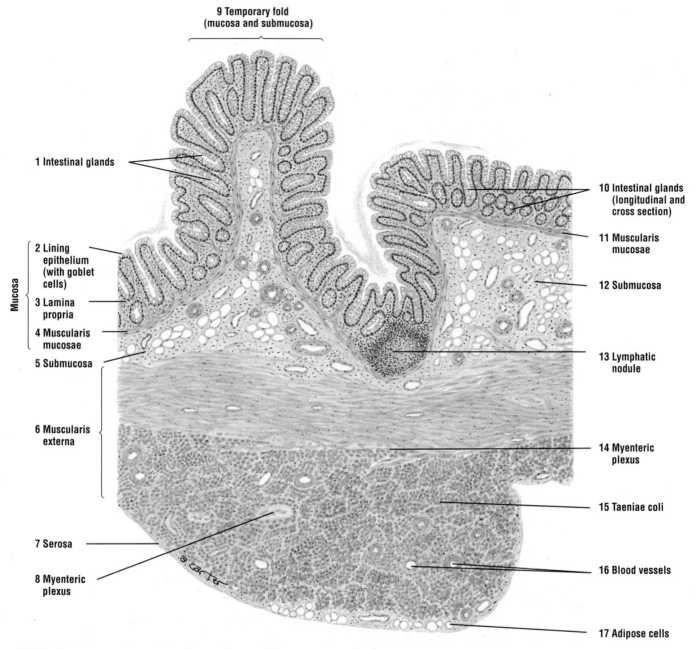

**9 Temporary fold
(mucosa and submucosa)**

1 Intestinal glands

Mucosa

**2 Lining
epithelium
(with goblet
cells)**

**3 Lamina
propria**

**4 Muscularis
mucosae**

5 Submucosa

**6 Muscularis
externa**

7 Serosa

**8 Myenteric
plexus**

**10 Intestinal glands
(longitudinal and
cross section)**

**11 Muscularis
mucosae**

12 Submucosa

**13 Lymphatic
nodule**

**14 Myenteric
plexus**

15 Taeniae coli

16 Blood vessels

17 Adipose cells

FIGURE 13.10 ■ Large intestine: colon wall (transverse section). Stain: hematoxylin and eosin. Medium magnification.

FIGURE 13.11 ▓ Appendix (Panoramic View, Transverse Section)

This figure illustrates a cross-section of the vermiform appendix at low magnification. Its morphology is similar to that of the colon, except for certain modifications.

In comparing the mucosa of the appendix with that of colon, the **lining epithelium (1)** contains numerous **goblet cells (1)**. In addition, the underlying **lamina propria (3)** shows **intestinal glands** (crypts of Lieberkühn) **(5)**, and there is a **muscularis mucosae (2)**. The intestinal glands (5) in the appendix are less developed, shorter, and often spaced farther apart than those in the colon. **Diffuse lymphatic tissue (6)** in the lamina propria (3) is abundant and often present in the **submucosa (8)**.

Lymphatic nodules with **germinal centers (4, 9)** are numerous and highly characteristic of the appendix. These nodules originate in the lamina propria (3) and may extend from the surface epithelium (1) to the submucosa (8).

The submucosa (8) has numerous **blood vessels (11)**. The **muscularis externa (7)** consists of the **inner circular layer (7a)** and the **outer longitudinal layer (7b)**. The **parasympathetic ganglia** of the **myenteric plexus (12)** are located between the inner (7a) and outer (7b) smooth muscle layers of the muscularis externa.

The outermost layer of the appendix is the **serosa (10)**, under which **adipose cells (13)** are seen.

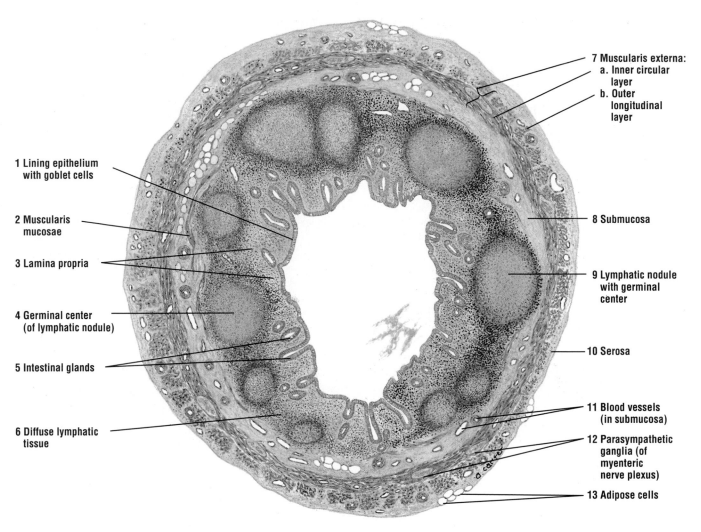

1 Lining epithelium with goblet cells

2 Muscularis mucosae

3 Lamina propria

4 Germinal center (of lymphatic nodule)

5 Intestinal glands

6 Diffuse lymphatic tissue

7 Muscularis externa:
  a. Inner circular layer
  b. Outer longitudinal layer

8 Submucosa

9 Lymphatic nodule with germinal center

10 Serosa

11 Blood vessels (in submucosa)

12 Parasympathetic ganglia (of myenteric nerve plexus)

13 Adipose cells

FIGURE 13.11 ■ Appendix (panoramic view, transverse section). Stain: hematoxylin and eosin. Low magnification.

FIGURE 13.12 ■ Rectum (Panoramic View, Transverse Section)

The histology of the upper rectum is similar to that of the colon.

The **surface epithelium (1)** of the **lumen (5)** is lined by simple columnar cells, with striated borders and goblet cells. The **intestinal glands (4), adipose cells (12),** and **lymphatic nodules (10)** in the **lamina propria (2)** are similar to those in the colon. The intestinal glands are longer, closer together, and filled with goblet cells. Beneath the lamina propria (2) is the **muscularis mucosae (11).**

The **longitudinal folds (3)** in the upper rectum and colon are temporary. These folds (3) contain a core of **submucosa (8)** that is covered by the mucosa. Permanent longitudinal folds (rectal columns) are found in the lower rectum and the anal canal.

Taeniae coli of the colon continue into the rectum, where the **muscularis externa (13)** acquire the typical **inner circular layer (13a)** and **outer longitudinal layer (13b)** of smooth muscle. Between these two smooth muscle layers are the **parasympathetic ganglia** of the **myenteric (Auerbach's) plexus (14).**

Adventitia (9) covers a portion of the rectum, and serosa covers the remainder. Numerous blood vessels, such as **arterioles (7, 15)** and **venules (6, 15),** are found in both the submucosa (8) and the adventitia (9).

FIGURE 13.13 ■ Anorectal Junction (Longitudinal Section)

The portion of the anal canal above the **anorectal junction (7)** represents the lowermost part of the rectum. The part of the anal canal below the anorectal junction (7) shows the transition from the **simple columnar epithelium (1)** to the **stratified squamous epithelium (8)** of the skin. The change from the rectal mucosa to the anal mucosa occurs at the anorectal junction (7).

The mucosa of the rectum is similar to the mucosa of the colon. The **intestinal glands (3)** are somewhat shorter, however, and are spaced farther apart. As a result, the **lamina propria (2)** is more prominent, diffuse lymphatic tissue more abundant, and solitary **lymphatic nodules (11)** more numerous.

The **muscularis mucosae (4)** and the intestinal glands (3) of the digestive tract terminate in the vicinity of the anorectal junction (7). The lamina propria (2) of the rectum is replaced by the dense irregular connective tissue of the **lamina propria** of the **anal canal (9).** The **submucosa (5)** of the rectum merges with the connective tissue in the lamina propria of the anal canal, a region that is highly vascular. The **internal hemorrhoidal plexus (10)** of veins lies in the mucosa of the anal canal. Blood vessels from this region continue into the submucosa (5) of the rectum.

The circular smooth muscle layer of the **muscularis externa (6)** increases in thickness in the upper region of the anal canal and forms the **internal anal sphincter (6).** Lower in the anal canal, the internal anal sphincter (6) is replaced by **skeletal muscles** of the **external anal sphincter (12).** External to the external anal sphincter (12) is the skeletal **levator ani muscle (13).**

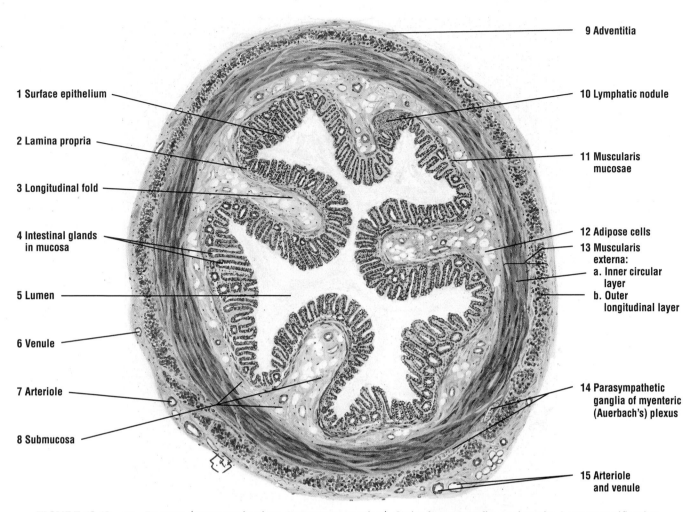

1 Surface epithelium

2 Lamina propria

3 Longitudinal fold

4 Intestinal glands
  in mucosa

5 Lumen

6 Venule

7 Arteriole

8 Submucosa

9 Adventitia

10 Lymphatic nodule

11 Muscularis
   mucosae

12 Adipose cells

13 Muscularis
   externa:
   a. Inner circular
      layer
   b. Outer
      longitudinal layer

14 Parasympathetic
   ganglia of myenteric
   (Auerbach's) plexus

15 Arteriole
   and venule

FIGURE 13.12 ■ Rectum (panoramic view, transverse section). Stain: hematoxylin and eosin. Low magnification.

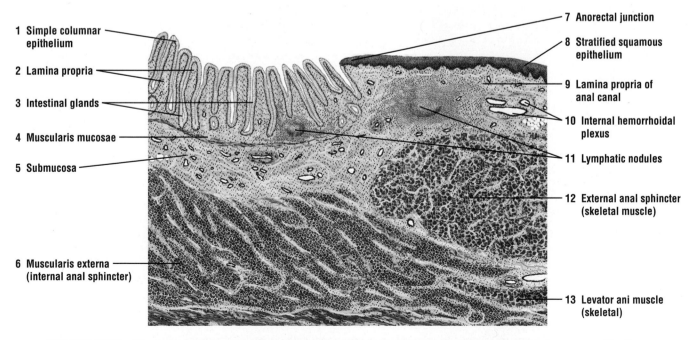

1 Simple columnar
  epithelium

2 Lamina propria

3 Intestinal glands

4 Muscularis mucosae

5 Submucosa

6 Muscularis externa
  (internal anal sphincter)

7 Anorectal junction

8 Stratified squamous
  epithelium

9 Lamina propria of
  anal canal

10 Internal hemorrhoidal
   plexus

11 Lymphatic nodules

12 External anal sphincter
   (skeletal muscle)

13 Levator ani muscle
   (skeletal)

FIGURE 13.13 ■ Anorectal junction (longitudinal section). Stain: hematoxylin and eosin. Low magnification.

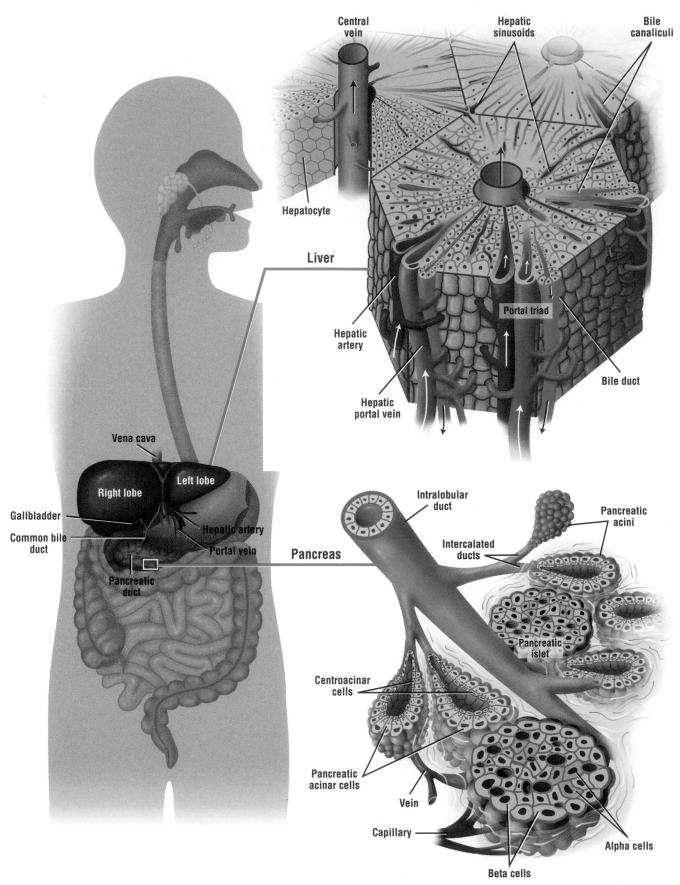

OVERVIEW FIGURE ■ A section from the liver and the pancreas is illustrated, with emphasis on the liver lobule and the duct system of the exocrine pancreas.

CHAPTER 14

Digestive System: Liver, Gallbladder, and Pancreas

In addition to the salivary glands that open into the oral cavity, the **liver, gallbladder,** and **pancreas** are also **accessory organs** of the digestive tract. These organs are located outside the digestive tract but are connected to the small intestine by excretory ducts. The **common bile duct** from the liver and the main pancreatic duct from the pancreas join in the duodenal loop to form a single duct that is common to both organs. This duct then penetrates the duodenal wall and enters the lumen of the small intestine. The gallbladder joins the common bile duct via the cystic duct. Therefore, **bile** from the gallbladder and **digestive enzymes** from the pancreas enter the duodenum via a common duct.

Liver

Absorbed food products and liquids from the digestive organs first percolate through liver capillaries, called **sinusoids.** Nutrient-rich blood in the **hepatic portal vein** is brought to the liver before it enters the general circulation. Because venous blood from the digestive organs is poor in oxygen, the **hepatic artery** from the aorta supplies liver cells with oxygenated blood, forming a dual blood supply to the liver.

The liver exhibits repeating hexagonal units, called **liver (hepatic) lobules** (see overview figure). In the center of each lobule is the **central vein,** from which plates of liver cells, called **hepatocytes,** and sinusoids radiate toward the periphery. Here, the connective tissue forms **portal triads** or **portal areas,** where branches of the hepatic artery, hepatic portal vein, and **bile duct** can be seen. Venous and arterial blood first mix in the liver sinusoids as they flow toward the central vein. From here, blood enters the general circulation through the hepatic veins that leave the liver.

The hepatic sinusoids are tortuous, dilated blood channels lined by a discontinuous layer of **fenestrated endothelial cells,** which are separated from the underlying hepatocytes by a **perisinusoidal space** (of Disse). As a result, ingested material carried in the sinusoids enters the discontinuous endothelial wall and comes in direct contact with the hepatocytes. The structure and path of the sinusoids through the liver allows an efficient exchange of materials between hepatocytes and blood.

Hepatocytes secrete bile into tiny channels, called **bile canaliculi,** that are located between individual hepatocytes. The canaliculi converge at the periphery of each liver lobule in the portal areas as **bile ducts.** The bile ducts then drain into larger hepatic ducts that carry bile out of the liver. Within the liver lobules, bile flows in bile canaliculi toward the bile duct in the portal area, whereas blood in the sinusoids flows toward the central vein. As a result, bile and blood do not mix.

Gallbladder

The gallbladder is a small, hollow organ attached to the inferior surface of the liver. Bile is produced by liver hepatocytes and then flows to and is stored in the gallbladder. Bile leaves the gallbladder via the cystic duct and enters the duodenum via the **common bile duct** through the **major duodenal papilla,** a finger-like protrusion of the duodenal wall into the lumen.

The gallbladder is not a gland. Its main function is to store and concentrate bile, which is released into the digestive tract as a result of hormonal stimulation after a meal. When the gallbladder is empty, the mucosa exhibits deep **folds.**

Exocrine Pancreas

The pancreas is a soft, elongated organ located posterior to the stomach. The **head** of the pancreas lies in the duodenal loop, and the **tail** extends across the abdominal cavity to the spleen. In contrast to the liver, the pancreas contains separate exocrine cells and endocrine cells. Most of the pancreas is an **exocrine gland.** The exocrine secretory units, or acini, contain pyramid-shaped **acinar cells,** the apices of which are filled with secretory granules. These granules contain the precursors of several pancreatic **digestive enzymes** that are secreted into the excretory ducts in an inactive form.

The secretory acini are subdivided into **lobules** and bound together by loose connective tissue. The **excretory ducts** in the exocrine pancreas start from within the center of individual acini as pale-staining, centroacinar cells that continue into the short **intercalated ducts.** The intercalated ducts merge to form **intralobular ducts** in the connective tissue, which in turn join to form larger **interlobular ducts** that empty into the **main pancreatic duct.**

Endocrine Pancreas

The endocrine units of the pancreas are scattered among the exocrine acini as isolated, pale-staining, vascularized units, called **pancreatic islets** (of Langerhans). Each islet is surrounded by fine fibers of reticular connective tissue. With special immunocytochemical processes, four cell types can be identified in each pancreatic islet: **alpha, beta, delta,** and **pancreatic polypeptide cells.**

Alpha cells comprise approximately 20% of the islets and are located primarily around the islet periphery. Beta cells are the most numerous, comprising approximately 70% of the islet cells, and are primarily concentrated in the center of the islet. The remaining cell types are few in number and are located in various places throughout the islets.

FIGURE 14.1 ■ Pig's Liver (Panoramic View, Transverse Section)

In the pig's liver, connective tissue from the hilus extends between the liver lobes as interlobular septa and defines the **hepatic lobules (7).** To illustrate the connective tissue boundaries of each hepatic lobule (7), a section of pig's liver was stained with Mallory-azan, which stains the connective septa dark blue.

A complete hepatic lobule (on the left) and parts of adjacent **hepatic lobules (7)** are illustrated. The blue-staining **interlobular septa (5, 9)** contain interlobular branches of the **portal vein (4, 11), bile duct (2, 12),** and **hepatic artery (3, 13),** which are collectively considered to be **portal areas,** or portal canals. At the periphery of each lobule can be seen several portal areas within the interlobular septa (5, 9). Within the interlobular septa (5, 9) are also found small lymphatic vessels and nerves, which only occasionally are seen.

In the center of each hepatic lobule (7) is the **central vein (1, 8).** Radiating from each central vein (1, 8) toward the lobule periphery are the **plates of hepatic cells (6).** Located between the hepatic plates (6) are blood channels, called **hepatic sinusoids (10).** Arterial and venous blood mix in the hepatic sinusoids (10) and then flow toward the central vein (1, 8) of each lobule (7).

Bile is produced by the liver cells. Bile flows through the very small bile canaliculi between the hepatocytes into the interlobular **bile ducts (2, 12)** (see Fig. 14-5).

The interlobular vessels and bile ducts (2, 3, 4, 11, 12, 13) are highly branched in the liver. In a cross-section of the liver lobule, more than one section of these structures can be seen within a portal area.

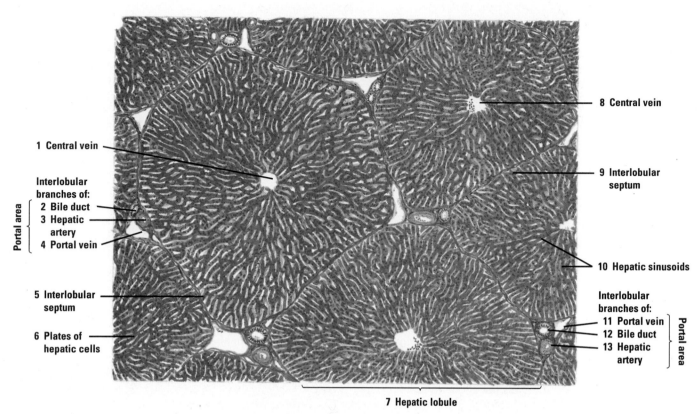

FIGURE 14.1 ■ Pig's liver (panoramic view, transverse section). Stain: mallory-azan. Low magnification.

FIGURE 14.2 ■ Primate Liver (Panoramic View, Transverse Section)

In the primate or human liver, the connective tissue septa between individual **hepatic lobules (8)** are not as conspicuous as in the pig, and the liver sinusoids are continuous between the lobules. Despite these differences, portal areas containing interlobular branches of the **portal veins (2, 11)**, **hepatic arteries (3, 13)**, and **bile ducts (1, 12)** are visible around the hepatic lobule (8) peripheries in the **interlobular septa (4, 10)**.

This figure illustrates numerous hepatic lobules (8). In the center of each hepatic lobule (8) is the **central vein (6, 9)**. The **hepatic sinusoids (5)** appear between the **plates of hepatic cells (7)** that radiate from the central veins (6, 9) toward the periphery of the hepatic lobule (8). As illustrated in Figure 14-1, branches of the interlobular vessels and bile ducts are seen within the portal areas of a hepatic lobule (8).

FUNCTIONAL CORRELATIONS

Liver

The liver performs hundreds of functions. Hepatocytes perform more functions than any other cell in the body, and they play both endocrine and exocrine roles.

Exocrine Functions

Hepatocytes perform many **exocrine functions.** One major exocrine function of hepatocytes is to synthesize and release 500 to 1,200 mL of **bile** into the **bile canaliculi** per day. Most of the bile enters the gallbladder, where it is stored and concentrated until its release when chyme enters the duodenum.

Bile salts in the bile **emulsify fats** in the small intestine (duodenum). This process allows more efficient digestion of fats by the fat-digesting **pancreatic lipase** that is produced by the pancreas. The digested fats are subsequently absorbed by cells in the small intestine and enter the blind-ending, lymphatic **lacteal** channels that are located in individual villi. From the lacteals, fats are carried into larger lymphatic ducts that eventually drain into the major veins.

Hepatocytes also excrete **bilirubin,** which is a toxic chemical formed in the body after degradation of worn-out erythrocytes by liver macrophages, called **Kupffer cells.** Bilirubin is taken up by hepatocytes from the blood and is excreted into bile.

Hepatocytes also have an important role in the immune system. **Antibodies** produced by plasma cells in the intestinal lamina propria are taken from blood by hepatocytes and are transported into bile canaliculi and bile. From here, antibodies enter the intestinal lumen, where they control the intestinal bacterial flora.

Endocrine Functions

Hepatocytes are also **endocrine cells.** The arrangement of hepatocytes in a liver lobule allows them to take up, metabolize, accumulate, and store numerous products from the blood. Hepatocytes then release many of the metabolized or secreted products back into the bloodstream as the blood flows through the sinusoids and comes in direct contact with individual hepatocytes.

The endocrine functions of the liver hepatocytes involve the synthesis of numerous **plasma proteins,** including albumin and the blood-clotting factors prothrombin and fibrinogen. The liver also stores fats, various vitamins, and carbohydrates as **glycogen.** When the cells of the body need **glucose,** the glycogen stored in the liver is converted back into glucose and released into the bloodstream.

Hepatocytes also **detoxify** the blood of drugs and harmful substances as the blood percolates through the sinusoids. **Kupffer cells** in the sinusoids are specialized liver phagocytes that are derived from blood monocytes. These large, branching cells filter and phagocytose particulate material, cellular debris, and worn-out or damaged erythrocytes that flow through the sinusoids.

The liver also performs vital functions early in life. In the fetus, the liver is the site of **hematopoiesis,** or blood cell production.

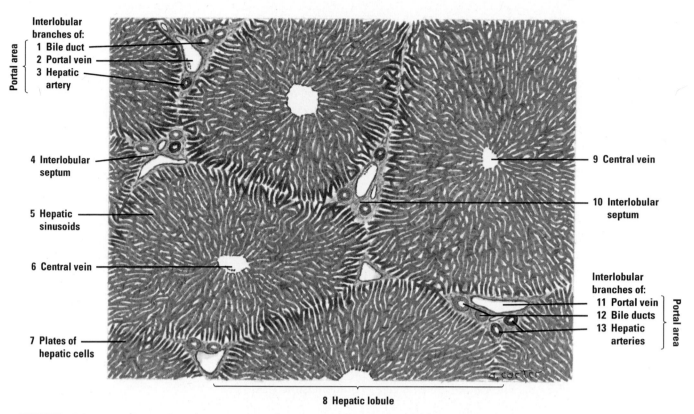

Interlobular
branches of:
1 Bile duct
2 Portal vein
**3 Hepatic
   artery**

Portal area

**4 Interlobular
   septum**

**5 Hepatic
   sinusoids**

6 Central vein

**7 Plates of
   hepatic cells**

9 Central vein

**10 Interlobular
    septum**

Interlobular
branches of:
11 Portal vein
12 Bile ducts
**13 Hepatic
    arteries**

Portal area

8 Hepatic lobule

FIGURE 14.2 ■ Primate liver (panoramic view, transverse section). Stain: hematoxylin and eosin. Low magnification.

FIGURE 14.3 ■ Bovine Liver: Liver Lobule (Transverse Section)

A lower-magnification photomicrograph of a bovine liver illustrates several hepatic (liver) lobules. The portal area of the hepatic lobule contains the branches of the **portal vein (5)**, **hepatic artery (6)**, and normally, a bile duct (not seen in this photomicrograph). From the **central vein (1)** radiate the **plates of hepatic cells (2)** toward the lobule periphery. Located between the plates of hepatic cells (2) are the blood channels, called **sinusoids (3)**. The sinusoids (3) convey blood from the portal vein (5) and the hepatic artery (6) to the central vein (1). Both the central vein (1) and the sinusoids (3) are lined by a discontinuous, fenestrated type of **endothelium (4)**.

FIGURE 14.4 ■ Hepatic (Liver) Lobule (Sectional View, Transverse Section)

A section of a hepatic lobule between the **central vein (9)** and the peripheral connective tissue **interlobular septum (1, 6)** of the portal area is illustrated in greater detail. In the interlobular septum (1, 6) are transverse sections of a **portal vein (4)**, **hepatic arteries (3)**, **bile ducts (5)**, and a **lymphatic vessel (2)**. Multiple cross-sections of hepatic arteries (3) and bile ducts (5) are the result of either their branching in the septum or their passage into and out of the septum.

Branches of the portal vein (4) and the hepatic artery (3) penetrate the interlobular septum (1, 6) and form the **sinusoids (8, 10)**. The sinusoids (8, 10) are situated between the **plates of hepatic cells (7)** and follow their branchings and anastomoses. Discontinuous **endothelial cells (10)** line the sinusoids (8, 10) and the central vein (9). **Blood cells** (erythrocytes and leukocytes) in the **sinusoids (8)** drain toward the central vein (9) of each lobule. Also in the sinusoids (10) are fixed macrophages, called the Kupffer cells (see Fig. 14-6).

FIGURE 14.5 ■ Bile Canaliculi in a Liver Lobule (Osmic Acid Preparation)

Preparation of a liver section with osmic acid and staining with hematoxylin and eosin reveals the **bile canaliculi (3, 5)**, which are tiny channels between individual liver (hepatic) cells in the **hepatic plates (4)**. The bile canaliculi (3, 5) follow an irregular course between the hepatic plates (4) and branch freely within the hepatic plates (4).

The **sinusoids (6)** are lined by discontinuous **endothelial cells (1)**. All sinusoids (6) drain toward and open into the **central vein (2)**.

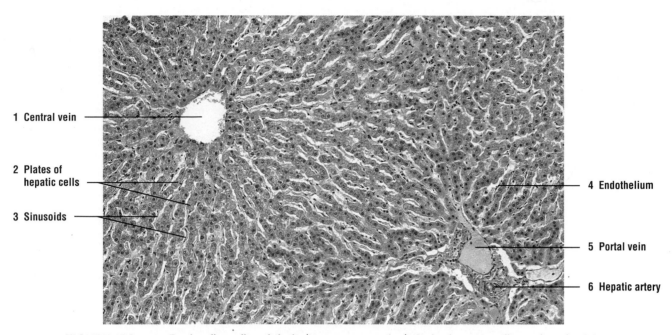

1 Central vein

2 Plates of hepatic cells

3 Sinusoids

4 Endothelium

5 Portal vein

6 Hepatic artery

FIGURE 14.3 ■ Bovine liver: liver lobule (transverse section). Stain: hematoxylin and eosin. 30×

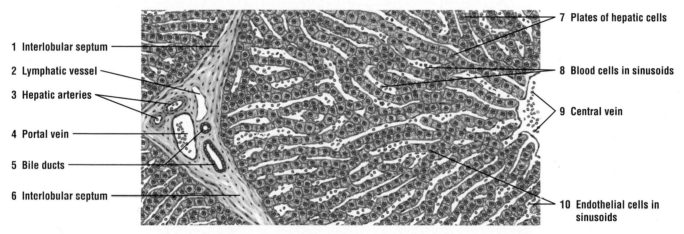

1 Interlobular septum

2 Lymphatic vessel

3 Hepatic arteries

4 Portal vein

5 Bile ducts

6 Interlobular septum

7 Plates of hepatic cells

8 Blood cells in sinusoids

9 Central vein

10 Endothelial cells in sinusoids

FIGURE 14.4 ■ Hepatic (liver) lobule (sectional view, transverse section). Stain: hematoxylin and eosin. High magnification.

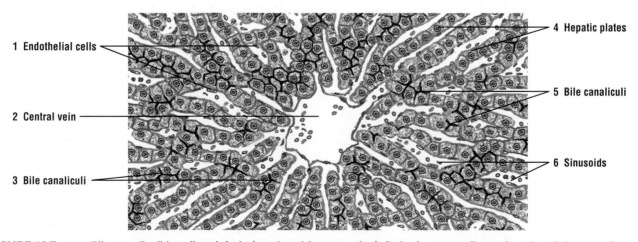

1 Endothelial cells

2 Central vein

3 Bile canaliculi

4 Hepatic plates

5 Bile canaliculi

6 Sinusoids

FIGURE 14.5 ■ Bile canaliculi in a liver lobule (osmic acid preparation). Stain: hematoxylin and eosin. High magnification.

FIGURE 14.6 ■ Kupffer Cells in Liver Lobule (India Ink Preparation)

The majority of cells that line the liver **sinusoids (5)** are **endothelial cells (2).** These small cells have an attenuated cytoplasm and a small nucleus. To demonstrate the phagocytic cells in the liver sinusoids (5), an animal was intravenously injected with India ink. The phagocytic **Kupffer cells (3, 7)** ingest the carbon particles from the ink, which fill their cytoplasm with dark deposits. As a result, Kupffer cells (3, 7) become prominent in the sinusoids (5) between the **hepatic plates (6).** Kupffer cells (3, 7) are large cells with several processes and an irregular or stellate outline that protrudes into the sinusoids (5). The nuclei of Kuppfer cells (3, 7) are obscured by the ingested carbon particles.

On the periphery of the lobule is a section of the connective tissue **interlobular septum (1)** and a part of the **bile duct (4)** that is lined with cuboidal cells.

FIGURE 14.7 ■ Glycogen Granules in Liver Cells (Hepatocytes)

The cytoplasm of liver cells varies in appearance depending on nutritional status. After a meal, liver **hepatocytes (1)** store increased amounts of glycogen in their cytoplasm. With periodic acid-Schiff staining, the **glycogen granules (2, 4)** in the hepatocyte (1) cytoplasm stain bright red and exhibit an irregular distribution.

Also visible in this illustration are hepatic **sinusoids (3)** and flattened **endothelial cells (5)** that line their lumina.

FIGURE 14.8 ■ Reticular Fibers in a Liver Lobule

Fine **reticular fibers (6, 8)** provide most of the supporting connective tissue of the liver. In this illustration, the reticular fibers stain black, and the liver cells stain pale pink/violet. The reticular fibers (6, 8) line the **sinusoids (8),** support the endothelial cells, and form a denser network of reticular fibers in the wall of the **central vein (7).** The reticular fibers (6, 8) also merge with the **collagen fibers** in the **interlobular septum (1),** where they surround the **portal vein (2)** and the **bile duct (3).**

Also visible in the reticular network are the pink-staining **nuclei of hepatocyes (4)** and the **hepatic plates (5)** that radiate from the central vein (7) toward the interlobular septum (1).

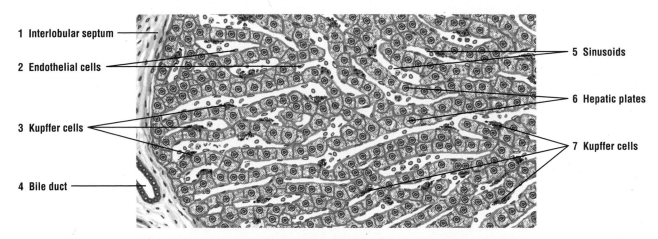

1 Interlobular septum

2 Endothelial cells

3 Kupffer cells

4 Bile duct

5 Sinusoids

6 Hepatic plates

7 Kupffer cells

FIGURE 14.6 ■ Kupffer cells in a liver lobule (India ink preparation). Stain: hematoxylin and eosin. High magnification.

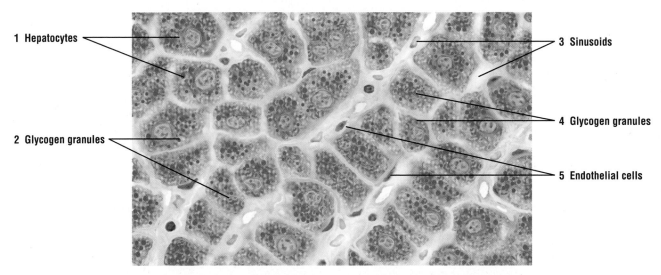

1 Hepatocytes

2 Glycogen granules

3 Sinusoids

4 Glycogen granules

5 Endothelial cells

FIGURE 14.7 ■ Glycogen granules in liver cells. Stain: periodic acid-Schiff with blue counterstain for nuclei. High magnification. Oil immersion.

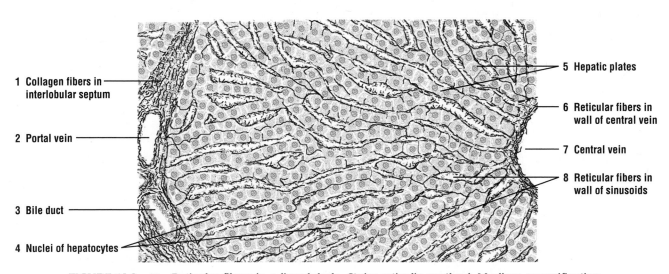

1 Collagen fibers in interlobular septum

2 Portal vein

3 Bile duct

4 Nuclei of hepatocytes

5 Hepatic plates

6 Reticular fibers in wall of central vein

7 Central vein

8 Reticular fibers in wall of sinusoids

FIGURE 14.8 ■ Reticular fibers in a liver lobule. Stain: reticulin method. Medium magnification.

FIGURE 14.9 ■ Wall of the Gallbladder

The gallbladder is a muscular sac. Its wall consists of mucosa, muscularis, and adventitia or serosa. The wall of the gallbladder does not contain a muscularis mucosae or submucosa.

The mucosa consists of a **simple columnar epithelium (1)** and the underlying connective tissue **lamina propria (2),** which contains loose connective tissue, some diffuse lymphatic tissue, and blood vessels (e.g., a **venule** and an **arteriole [9]**). In the nondistended state, the gallbladder wall shows temporary **mucosal folds (7)** that disappear when the gallbladder becomes distended with bile. The mucosal folds (7) resemble the villi in the small intestine. However, they vary in size and shape, and they display an irregular arrangement. Between the mucosal folds (7) are **diverticula** or **crypts (3, 8)** that often form deep indentations in the mucosa. In cross-section, the diverticula or crypts (3, 8) in the lamina propria (2) resemble tubular glands. However, the gallbladder proper contains no glands, except in the neck region of the organ.

External to the lamina propria (2) is the muscularis of the gallbladder, with bundles of randomly oriented **smooth muscle fibers (10),** which do not show distinct layers, and interlacing **elastic fibers (4).**

Surrounding the bundles of smooth muscle fibers (10) is a thick layer of dense **connective tissue (6)** that contains large blood vessels (e.g., an **artery** and a **vein [11]**), lymphatics, and **nerves (5).**

Serosa (12) covers all the unattached gallbladder surface. Where the gallbladder is attached to the liver surface, this connective tissue layer is the adventitia.

FUNCTIONAL CORRELATIONS

The Gallbladder

The primary functions of the gallbladder are to collect, store, concentrate, and expel **bile** when it is needed for the emulsification of fat. Bile is continually produced by the liver hepatocytes and is transported via the excretory ducts to the gallbladder for storage. Here, sodium is actively transported through the simple columnar epithelium of the gallbladder into the extracellular connective tissue, creating a strong osmotic pressure. Water and chloride ions passively follow, producing concentrated bile.

Release of bile into the duodenum is under hormonal control. Responding to the entrance of dietary fats into the proximal duodenum, the hormone **cholecystokinin** is released into the bloodstream by **enteroendocrine cells** in the intestinal mucosa. Cholecystokinin is carried in the bloodstream to the gallbladder, where it causes strong rhythmic contractions of the smooth muscle in its wall. At the same time, the smooth **sphincter muscles** around the neck of the gallbladder relax. The combination of these two actions forces the bile into the duodenum via the **common bile duct.**

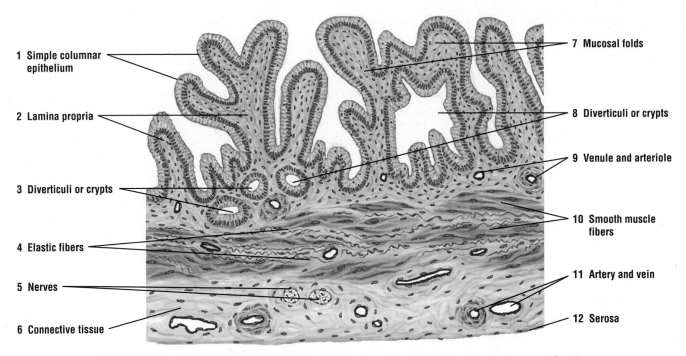

1 Simple columnar epithelium

2 Lamina propria

3 Diverticuli or crypts

4 Elastic fibers

5 Nerves

6 Connective tissue

7 Mucosal folds

8 Diverticuli or crypts

9 Venule and arteriole

10 Smooth muscle fibers

11 Artery and vein

12 Serosa

FIGURE 14.9 ■ Wall of the gallbladder. Stain: hematoxylin and eosin. Low magnification.

FIGURE 14.10 ■ Pancreas (Sectional View)

The pancreas has both endocrine and exocrine components. The exocrine component forms the majority of the pancreas and consists of closely packed, secretory **serous acini** and **zymogenic cells (1)** arranged into small lobules. The lobules are surrounded by thin intralobular and **interlobular connective tissue septa (4, 13)** that contain **blood vessels (5, 9), interlobular ducts (12),** nerves, and occasionally, a sensory receptor, called a **Pacinian corpuscle (11).** Within the serous acini (1) are the isolated **pancreatic islets** (of Langerhans) **(3, 7).** The pancreatic islets (3, 7) represent the endocrine portion and are the characteristic features of the pancreas.

Each pancreatic serous acinus (1) consists of pyramid-shaped, protein-secreting zymogenic cells (1) that surround a small central lumen. The excretory ducts of the individual acini are visible as pale-staining, **centroacinar cells (6, 10)** within their lumina. The secretory products leave the acini via **intercalated** (intralobular) **ducts (2)** that have small lumina lined with low cuboidal epithelium. The centroacinar cells (6, 10) are continuous with the epithelium of the intercalated ducts (2).

The intercalated ducts (2) drain into interlobular ducts (12) in the interlobular connective tissue septa (4, 13). The interlobular ducts (12) are lined by a simple cuboidal epithelium that becomes taller and is stratified in larger ducts.

Pancreatic islets (3, 7) are demarcated from the surrounding exocrine acini (1) tissue by a thin layer of reticular fibers. The islets (3, 7) are larger than the acini and are compact clusters of epithelial cells that are permeated by **capillaries (8).** The cells of a pancreatic islet (3, 7) are illustrated at higher magnification in Figures 14-11 and 14-12.

FUNCTIONAL CORRELATIONS

Exocrine Pancreas

The exocrine and endocrine functions of the pancreas are performed separately by exocrine and endocrine cells. The pancreas produces numerous digestive enzymes that exit the gland through a major excretory duct, whereas the different hormones are transported via blood vessels.

Both hormones and vagal stimulation regulate pancreatic exocrine secretions. Two intestinal hormones, **secretin** and **cholecystokinin,** which are secreted by the **enteroendocrine (APUD) cells** in the duodenal mucosa into the bloodstream, regulate pancreatic secretions.

In response to the presence of acidic chyme in the small intestine (duodenum), release of the hormone secretin stimulates exocrine pancreatic cells to produce large amounts of a watery fluid that is rich in **sodium bicarbonate ions.** This fluid, which has little or no enzymatic activity, is primarily produced by **centroacinar cells** in the acini and by cells that line the smaller **intercalated ducts.** The main function of this bicarbonate fluid is to neutralize the acidic chyme, to stop the action of pepsin from the stomach, and to create a neutral pH in the duodenum for the action of digestive pancreatic enzymes.

In response to the presence of fats and proteins in the small intestine, cholecystokinin is released into the bloodstream. Cholecystokinin stimulates the acinar cells in the pancreas to secrete large amounts of digestive enzymes: **pancreatic amylase** for carbohydrate digestion, **pancreatic lipase** for lipid digestion, **deoxyribonuclease** and **ribonuclease** for nuclei acid digestion, and the proteolytic enzymes **trypsinogen, chymotrypsinogen,** and **procarboxypeptidase.**

Pancreatic enzymes are first produced in the acinar cells as an inactive form. They are only activated in the duodenum by the hormone **enterokinase,** which is secreted by the intestinal mucosa. This hormone converts trypsinogen to trypsin, which then converts all other pancreatic enzymes into active digestive enzymes.

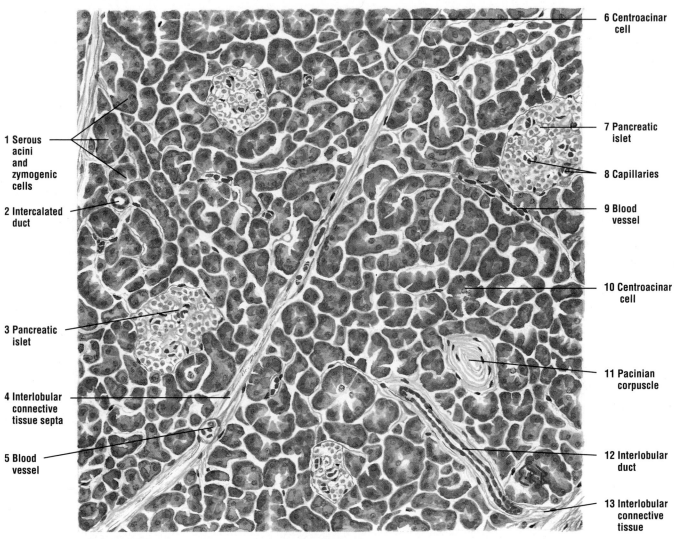

6 Centroacinar cell

7 Pancreatic islet

8 Capillaries

9 Blood vessel

10 Centroacinar cell

11 Pacinian corpuscle

12 Interlobular duct

13 Interlobular connective tissue

1 Serous acini and zymogenic cells

2 Intercalated duct

3 Pancreatic islet

4 Interlobular connective tissue septa

5 Blood vessel

FIGURE 14.10 ■ Pancreas (sectional view). Stain: hematoxylin and eosin. Low magnification.

FIGURE 14.11 ■ Pancreatic Islet

A pale-staining, **pancreatic islet** (of Langerhans) **(2)** is illustrated at a higher magnification. The endocrine cells of the islet (2) are arranged in cords and clumps, between which are connective tissue fibers and a **capillary (3)** network. A thin **connective tissue capsule (4)** separates the endocrine pancreas from the exocrine **serous acini (5).** Some serous acini (5) contain pale-staining, **centroacinar cells (5)** that are the initial part of the duct system that then connect to the **intercalated duct (1).** Myoepithelial cells do not surround the secretory acini in the pancreas.

In routine histologic preparations, the individual hormone-secreting cells of the pancreatic islet (1) cannot be identified.

FIGURE 14.12 ■ Pancreatic Islet (Special Preparation)

This pancreas has been prepared with a special stain to distinguish the glucagon-secreting **alpha cells (1)** from the insulin-secreting **beta cells (3).** The cytoplasm of the alpha cells (1) stains pink, whereas the cytoplasm of beta cells (3) stains blue. The alpha cells (1) are situated more peripherally in the islet, and the beta cells (3) are situated more in the center. Also, beta cells (3) predominate, constituting approximately 70% of the islet. Delta cells (not illustrated) are also present in the islets. These cells are the least abundant, have a variable shape, and may occur anywhere in the pancreatic islet.

Capillaries (2) around the endocrine cells demonstrate the rich vascularity of the pancreatic islets. The thin **connective tissue capsule (4)** separates the islet cells from the **serous acini (6). Centroacinar cells (5)** are visible in some of the acini.

FUNCTIONAL CORRELATIONS

Endocrine Pancreas

The endocrine components of the pancreas are scattered throughout the organ as islands of endocrine cells, called **pancreatic islets** (of Langerhans). Pancreatic islets secrete two major hormones that regulate blood glucose levels and glucose metabolism. **Alpha cells** in the pancreatic islets produce the hormone **glucagon,** which is released in response to low levels of glucose in the blood. Glucagon elevates blood glucose levels by accelerating the conversion of glycogen, amino acids, and fatty acids in the liver cells into glucose.

Beta cells in pancreatic islets produce the hormone **insulin,** the release of which is stimulated by elevated blood glucose levels after a meal. Insulin lowers blood glucose levels by accelerating membrane transport of glucose into liver cells, muscle cells, and adipose cells. Insulin also accelerates the conversion of glucose into glycogen in liver cells. The effects of insulin on blood glucose levels are opposite those of glucagon.

Delta cells secrete the hormone **somatostatin.** This hormone decreases and inhibits secretory activities of both alpha (glucagon-secreting) and beta (insulin-secreting) cells through local action within the pancreatic islets.

Pancreatic polypeptide cells produce the hormone **pancreatic polypeptide,** which inhibits production of pancreatic enzymes and alkaline secretions.

FIGURE 14.13 ■ Pancreas: Endocrine (Pancreatic Islet) and Exocrine Regions

A higher-magnification photomicrograph of the pancreas illustrates both exocrine and endocrine components. In the center is the light-staining, endocrine **pancreatic islet (3).** A thin **connective tissue capsule (2)** separates the pancreatic islet (3) from the exocrine **secretory acini (5).** The pancreatic islet (3) is vascularized by blood vessels and **capillaries (6).** The exocrine secretory acini (5) consist of pyramid-shaped cells arranged around small lumina, in the centers of which are seen one or more light-staining, **centroacinar cells (4).**

The smallest excretory duct in the pancreas is the **intercalated duct (1),** which is lined by a simple cuboidal epithelium.

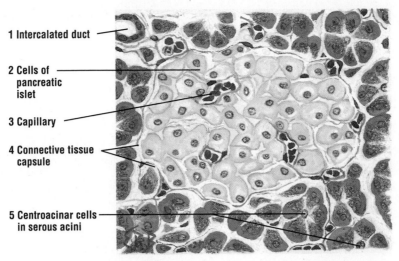

1 Intercalated duct

2 Cells of pancreatic islet

3 Capillary

4 Connective tissue capsule

5 Centroacinar cells in serous acini

FIGURE 14.11 ■ Pancreatic islet. Stain: hematoxylin and eosin. High magnification.

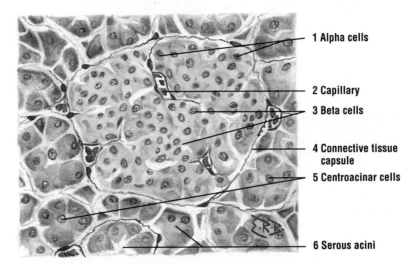

1 Alpha cells

2 Capillary

3 Beta cells

4 Connective tissue capsule

5 Centroacinar cells

6 Serous acini

FIGURE 14.12 ■ Pancreatic islet (special preparation). Stain: Gomori's chrome alum hematoxylin-phloxine. High magnification.

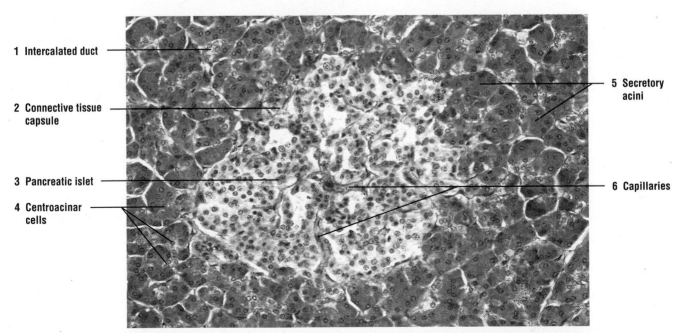

1 Intercalated duct

2 Connective tissue capsule

3 Pancreatic islet

4 Centroacinar cells

5 Secretory acini

6 Capillaries

FIGURE 14.13 ■ Pancreas: endocrine (pancreatic islet) and exocrine regions. Stain: periodic acid-Schiff and hematoxylin. 80×

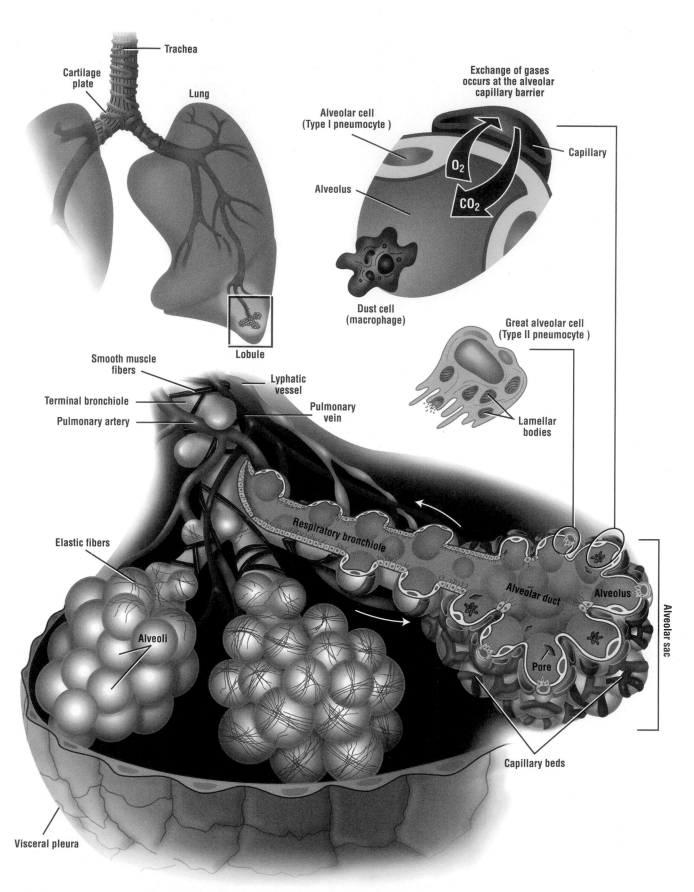

Trachea

Cartilage plate

Lung

Exchange of gases occurs at the alveolar capillary barrier

Alveolar cell (Type I pneumocyte)

O_2

CO_2

Capillary

Alveolus

Dust cell (macrophage)

Great alveolar cell (Type II pneumocyte)

Lobule

Smooth muscle fibers

Lyphatic vessel

Terminal bronchiole

Pulmonary artery

Pulmonary vein

Lamellar bodies

Respiratory bronchiole

Elastic fibers

Alveolar duct

Alveolus

Alveolar sac

Alveoli

Pore

Capillary beds

Visceral pleura

OVERVIEW FIGURE ■ A section of the lung illustrated in three dimensions and in transverse section, with an emphasis on the internal structure of the respiratory bronchiole and alveolar cells.

CHAPTER 15

Respiratory System

Components of the Respiratory System

The respiratory system consists of the **lungs** and numerous **air passages,** or tubes, of various sizes that lead to and from each lung.

The **conducting portion** of the respiratory system consists of passageways outside and inside the lungs that conduct air to and from the lungs. In contrast, the **respiratory portion** consists of passagways within the lungs that not only conduct the air but also allow **respiration,** or gaseous exchange.

The extrapulmonary passages (i.e., those outside the lungs), which include the trachea, bronchi, and larger bronchioles, are lined by a distinct, **pseudostratified ciliated epithelium** containing numerous **goblet cells.** As the passageways enter the lungs, they continue to branch, and their diameters become progressively smaller. Also the height of the lining epithelium, the amount of cilia, and the number of goblet cells in these tubules gradually decrease.

Gaseous exchange in the lungs takes place in the **alveoli,** which are the terminal air spaces of the respiratory system. In the alveoli, goblet cells are absent, and the lining epithelium is thin **simple squamous.**

Olfactory Epithelium

Air that enters the lungs first passes by the roof or superior region of the nasal cavity. Located in the roof of the nose is a highly specialized epithelium, called the **olfactory epithelium,** for the detection and transmission of odors. This epithelium consists of three cell types: supportive (sustentacular), basal, and olfactory (sensory).

Olfactory cells are the **sensory bipolar neurons** that are distributed between the more apical supportive cells and the basal cells of the olfactory epithelium. The olfactory cells end at the surface of the olfactory epithelium as small, round structures, called the **olfactory bulbs.** Radiating from each olfactory bulb are long, **nonmotile olfactory cilia** that lie parallel to the epithelial surface; these nonmotile cilia function as odor receptors. In contrast to respiratory epithelium, the olfactory epithelium has no goblet cells or motile cilia. In the connective tissue directly below the olfactory epithelium are **olfactory nerves** and **olfactory (Bowman's) glands.** The olfactory (Bowman's) glands produce a serous fluid that bathes the olfactory cilia and dissolves the odor molecules for detection by the olfactory cells.

Conducting Portion of the Respiratory System

The conducting portion of the respiratory system consists of the nasal cavities, pharynx, larynx, trachea, extrapulmonary bronchi, and a series of intrapulmonary bronchi and bronchioles with decreasing diameters that end as **terminal bronchioles. Hyaline cartilage** provides structural support and insures that the larger air passageways are always patent (i.e., open). Incomplete, C-shaped **hyaline cartilage rings** encircle the **trachea.** As the trachea divides into smaller **bronchi** and the bronchi enter the lungs, the hyaline cartilage rings are replaced by **hyaline cartilage plates.** In smaller bronchi, the cartilage plates decrease in size and number. When the diameters of bronchioles decrease to approximately 1 mm, cartilage plates completely disappear from conducting passageways. Terminal bronchioles represent the final conducting passageways and have diameters ranging from 0.5 to 1.0 mm.

The larger bronchioles are lined by a **ciliated pseudostratified epithelium** that is similar to that of the trachea and bronchi. As the diameter of the tubule decreases, the height of the epithelium is gradually reduced, and the epithelium becomes **simple ciliated epithelium.** The epithelium of larger bronchioles also contains numerous **goblet cells.** The number of these cells gradually decreases, and goblet cells are not present in the epithelium of terminal bronchioles.

Smaller bronchioles are lined only by **simple cuboidal epithelium.** Also, the epithelium of terminal bronchioles contains nonciliated cuboidal cells, called **Clara cells.** These cells increase in number as the number of ciliated cells decreases.

Respiratory Portion of the Respiratory System

The respiratory portion of the respiratory system is the distal continuation of the conducting portion, and it consists of air passageways where respiration or gaseous exchange occurs. Terminal bronchioles of the conducting system give rise to **respiratory bronchioles,** which end in thin-walled outpocketings, called **alveoli.** The respiratory bronchioles also represent the **transitional zone** between air conduction and air exchange, or respiration.

Respiration can only occur in alveoli, because the barrier between inspired air in the alveoli and venous blood in the capillaries is extremely thin. Other intrapulmonary structures where respiration occurs are the **alveolar ducts** and the **alveolar sacs.**

The lungs also contain different cell types; in the alveoli, two cell types are found. The most abundant cells are the **squamous alveolar cells (type I pneumocytes).** These thin cells line all the alveolar surfaces. Interspersed among the squamous alveolar cells, either singly or in small groups, are the **great alveolar cells (type II pneumocytes).** Lung **macrophages,** which are derived from circulating blood monocytes, are also found both in the connective tissue of alveolar walls or interalveolar septa (**alveolar macrophages**) and in the alveoli (**dust cells**). Also present in the interalveolar septa are extensive capillary networks, pulmonary arteries, pulmonary veins, lymphatic ducts, and nerves (see overview figure).

FIGURE 15.1 ■ Olfactory Mucosa and Superior Concha (Panoramic View)

The **olfactory mucosa (2, 5)** is located in the roof of the nasal cavity, on each side of the dividing septum, and on the surface of the **superior concha (1),** which is one of the bony shelves in the nasal cavity.

The **olfactory epithelium (2, 5)** (see Fig. 15-2) is specialized for the reception of smell. As a result, it appears different from the respiratory epithelium. Olfactory epithelium (2, 5) is pseudostratified tall columnar epithelium without goblet cells and without motile cilia, in contrast to the respiratory epithelium.

The underlying **lamina propria (2)** contains the branched tubuloacinar **olfactory (Bowman's) glands (3, 6).** These glands produce a serous secretion, in contrast to the mixed mucous and serous secretions the glands in the rest of the nasal cavity produce. The small nerves in the lamina propria (2) are the olfactory nerves, or **fila olfactoria (4, 7).** The fila olfactoria (4, 7) represent the aggregated axons that leave the olfactory cells and continue into the cranial cavity, where they synapse in the olfactory (cranial) nerves.

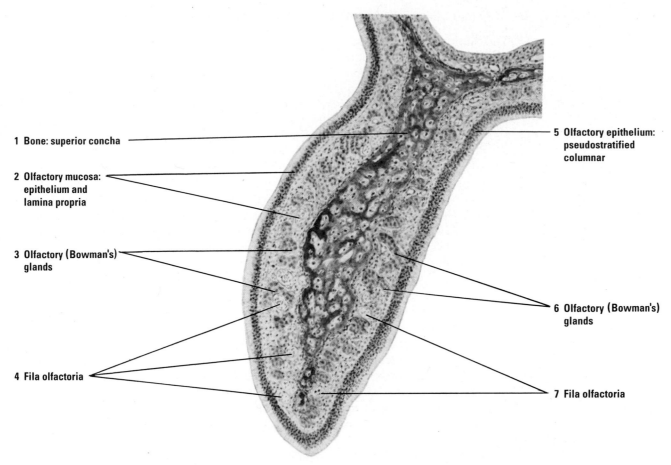

1 Bone: superior concha

2 Olfactory mucosa: epithelium and lamina propria

3 Olfactory (Bowman's) glands

4 Fila olfactoria

5 Olfactory epithelium: pseudostratified columnar

6 Olfactory (Bowman's) glands

7 Fila olfactoria

FIGURE 15.1 ■ Olfactory mucosa and superior concha (panoramic view). Stain: hematoxylin and eosin. Low magnification.

FIGURE 15.2 ■ Olfactory Mucosa: Detail of a Transitional Area

This illustration depicts a transition between the **olfactory epithelium (1)** and the **respiratory epithelium (9)**. In the transition region, the histologic differences between these epithelia are obvious. The olfactory epithelium (1) is tall pseudostratified columnar epithelium and is composed of three different cell types: supportive, basal, and neuroepithelial olfactory cells. The individual cell outlines are difficult to distinguish in a routine histologic preparation; however, the location and shape of the nuclei allow identification of the cell types.

The **supportive,** or sustentacular, **cells (3)** are elongated, with oval nuclei that are situated more apically or superficially in the epithelium. The **olfactory cells (4)** have oval or round nuclei that are located between the nuclei of the supportive cells (3) and the **basal cells (5).** The apices and bases of the olfactory cells (4) are slender. The apical surfaces of the olfactory cells (4) contain slender, nonmotile microvilli that extend into the **mucus (2)** that covers the epithelial surface. The basal cells (5) are short cells at the base of the epithelium between the supportive cells (3) and the olfactory cells (4).

Extending from the bases of the olfactory cells (4) are axons that pass into the **lamina propria (6)** as bundles of unmyelinated **olfactory nerves (fila olfactoria) (14)**. The olfactory nerves (14) leave the nasal cavity and pass into the olfactory bulbs at the base of the brain.

The transition from the olfactory epithelium (1) to the respiratory epithelium (9) is abrupt. The respiratory epithelium (9) is pseudostratified columnar epithelium with distinct **cilia (10)** and many **goblet cells (11)**. Also, in the illustrated transition area, the height of the respiratory epithelium (9) is similar to that of the olfactory epithelium (1). In other regions of the tract, the respiratory epithelium (9) is reduced in comparison to the olfactory epithelium (1).

The underlying **lamina propria (6)** contains capillaries, lymphatic vessels, **arterioles (8), venules (13),** and branched, tubuloacinar serous **olfactory (Bowman's) glands (7).** The olfactory glands (7) deliver their secretions through narrow excretory **ducts (12)** that penetrate the olfactory epithelium (1). The secretions from the olfactory glands (7) moisten the epithelial surface, dissolve the molecules of odoriferous substances, and stimulate the olfactory cells (4).

FIGURE 15.3 ■ Olfactory Mucosa in the Nose: Transition Area

In the superior region of the nasal cavity, the **respiratory epithelium** changes abruptly into the **olfactory epithelium,** as shown in this higher-power photomicrograph.

The respiratory epithelium is lined by motile **cilia (1)** and contains **goblet cells (2)**. In contrast, the olfactory epithelium lacks cilia (1) and goblet cells (2). Instead, the olfactory epithelium exhibits nuclei of **supportive cells (5),** located near the epithelial surface; nuclei of odor-receptive **olfactory cells (6),** located more in the center of the epithelium; and **basal cells (7),** located close to the **basement membrane (3).**

Below the olfactory epithelium in the connective tissue **lamina propria (4)** are **blood vessels (9), olfactory nerves (10),** and **olfactory (Bowman's) glands (8).**

FUNCTIONAL CORRELATIONS

Olfactory Epithelium

To detect odors, odoriferous substances must first be dissolved. The dissolved odor molecules then bind to odor-receptor molecules on **olfactory cilia** and stimulate the **receptors cells** in the olfactory epithelium to conduct impulses. The unmyelinated afferent axons of olfactory cells leave the olfactory epithelium and form numerous small **olfactory nerve bundles** in the lamina propria. Impulses from olfactory cells are conducted in the nerves that pass through the ethmoid bone in the skull and that synapse in the **olfactory bulbs** of the brain. Olfactory bulbs are located in the cranial cavity of the skull above the nasal cavity. From here, neurons relay the information to higher centers in the cortex for odor interpretation.

Olfactory epithelium is kept moist by a watery secretion that is produced by serous tubuloacinar **olfactory (Bowman's) glands** directly below the epithelium in the lamina propria. This secretion, delivered via ducts, continually washes the surface of the olfactory epithelium. In this manner, odor molecules dissolve in the secreted fluid and are continually washed away by new fluid, allowing the receptor cells to again detect and respond to new odors.

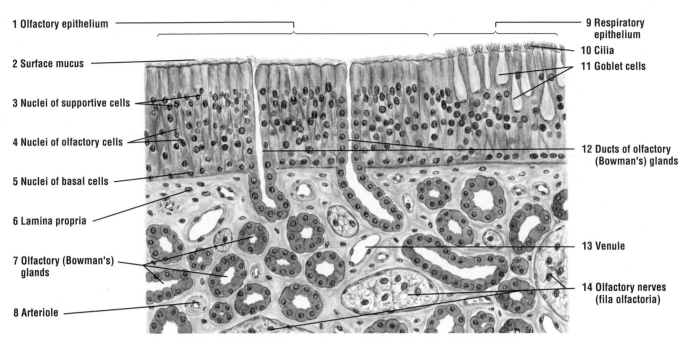

1 Olfactory epithelium

2 Surface mucus

3 Nuclei of supportive cells

4 Nuclei of olfactory cells

5 Nuclei of basal cells

6 Lamina propria

7 Olfactory (Bowman's) glands

8 Arteriole

9 Respiratory epithelium

10 Cilia

11 Goblet cells

12 Ducts of olfactory (Bowman's) glands

13 Venule

14 Olfactory nerves (fila olfactoria)

FIGURE 15.2 ■ Olfactory mucosa: details of a transitional area. Stain: hematoxylin and eosin. High magnification.

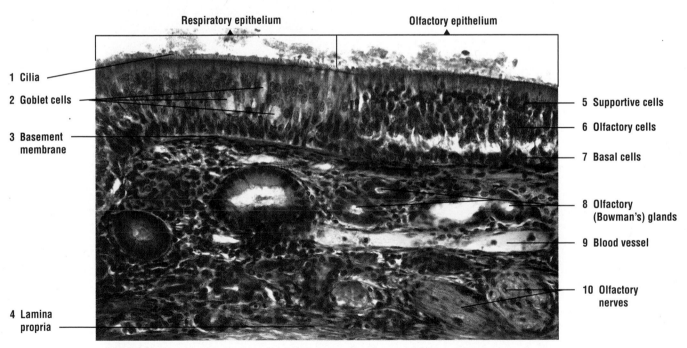

Respiratory epithelium   Olfactory epithelium

1 Cilia

2 Goblet cells

3 Basement membrane

4 Lamina propria

5 Supportive cells

6 Olfactory cells

7 Basal cells

8 Olfactory (Bowman's) glands

9 Blood vessel

10 Olfactory nerves

FIGURE 15.3 ■ Olfactory mucosa in the nose: transition area. Stain: mallory-azan. 80×

FIGURE 15.4 ■ Epiglottis (Longitudinal Section)

The epiglottis is the superior portion of the larynx that projects upward from the larynx's anterior wall.

A central **epiglottic (elastic) cartilage (7)** forms the framework of the epiglottis. Its **lingual (anterior) mucosa (6)** is covered with a nonkeratinized **stratified squamous epithelium (9).** The underlying **lamina propria (4)** merges with the **perichondrium (8)** of the epiglottic cartilage (7).

The lingual mucosa (6), with a **stratified squamous epithelium (3),** covers the apex of the epiglottis and approximately half the **laryngeal (posterior) mucosa (2).** At the transition area, the connective tissue papillae from the lingual mucosa disappear, and a **pseudostratified ciliated columnar epithelium (5)** covers the epiglottis.

Tubuloacinar mucous, serous, or mixed glands are present in the lamina propria (4). Occasional **taste buds (1)** in the epithelium and solitary lymphatic nodules may be present in the lingual mucosa (6) or the laryngeal mucosa (2).

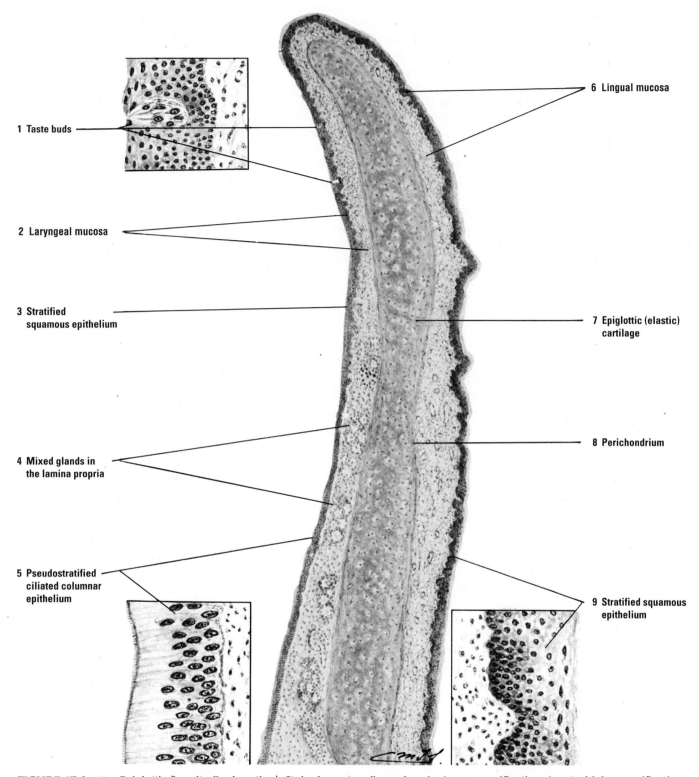

1 Taste buds

2 Laryngeal mucosa

3 Stratified squamous epithelium

4 Mixed glands in the lamina propria

5 Pseudostratified ciliated columnar epithelium

6 Lingual mucosa

7 Epiglottic (elastic) cartilage

8 Perichondrium

9 Stratified squamous epithelium

FIGURE 15.4 ■ Epiglottis (longitudinal section). Stain: hematoxylin and eosin. Low magnification. Insets: high magnification.

FIGURE 15.5 ■ Larynx (Frontal Section)

A vertical section through the larynx shows the two **vocal folds (13, 18, 19, 20)**, supporting **cartilages (8, 11)**, and **muscles (10, 20)**.

The **false (superior) vocal fold (13)** is formed by the mucosa and is continuous with the **posterior surface** of the **epiglottis (12)**. The lumen is lined by **pseudostratified ciliated columnar epithelium (14)** with goblet cells. In the **lamina propria (3)** are **mixed glands (15)** that are predominantly mucous. **Excretory ducts (16)** from these mixed glands (15) open onto the epithelial surface (15). **Lymphatic nodules (7)** are located in the lamina propria (3) on the ventricular side of the vocal fold.

The **ventricle (17)** is a deep indentation and recess that separates the false vocal fold (13) from the **true (inferior) vocal fold (18, 19, 20)**. The mucosa in the wall (3, 4, 5, 6) of the ventricle (17) is similar to that of the false vocal fold (13). Lymphatic nodules are more numerous in this area and are sometimes called the **laryngeal tonsils (7)**. The lamina propria (3) blends with the **perichondrium (9)** of the **thyroid cartilage (hyaline) (8)**. No distinct submucosa is found. The lower wall of the ventricle makes the transition to a true vocal fold (18, 19, 20).

The mucosa of the true vocal fold (18, 19, 20) is lined by nonkeratinized **stratified squamous epithelium (18)** and a thin, dense lamina propria that is devoid of glands, lymphatic tissue, and blood vessels. At the apex of the true vocal fold is the **vocal ligament (19)**, with dense elastic fibers that extend into the adjacent lamina propria and the skeletal **vocalis muscle (20)**. The skeletal **thyroarytenoid muscle (10)** and the thyroid cartilage (8) comprise the remaining wall.

The epithelium in the lower larynx changes to **pseudostratified ciliated columnar epithelium (21)**, and the **lamina propria** contains **mixed glands (22)**. The **cricoid cartilage (hyaline) (11)** is the lowermost cartilage of the larynx.

1 Adipose tissue

2 Arteriole and venule

3 Lamina propria of ventricular wall

4 Serous acini

5 Mucous acini

6 Excretory duct

7 Lymphatic nodules (laryngeal tonsils)

8 Thyroid cartilage (hyaline)

9 Perichondrium

10 Thyroarytenoid muscle (skeletal)

11 Cricoid cartilage (hyaline)

12 Posterior surface of the epiglottis

13 False (superior) vocal fold

14 Pseudostratified ciliated columnar epithelium

15 Mixed glands

16 Excretory duct

17 Ventricle

18 Stratified squamous epithelium

19 Vocal ligament

20 Vocalis muscle (skeletal)

True (inferior) vocal fold

21 Pseudostratified ciliated columnar epithelium

22 Mixed glands in lamina propria (lower larynx)

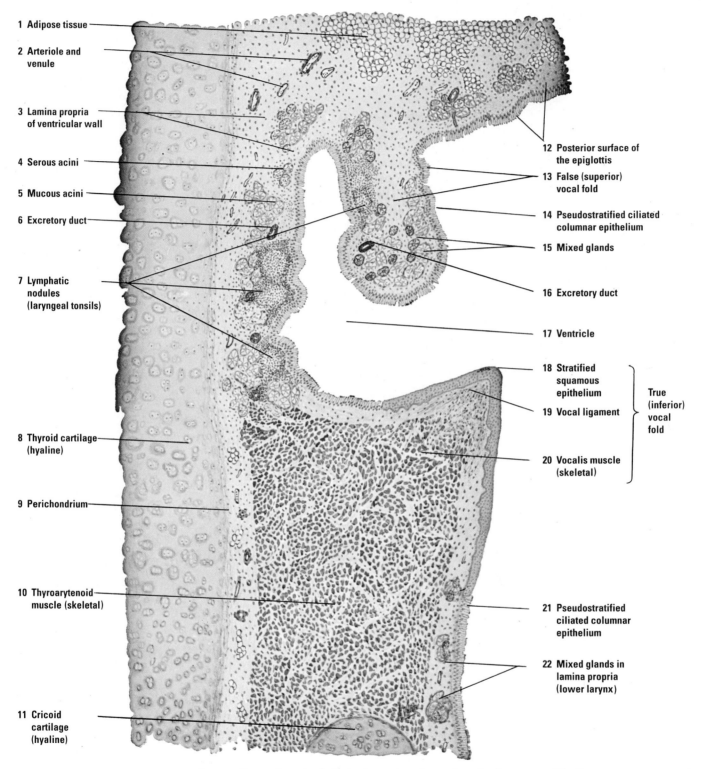

FIGURE 15.5 ■ Larynx (frontal section). Stain: hematoxylin and eosin. Low magnification.

FIGURE 15.6 ■ Trachea (Panoramic View, Transverse Section)

The wall of the trachea consists of mucosa, submucosa, hyaline cartilage, and adventitia. The trachea is kept patent (i.e., open) by C-shaped **hyaline cartilage (3)** rings. Hyaline cartilage (3) is surrounded by the dense connective tissue **perichondrium (9),** which merges with the **submucosa (4)** on one side and with the **adventitia (1)** on the other. Numerous **nerves (6), blood vessels (8),** and **adipose tissue (2)** are located in the adventitia.

The gap between the posterior ends of the hyaline cartilage (3) is filled by the smooth **trachealis muscle (7).** The trachealis muscle (7) lies in the connective tissue deep to the **elastic membrane (14)** of the mucosa. Most of the fibers of the trachealis muscle (7) insert into the perichondrium (9) that covers the hyaline cartilage (3).

The lumen of the trachea is lined by **pseudostratified ciliated columnar epithelium (12)** with goblet cells. The underlying **lamina propria (13)** contains fine connective tissue fibers, diffuse lymphatic tissue, and occasional solitary lymphatic nodules. Located deeper in the lamina propria (13) is the longitudinal elastic membrane (14) that is formed by elastic fibers. The elastic membrane (14) divides the lamina propria (13) from the submucosa (4), which contains loose connective tissue similar to that of the lamina propria (13). In the submucosa (4) are the tubuloacinar **seromucous tracheal glands (10),** the **excretory ducts (11)** of which pass through the lamina propria (13) to the tracheal lumen.

The mucosa exhibits **mucosal folds (5)** along the posterior wall of the trachea, where the hyaline cartilage (3) is absent. The seromucous tracheal glands (10) in the submucosa can extend to and be seen in the adventitia (1).

FIGURE 15.7 ■ Tracheal Wall (Sectional View)

A section of tracheal wall between the **hyaline cartilage (1)** and the lining **pseudostratified ciliated columnar epithelium (8)** with **goblet cells (10)** is illustrated at a higher magnification. A thin **basement membrane (9)** separates the lining epithelium (8) from the **lamina propria (11).**

Below the lamina propria (11) is the connective tissue **submucosa (6),** where the **seromucous tracheal glands (3)** are found. A **serous demilune (7)** surrounds a mucous acinus of the seromucous tracheal glands (3). The **excretory duct (5)** of the seromucous tracheal glands (3) is lined by simple cuboidal epithelium and extends through the lamina propria (11) to the epithelial surface (8).

The adjacent hyaline cartilage (1) is surrounded by the connective tissue **perichondrium (2).** The larger **chondrocytes** in **lacunae (4)** that are located in the interior of the hyaline cartilage (1) become progressively flatter toward the perichondrium (2), which gradually blends with the surrounding connective tissue of the submucosa (6). An **arteriole** and **venule (12)** supply the connective tissue of the submucosa (6) and the lamina propria (11).

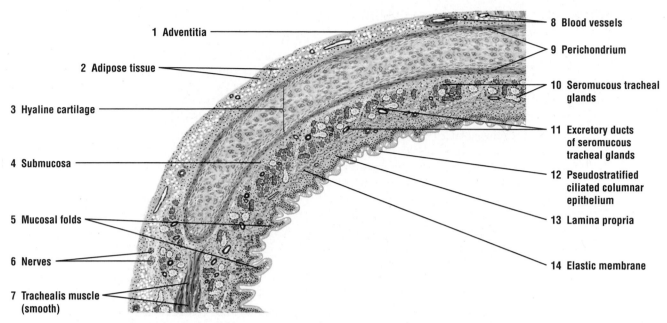

1 Adventitia

2 Adipose tissue

3 Hyaline cartilage

4 Submucosa

5 Mucosal folds

6 Nerves

7 Trachealis muscle (smooth)

8 Blood vessels

9 Perichondrium

10 Seromucous tracheal glands

11 Excretory ducts of seromucous tracheal glands

12 Pseudostratified ciliated columnar epithelium

13 Lamina propria

14 Elastic membrane

FIGURE 15.6 ■ Trachea (transverse section). Stain: hematoxylin and eosin. Low magnification.

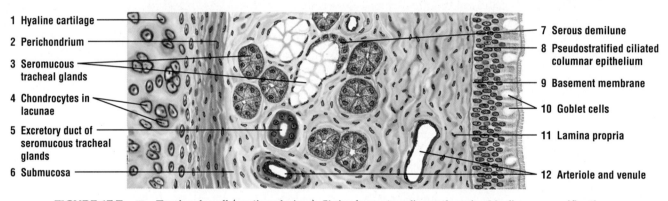

1 Hyaline cartilage

2 Perichondrium

3 Seromucous tracheal glands

4 Chondrocytes in lacunae

5 Excretory duct of seromucous tracheal glands

6 Submucosa

7 Serous demilune

8 Pseudostratified ciliated columnar epithelium

9 Basement membrane

10 Goblet cells

11 Lamina propria

12 Arteriole and venule

FIGURE 15.7 ■ Tracheal wall (sectional view). Stain: hematoxylin and eosin. Medium magnification.

FIGURE 15.8 ■ Lung (Panoramic View)

This illustration shows the major structures in the lung for air conduction and gaseous exchange (i.e., respiration). The histology of the intrapulmonary bronchi is similar to that of the trachea and extrapulmonary bronchi, except that in the intrapulmonary bronchi, the C-shaped cartilage rings of the trachea are replaced by cartilage plates. All cartilage in the trachea and lung is hyaline cartilage.

The wall of an **intrapulmonary bronchus (5)** is identified by the surrounding **hyaline cartilage plates (7).** The bronchus (5) is also lined by pseudostratified columnar ciliated epithelium with goblet cells. The wall in the intrapulmonary brochus (5) consists of a thin **lamina propria (4),** a narrow layer of **smooth muscle (3),** a **submucosa (2)** with **bronchial glands (6),** hyaline cartilage plates (7), and **adventitia (1).**

As the intrapulmonary bronchus (5) branches into smaller bronchi and bronchioles, the epithelial height and the cartilage around the bronchi decrease, until only an occasional piece of cartilage is seen. Cartilage disappears from the bronchi and bronchioles walls when the diameter decreases to approximately 1 mm.

In the **bronchiole (17),** pseudostratified columnar ciliated epithelium with occasional goblet cells lines the lumen. The lumen shows **mucosal folds (18)** because of the contractions of the surrounding **smooth muscle (19)** layer. Bronchial glands and cartilage plates are no longer present, and the bronchiole (17) is surrounded by the **adventitia (16).** In this illustration, a **lymphatic nodule (15)** and a **vein (15)** adjacent to the adventitia (16) accompany the bronchiole (17).

The **terminal bronchioles (8, 10)** exhibit **mucosal folds (10)** and are lined by a columnar ciliated epithelium that lacks goblet cells. A thin layer of lamina propria and **smooth muscle (11)** and an adventitia surround the terminal bronchioles (8, 10).

The **respiratory bronchioles (12, 22)** with alveoli outpocketings are directly connected to the **alveolar ducts (13, 20)** and the **alveoli (23).** In the respiratory bronchioles (12, 22), the epithelium is low columnar or cuboidal, and it may be ciliated in the proximal portion of the tubules. A thin connective tissue layer supports the smooth muscle, the elastic fibers of the lamina propria, and the accompanying **blood vessels (21).** The **alveoli (12)** in the walls of the respiratory bronchioles (12, 22) appear as small evaginations or outpockets.

Each respiratory bronchiole (12, 22) divides into several alveolar ducts (13, 20). The walls of the alveolar ducts (13, 20) are lined by alveoli (23) that directly open into the alveolar duct. Clusters of alveoli (23) that surround and open into alveolar ducts (13, 20) are called **alveolar sacs (24).** In this illustration, the plane of section passes from a terminal bronchiole (8) to the respiratory bronchiole and into the alveolar ducts (20).

The **pulmonary vein (9)** and **pulmonary artery (9)** also branch as they accompany the bronchi and bronchioles into the lung. In addition, small blood vessels are seen in the connective tissue **trabecula (25)** that separates the lungs into different segments.

The **serosa (14),** or visceral pleura, surrounds the lungs. Serosa (14) consists of a thin layer of pleural **connective tissue (14a)** and a simple squamous layer of pleural **mesothelium (14b).**

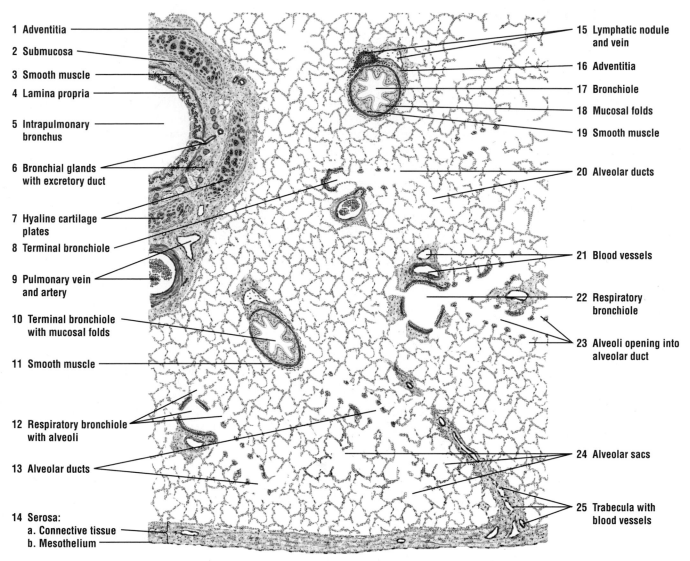

1 Adventitia

2 Submucosa

3 Smooth muscle

4 Lamina propria

5 Intrapulmonary bronchus

6 Bronchial glands with excretory duct

7 Hyaline cartilage plates

8 Terminal bronchiole

9 Pulmonary vein and artery

10 Terminal bronchiole with mucosal folds

11 Smooth muscle

12 Respiratory bronchiole with alveoli

13 Alveolar ducts

14 Serosa:
   a. Connective tissue
   b. Mesothelium

15 Lymphatic nodule and vein

16 Adventitia

17 Bronchiole

18 Mucosal folds

19 Smooth muscle

20 Alveolar ducts

21 Blood vessels

22 Respiratory bronchiole

23 Alveoli opening into alveolar duct

24 Alveolar sacs

25 Trabecula with blood vessels

FIGURE 15.8 ■ Lung (panoramic view). Stain: hematoxylin and eosin. Low magnification.

FIGURE 15.9 ■ Intrapulmonary Bronchus (Transverse Section)

The trachea divides outside the lungs and gives rise to the primary, or extrapulmonary, bronchi. On entering the lungs, the primary bronchi divide and give rise to a series of smaller, or intrapulmonary, bronchi.

The intrapulmonary bronchi are lined by pseudostratified columnar ciliated **bronchial epithelium (6),** which is supported by a thin layer of **lamina propria (7)** of fine connective tissue with elastic fibers (not illustrated) and a few lymphocytes. A thin layer of **smooth muscle (10, 16)** surrounds the lamina propria (7) and separates it from the **submucosa (8).** The submucosa (8) contains numerous **seromucous bronchial glands (5, 18).** An **excretory duct (18)** from the bronchial gland (5, 18) passes through the lamina propria (7) and opens into the bronchial lumen. In mixed seromucous bronchial glands (5, 18), serous demilunes may be seen.

In the lung, the hyaline cartilage rings of the trachea are replaced by the **hyaline cartilage plates (11, 14)** that surround the bronchus. A connective tissue **perichondrium (12, 15)** covers each cartilage plate (11, 14). The hyaline cartilage plates (11, 14) become smaller and farther apart as the bronchi continue to divide and to decrease in size. Between the cartilage plates (11, 14), the submucosa (8) blends with the **adventitia (3).** Bronchial glands (5, 18) and **adipose cells (2)** are present in the submucosa (8) of larger bronchi.

Bronchial blood vessels (19) and a **bronchial arteriole (4)** are visible in the connective tissue around the bronchus. Also accompanying the bronchus are a larger **vein (9)** and an **artery (17).**

Surrounding the intrapulmonary bronchus, its connective tissue, and the hyalinge cartilage plates (11, 14) are the lung **alveoli (1, 13).**

FIGURE 15.10 ■ Terminal Bronchiole (Transverse Section)

The bronchioles subdivide into smaller, terminal bronchioles, the diameters of which are approximately 1 mm or less. The terminal bronchioles are lined by **simple columnar epithelium (3).** In the smallest bronchioles, the epithelium may be simple cuboidal. The cartilage plates, bronchial glands, and goblet cells are absent from the terminal bronchioles. The terminal bronchioles represent the smallest passageways for conducting air.

Because of smooth muscle contractions, **mucosal folds (7)** are prominent in the brochioles. A well-developed **smooth muscle (5)** layer surrounds the thin **lamina propria (6),** which in turn is surrounded by the **adventitia (8).**

Adjacent to the bronchiole is a small branch of the **pulmonary artery (2).** The terminal bronchiole is surrounded by the lung **alveoli (1).** Surrounding the alveoli are the **thin interalveolar septa** with **capillaries (4).**

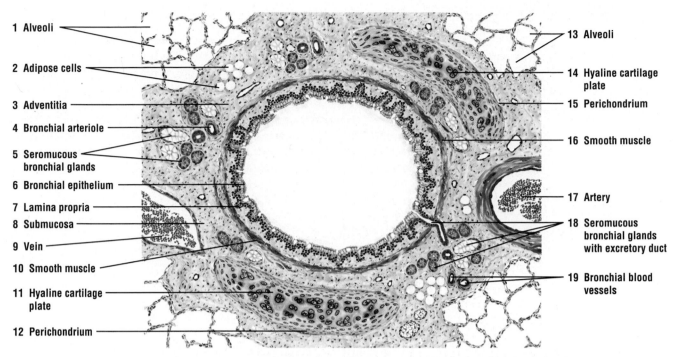

1 Alveoli

2 Adipose cells

3 Adventitia

4 Bronchial arteriole

5 Seromucous bronchial glands

6 Bronchial epithelium

7 Lamina propria

8 Submucosa

9 Vein

10 Smooth muscle

11 Hyaline cartilage plate

12 Perichondrium

13 Alveoli

14 Hyaline cartilage plate

15 Perichondrium

16 Smooth muscle

17 Artery

18 Seromucous bronchial glands with excretory duct

19 Bronchial blood vessels

FIGURE 15.9 ■ Intrapulmonary bronchus (transverse section). Stain: hematoxylin and eosin. Low magnification.

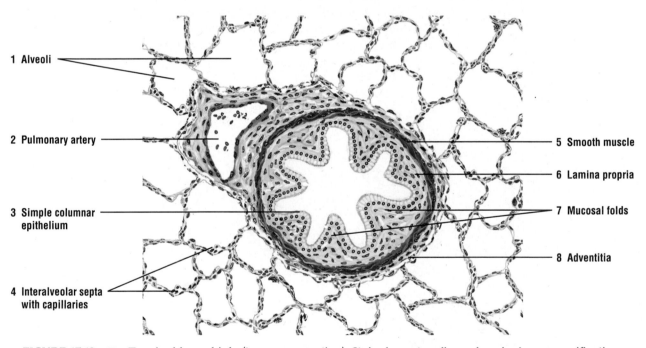

1 Alveoli

2 Pulmonary artery

3 Simple columnar epithelium

4 Interalveolar septa with capillaries

5 Smooth muscle

6 Lamina propria

7 Mucosal folds

8 Adventitia

FIGURE 15.10 ■ Terminal bronchiole (transverse section). Stain: hematoxylin and eosin. Low magnification.

FIGURE 15.11 ■ Respiratory Bronchiole, Alveolar Duct, and Lung Alveoli

The terminal bronchioles give rise to the **respiratory bronchioles (2),** which represent a transition zone between the conducting and respiratory portions of the respiratory system.

The wall of the respiratory bronchiole (2) is lined by **simple cuboidal epithelium (3).** Single **alveolar outpocketings (1, 6)** are found in the wall of each respiratory bronchiole (2). Cilia may be present in the epithelium of the proximal portion of the respiratory bronchiole (2) but disappear in the distal portion. A thin layer of **smooth muscle (7)** surrounds the epithelium. A small branch of the **pulmonary artery (4)** accompanies the respiratory bronchiole (2) into the lung. Each respiratory bronchiole (2) gives rise to an **alveolar duct (9),** into which open numerous **alveoli (8).** In the lamina propria that surround the rim of alveoli (8) in the alveolar duct (8) are **smooth muscle bundles (5).** These smooth muscle bundles (5) appear as knobs between adjacent alveoli.

FIGURE 15.12 ■ Alveolar Walls and Alveolar Cells

The **alveoli (3)** are evaginations, or outpocketings, of the respiratory bronchioles, alveolar ducts, and alveolar sacs, which are the terminal ends of the alveolar ducts. The alveoli (3) are lined by a layer of thin, simple squamous **alveolar cells (type I pneumocytes) (7).** The adjacent alveoli (3) share common **interalveolar septa (4),** or alveolar walls.

The interalveolar septa (4) consist of simple squamous alveolar cells (7), fine connective tissue fibers and fibroblasts, and numerous **capillaries (1).** The thin interalveolar septa (4) bring the capillaries (1) close to the squamous alveolar cells (7) of the adjacent alveoli (3).

In addition, the alveoli (3) also contain **alveolar macrophages (dust cells) (6).** Normally, the alveolar macrophages (6) contain several carbon or dust particles in their cytoplasm. Also found in the alveoli (3) are the **great alveolar cells (type II pneumocytes) (2, 5).** The great alveolar cells (2, 5) are interspersed among the simple squamous alveolar macrophages (6) in the alveoli (3).

At the free ends of the interalveolar septa (4) and around the open ends of the alveoli (3) are narrow bands of **smooth muscle fibers (8).** These muscle fibers are continuous with the muscle layer that lined the respiratory bronchioles.

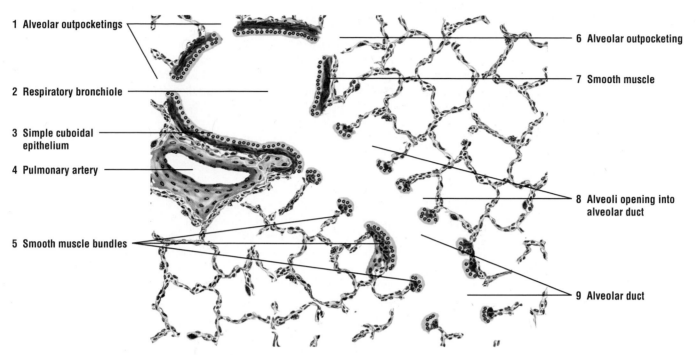

1 Alveolar outpocketings

2 Respiratory bronchiole

3 Simple cuboidal epithelium

4 Pulmonary artery

5 Smooth muscle bundles

6 Alveolar outpocketing

7 Smooth muscle

8 Alveoli opening into alveolar duct

9 Alveolar duct

FIGURE 15.11 ■ Respiratory bronchiole, alveolar duct, and lung alveoli. Stain: hematoxylin and eosin. Low magnification.

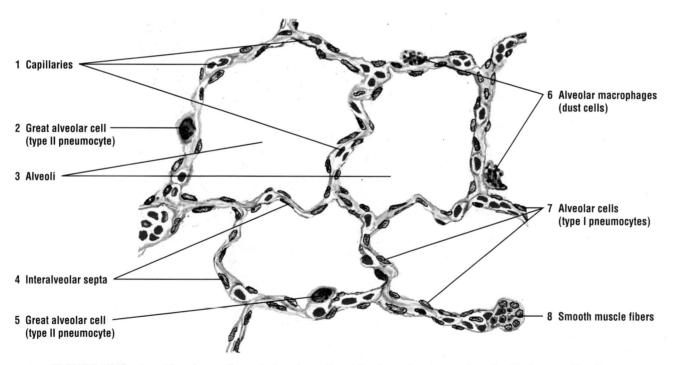

1 Capillaries

2 Great alveolar cell (type II pneumocyte)

3 Alveoli

4 Interalveolar septa

5 Great alveolar cell (type II pneumocyte)

6 Alveolar macrophages (dust cells)

7 Alveolar cells (type I pneumocytes)

8 Smooth muscle fibers

FIGURE 15.12 ■ Alveolar walls and alveolar cells. Stain: hematoxylin and eosin. High magnification.

FIGURE 15.13 ■ Lung: Terminal Bronchiole, Respiratory Bronchiole, and Alveoli

This photomicrograph of the lung shows the smallest air-conducting passage, the **terminal bronchiole (1)**. The terminal bronchiole (1) gives rise to thinner **respiratory bronchioles (4, 9)**, the walls of which are characterized by numerous **alveoli (2, 5, 8)**. Each respiratory bronchiole (4, 9) gives rise to an **alveolar duct (3)** that continues into the **alveolar sacs (6)**. The terminal bronchiole (1) and the adjacent **blood vessel (7)** are surrounded by the alveoli (2, 5, 8).

FUNCTIONAL CORRELATIONS

Conducting Portion

The conducting portions of the respiratory system condition the inhaled air. **Mucus** is continuously produced by **goblet cells** in respiratory epithelium and by **mucous glands** in the lamina propria. These secretions form a mucous layer that covers the luminal surfaces in most conducting tubes. As a result, the **moist mucosa** in the conducting portion of the respiratory system **humidifies** the air. The mucus and ciliated epithelium also filter and clean the air of particulate matter, infectious microorganisms, and other airborne matter. In addition, a rich and extensive **capillary network** beneath the epithelium in the connective tissue **warms** the inspired air as it passes the conducting portion and before it reaches the respiratory portion in the lungs.

Lung Cells

Type I alveolar cells, also called **type I pneumocytes,** are extremely thin, simple squamous cells that line the alveoli in the lung and are the main sites of gaseous exchange. A thin **interalveolar septum** is located between adjacent alveoli. Here, delicate reticular and elastic fibers and a network of capillaries are found. Alveolar cells are in close contact with the endothelial lining of the capillaries and form a thin **blood-air barrier** for respiration.

　　Great alveolar cells, also called **type II pneumocytes** or **septal cells,** are fewer in number and cuboidal in shape. They are found, either singly or in groups, adjacent to the squamous type I alveolar cells within the alveoli. Their rounded apices project into the alveoli above the type I alveolar cells. Great alveolar cells are secretory and contain dense-staining **lamellar bodies** in their apical cytoplasm. These cells synthesize and secrete a phospholipid-rich product, called pulmonary **surfactant.** When released into the alveoli, surfactant spreads as a thin layer over the surfaces of type I alveolar cells, lowering the alveolar **surface tension.** The reduced surface tension in the alveoli decreases the force that is needed to inflate alveoli during inspiration. Therefore, surfactant stabilizes the alveolar diameters, facilitates their expansion, and prevents their collapse during respiration by minimizing the collapsing forces. During fetal development, the great alveolar cells secrete a sufficient amount of surfactant for respiration during the last 28 to 32 weeks of gestation. In addition to producing surfactant, the great alveolar cells can divide and function as **stem cells** for type I squamous alveolar cells in the alveoli. Surfactant is also believed to have some **bactericidal** effects in the alveoli that counteract potentially dangerous inhaled pathogens.

　　Alveolar macrophages, or **dust cells,** are monocytes that have entered the pulmonary connective tissue and alveoli. The primary function of these macrophages is to clean the alveoli of invading microorganisms and inhaled particulate matter by **phagocytosis.** These cells are seen either in the individual alveoli or in the thin alveolar septa. Their cytoplasm normally contains phagocytosed particulate matter.

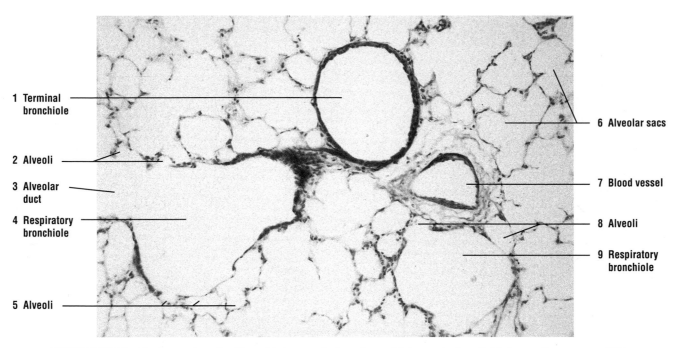

1 Terminal bronchiole

2 Alveoli

3 Alveolar duct

4 Respiratory bronchiole

5 Alveoli

6 Alveolar sacs

7 Blood vessel

8 Alveoli

9 Respiratory bronchiole

FIGURE 15.13 ■ Lung: terminal brochiole, respiratory bronchiole, and alveoli. Stain: mallory-azan. 40×

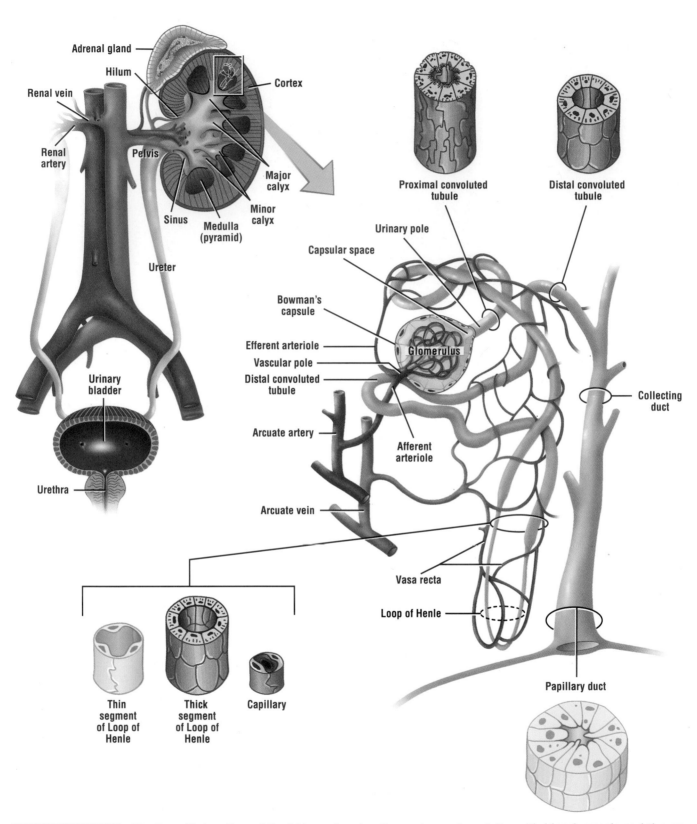

OVERVIEW FIGURE ■ A sagittal section of the kidney showing the cortex and medulla, with blood vessels and the excretory ducts, including the pelvis and the ureter and a histologic comparison of the blood vessels, the different tubules of the nephron, and the collecting ducts.

CHAPTER 16

Urinary System

The Kidney

The urinary system consists of two **kidneys,** two **ureters** that lead to a single urinary **bladder,** and a single **urethra.** The kidneys are large, bean-shaped organs located retroperitoneally on the posterior body wall. Superior to each kidney is the **adrenal gland,** which is embedded in renal fat and connective tissue. The concave, medial border of the kidney is the **hilum,** which contains three large structures: the **renal artery,** the **renal vein,** and the funnel-shaped **renal pelvis.** Surrounding these structures is loose connective tissue and a fat-filled space, called the **renal sinus.**

Each kidney is covered by a dense irregular connective tissue capsule. A sagittal section through the kidney shows a darker, outer **cortex** and a lighter, inner **medulla,** which consists of numerous cone-shaped **renal pyramids.** The base of each pyramid faces the cortex and forms the corticomedullary boundary. The round apex of each pyramid extends downward to the renal pelvis to form the **renal papilla.** A portion of the cortex also extends on each side of the renal pyramids to form the **renal columns.**

Each renal papilla is surrounded by a funnel-shaped **minor calyx,** which collects urine from the papilla. The minor calyces join in the renal sinus to form a **major calyx.** In turn, major calyces join to form the larger, funnel-shaped renal pelvis. The renal pelvis leaves each kidney through the hilum, narrows to become a muscular **ureter,** and descends toward the bladder on each side of the posterior body wall.

Uriniferous Tubules and Nephrons of the Kidney

The functional unit of each kidney is the microscopic **uriniferous tubule,** which consists of a **nephron** and a **collecting duct** into which empty the filtered contents of the nephron. Millions of nephrons are present in each kidney cortex. The nephron is subdivided into two components, a renal corpuscle and renal tubules.

There are two types of nephrons. **Cortical nephrons** are located in the cortex of the kidney, whereas the **juxtamedullary nephrons** are situated near the junction of the cortex and medulla of the kidney. All nephrons participate in urine formation, but juxtamedullary nephrons produce a hypertonic environment in the interstitium of the kidney medulla that is necessary for the production of concentrated (i.e., hypertonic) urine.

Renal Corpuscles

The renal corpuscle consists of a tuft of capillaries, called the **glomerulus,** surrounded by a double layer of epithelial cells, called the **glomerular (Bowman's) capsule.** The inner or **visceral layer** of the capsule consists of highly modified, branching epithelial cells, called **podocytes.** These cells are adjacent to and completely invest the glomerular capillaries. The outer or **parietal layer** of the capsule consists of simple squamous epithelium. Leaving each renal corpuscle are twisted, or convoluted, renal tubules.

The renal corpuscle is the initial segment of each nephron. Blood is filtered in renal corpuscles through the capillaries of the glomerulus, and the filtrate enters the **capsular (urinary) space** between the parietal and visceral cell layers of the glomerular capsule. Each renal corpuscle has a **vascular pole,** where arterial blood vessels that form the glomerulus enter and exit. On the op-

posite end of the renal corpuscle is the **urinary pole.** Filtrate that is produced by the glomerulus leaves each renal corpuscle at the urinary pole and enters the convoluted renal tubule.

Filtration of blood in renal corpuscles is facilitated by the glomerular endothelium. The endothelium in glomerular capillaries is **porous** (i.e., fenestrated) and highly permeable to many substances in the blood; however it is not permeable to the formed blood elements or plasma proteins. Thus, glomerular filtrate that enters the capsular space is not urine. Instead, it is an ultrafiltrate that is similar to plasma, except for the absence of proteins.

Renal Tubules

As the glomerular filtrate leaves the renal corpuscle at the urinary pole, it flows through different parts of the nephron before reaching the renal tubules, called the collecting tubules. The glomerular filtrate first enters the **renal tubule,** which extends from the glomerular capsule to the collecting tubule. This renal tubule has several distinct histologic and functional regions.

The portion of the renal tubule that begins at the renal corpuscle is highly twisted or tortuous and therefore is called the **proximal convoluted tubule.** Initially, this tubule is located in the cortex and then descends into the medulla to become continuous with the loop of Henle. The **loop of Henle** consists of several parts: a thick, descending portion of the proximal convoluted tubule; a thin, descending and ascending segment; and a thick, ascending portion, called the **distal convoluted tubule.** The distal convoluted tubule is shorter and less convoluted than the proximal convoluted tubule, and it ascends into the kidney cortex. Glomerular filtrate then flows from the distal convoluted tubule to the **collecting tubule.** In juxtamedullary nephrons, the loop of Henle is very long; it descends from the kidney cortex deep into the medulla and then loops back to ascend into the cortex (see overview figure).

The collecting tubule is not part of the nephron. A number of short collecting tubules join to form several larger **collecting ducts.** As the collecting ducts become larger and descend toward the papillae of the medulla, they are called **papillary ducts.** Smaller collecting ducts are lined by light-staining cuboidal epithelium. Deeper in the medulla, the epithelium in these ducts changes to columnar epithelium. At the tip of each papilla, the papillary ducts empty their contents into the minor calyx. The area on the papilla that exhibits the openings of papillary ducts is called the **area cribrosa** (see overview figure).

The kidney cortex also exhibits numerous lighter-staining **medullary rays** that extend vertically from the bases of the pyramids into the cortex. Medullary rays consist primarily of collecting ducts, blood vessels, and straight portions of a number of nephrons.

FIGURE 16.1 ■ Kidney: Cortex, Medulla, and Pyramid (Panoramic View)

The kidney is subdivided into an outer **cortex (20)** and an inner **medulla (21)**. Externally, the cortex is covered with a connective tissue **capsule (19)** and the **perirenal adipose tissue (18)**.

The cortex contains **convoluted tubules (3)**, **glomeruli (2, 8)**, **straight tubules (4)**, and **medullary rays (5)**. Also in the cortex are the **interlobular arteries (6)** and **interlobular veins (7)**. The medullary rays (5) are formed by the straight portions of nephrons and collecting tubules. The medullary rays do not extend to the kidney capsule because of the **subcapsular convoluted tubules (1)**.

The medulla comprises a number of renal pyramids. The **base (11)** of each pyramid is adjacent to the cortex (20), and its apex is directed inward. The apex of a renal pyramid forms the pointed **renal papilla (16)** that projects into the **minor calyx (14)**.

The papilla (16) is usually covered with a simple **columnar epithelium (12)**. As the epithelium reflects onto the outer wall of the minor calyx, it becomes a **transitional epithelium (13)**. A thin layer of connective tissue and smooth muscle (not illustrated) under this epithelium then merges with the **connective tissue** of the **renal sinus (17)**.

In the renal sinus (17) between the pyramids are branches of the renal artery and vein, called the **interlobar artery and vein (15)**, or the interlobar vessels. The interlobar vessels (15) enter the kidney and arch over the base of the pyramid at the corticomedullary junction as the **arcuate arteries (9)**. The arcuate arteries (9) give rise to smaller **interlobular arteries and veins (6, 7, 10)** that pass radially into the kidney cortex (20) and give rise to the afferent glomerular arteries that form the glomeruli (2, 8).

FUNCTIONAL CORRELATIONS

Kidney

The kidneys are vital organs for maintaining **homeostasis.** They regulate blood pressure, blood composition, and fluid volume of the body. They also produce urine and maintain the acid-base balance. Urine formation in the kidneys involves three main processes: **filtration** of blood in the glomeruli, **reabsorption** of nutrients and other valuable substances from the filtrate, and **secretion** or **excretion** of metabolic waste products and/or unwanted chemicals or substances into the filtrate. Approximately 99% of the glomerular filtrate produced by the kidneys is reabsorbed into the system in the nephrons; the remaining 1% enters the bladder to be voided as urine.

In addition, kidney cells produce two important hormones, renin and erythropoietin. **Renin** regulates blood pressure to maintain proper filtration pressure in the kidney glomeruli. **Erythropoietin,** which is believed to be produced and released by the endothelial cells of the peritubular capillary network, stimulates erythrocyte production in red bone marrow.

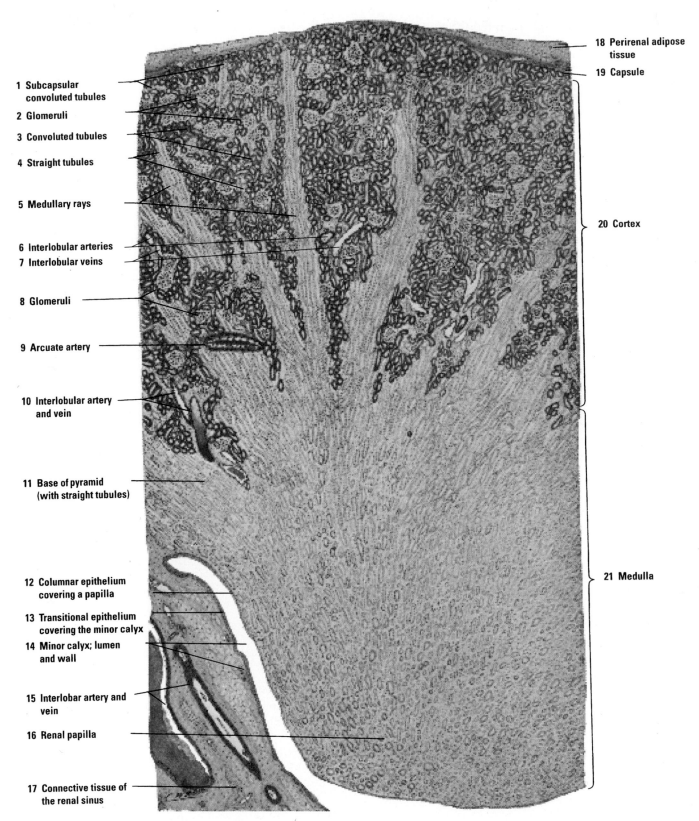

1 Subcapsular convoluted tubules

2 Glomeruli

3 Convoluted tubules

4 Straight tubules

5 Medullary rays

6 Interlobular arteries

7 Interlobular veins

8 Glomeruli

9 Arcuate artery

10 Interlobular artery and vein

11 Base of pyramid (with straight tubules)

12 Columnar epithelium covering a papilla

13 Transitional epithelium covering the minor calyx

14 Minor calyx; lumen and wall

15 Interlobar artery and vein

16 Renal papilla

17 Connective tissue of the renal sinus

18 Perirenal adipose tissue

19 Capsule

20 Cortex

21 Medulla

FIGURE 16.1 ■ Kidney: cortex, medulla, and pyramid (panoramic view). Stain: hematoxylin and eosin. Low magnification.

FIGURE 16.2 ■ Kidney Cortex and Upper Medulla

A higher magnification of the kidney shows the cortex in greater detail. The **renal corpuscles (5, 9)** consist of a **glomerulus (5a)** and a **glomerular (Bowman's) capsule (5b).** The glomerulus (5a) is a tuft of capillaries formed from the afferent **glomerular arteriole (11).** It is supported by fine connective tissue and is surrounded by the glomerular (Bowman's) capsule (5b).

The internal or **visceral layer (9a)** of the glomerular capsule (5b) surrounds the glomerular capillaries with modified epithelial cells, called podocytes. At the **vascular pole (8)** of the renal corpuscle (9), the epithelium of the visceral layer (9a) reflects to form the simple squamous **parietal layer (9b)** of the glomerular capsule (5b). The space between the visceral layer (9a) and the parietal layer (9b) of the renal corpuscle (9) is called the **capsular space (10).**

Two types of convoluted tubules, which are sectioned here in various planes, surround the renal corpuscles (5, 9). These are the **proximal convoluted tubules (1)** and the **distal convoluted tubules (2, 4).** The convoluted tubules are the initial and terminal segments of the nephron. The proximal convoluted tubules (1) are longer than the distal convoluted tubules (2, 4) and therefore more numerous in the cortex. The proximal convoluted tubules (1) exhibit a small, uneven lumen and a single layer of cuboidal cells with eosinophilic, granular cytoplasm. A brush border (microvilli) lines the cells, but it is not always well preserved in the sections. Also, the cell boundaries in the proximal convoluted tubules (1) are not distinct because of extensive basal and lateral cell membrane interdigitations with neighboring cells.

The capsular space (10) in the renal corpuscle (5, 9) is continuous with the lumen of the proximal convoluted tubule at the urinary pole (see Fig. 16-3). At the urinary pole, the squamous epithelium of the parietal layer (9b) of the glomerular capsule (5b) changes to cuboidal epithelium of the proximal convoluted tubule.

The distal convoluted tubules (2, 4) are shorter and fewer in number in the cortex. The distal convoluted tubules (2, 4) also exhibit larger lumina with smaller, cuboidal cells. Their cytoplasm stains less intensely than that of the proximal convoluted tubules (1), and the brush border is not present on the cells. Similar to the proximal convoluted tubules (1), however, the distal convoluted tubules (2, 4) show deep basal and lateral cell membrane infoldings and interdigitations.

Also in the cortex are the medullary rays, which include three types of tubules: **straight (descending) segments** of the **proximal tubules (14), straight (ascending) segments** of the **distal tubules (6),** and the **collecting tubules (12).** The straight (descending) segments of the proximal tubules (14) are similar to the proximal convoluted tubules (1), and the straight (ascending) segments of the distal tubules (6) are similar to the distal convoluted tubules (2, 4). The collecting tubules (12) in the cortex are distinct because of their lightly stained cuboidal cells and cell membranes.

The medulla contains only straight portions of the tubules and segments of the loop of Henle (thick and thin descending segments as well as thin and thick ascending segments). The **thin segments** of the **loop of Henle (15)** are lined by simple squamous epithelium and resemble the **capillaries (13).** The distinguishing features of the thin segments of the loop of Henle (15) are the thicker epithelial lining and the absence of blood cells in their lumina. In contrast, most capillaries (13) have blood cells in the lumina.

Also visible in the cortex are the **interlobular blood vessels (3)** and the larger **interlobular vein and artery (7).** The interlobular blood vessels (3) give rise to the afferent glomerular arteriole (11) that enters the glomerular capsule (5b) at the vascular pole (8) and forms the capillary tuft of the glomerulus (5a).

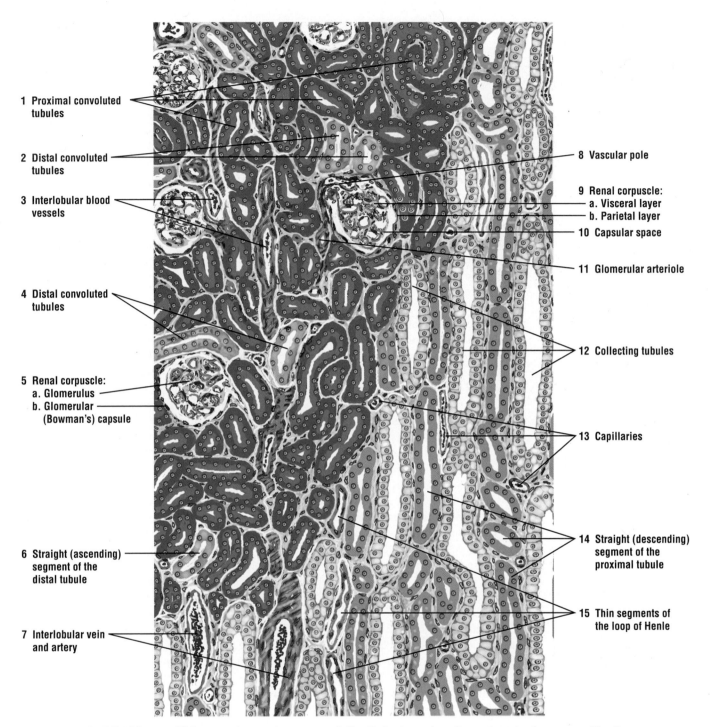

1 Proximal convoluted tubules

2 Distal convoluted tubules

3 Interlobular blood vessels

4 Distal convoluted tubules

5 Renal corpuscle:
   a. Glomerulus
   b. Glomerular (Bowman's) capsule

6 Straight (ascending) segment of the distal tubule

7 Interlobular vein and artery

8 Vascular pole

9 Renal corpuscle:
   a. Visceral layer
   b. Parietal layer

10 Capsular space

11 Glomerular arteriole

12 Collecting tubules

13 Capillaries

14 Straight (descending) segment of the proximal tubule

15 Thin segments of the loop of Henle

FIGURE 16.2 ■ Kidney cortex and upper medulla. Stain: hematoxylin and eosin. Low magnification.

FUNCTIONAL CORRELATIONS

Kidney Tubules

All nephrons participate in urine formation. Resorption of most substances from the glomerular filtrate takes place in the **proximal convoluted tubules.** Cells in the proximal convoluted tubules show numerous deep infoldings of the basal cell membrane, between which are numerous elongated mitochondria. These features characterize cells that are involved in the active transport of molecules and/or electrolytes. The mitochondria supply the necessary ATP (i.e., energy) for pumping ions, such as sodium, from the filtrate across the cell membrane into the interstitium.

In addition to podocytes and endothelial cells, glomerular capillaries also contain specialized cells, called **mesangial cells.** As urine is filtered, numerous macromolecules are trapped in the basal lamina of the glomerulus, and these trapped macromolecules could clog the filtering membrane. Mesangial cells act as **macrophages** in the intraglomerular regions; they phagocytose particulate material that accumulates on the basal lamina during filtration.

As the glomerular filtrate enters the proximal convoluted tubules, all **glucose, proteins, and amino acids;** almost all carbohydrates; and approximately 75% to 80% of water and sodium chloride ions are absorbed from the glomerular filtrate into the surrounding **peritubular capillaries.** The presence of **microvilli** (brush border) on the proximal convoluted tubule cells greatly increases their surface area and facilitates the absorption of filtered material. In addition, proximal convoluted tubules secrete certain metabolites, hydrogen, ammonia, dyes, and drugs (e.g., penicillin) from the body into the glomerular filtrate. The metabolic waste products urea and uric acid remain in the proximal convoluted tubules and are eliminated from the body in the urine.

The **loops of Henle** produce **hypertonic urine** by creating an osmotic gradient from the cortex of the kidney to the tips of the renal papillae. Sodium chloride and urea are transported and concentrated in the interstitial tissue of the kidney medulla by a complex, countercurrent multiplier system that creates a high interstitial osmolarity deep in the medulla. The hypertonicity (i.e., high osmotic pressure) of extracellular fluid in the medulla removes water from the glomerular filtrate as it flows through these tubules. In the juxtamedullary nephrons, the loops of Henle are very long, extend deep into the medulla, and assist in maintaining the high osmotic gradient that is necessary for removing water from the filtrate into the interstitium.

The **distal convoluted tubules** are shorter and less convoluted than the proximal convoluted tubules. The basolateral membranes of distal convoluted tubule cells show increased interdigitations and the presence of elongated mitochondria within these infoldings. The main function of the distal convoluted tubules is to actively resorb sodium ions from the tubular filtrate. This activity is directly linked with the excretion of hydrogen and potassium ions into the tubular fluid.

Sodium reabsorption in the distal convoluted tubules is controlled by the hormone **aldosterone,** which is secreted by the adrenal cortex. In the presence of aldosterone, cells of the distal convoluted tubules actively absorb sodium and chloride ions from the filtrate and transport them across the cell membrane into the interstitium, where they are absorbed by the **peritubular capillaries** and returned to the body. Thus, the functions of distal convoluted tubules are vital for maintaining the acid-base balance of body fluids.

FIGURE 16.3 ■ Kidney Cortex: Juxtaglomerular Apparatus

A higher magnification of the kidney cortex illustrates the renal corpuscle, convoluted tubules, and juxtaglomerular apparatus.

The renal corpuscle exhibits **glomerular capillaries (2)**, the **parietal layer (10a)** and **visceral layer (10b)** epithelium of the **glomerular (Bowman's) capsule (10)**, and the **capsular space (13)**. Brush borders and acidophilic cells distinguish the **proximal convoluted tubules (6, 14)** from the **distal convoluted tubules (1, 15)**, the smaller, less intensely stained cells of which lack brush borders. The cuboidal cells of the **collecting tubules (8)** exhibit cell outlines and pale cytoplasm. Distinct **basement membranes (9)** surround these tubules.

An interlobular **arteriole (7b)** ascends the kidney cortex and gives rise to **afferent glomerular arteriole (12)**. Each renal corpuscle exhibits a vascular pole, where the afferent glomerular arteriole (12) enters and the efferent glomerular arterioles exit. The interlobular **venule (7a)** collects blood from the efferent glomerular arteriole. On the opposite side of the renal corpuscle is the **urinary pole (11)**. Here, the capsular space (13) becomes continuous with the lumen of the proximal convoluted tubule (6, 14). The plane of section through both the vascular and urinary poles is only occasionally seen in the kidney cortex. However, this section shows the renal corpuscle, where blood is filtered and glomerular filtrate is accumulated.

At the vascular pole, the smooth muscle cells in the tunica media of the afferent glomerular arteriole (12) are replaced by modified epithelioid-like cells with cytoplasmic granules. These cells are the **juxtaglomerular cells (4)**. In the adjacent distal convoluted tubule, the cells that border the juxtaglomerular cells (4) are narrow and more columnar. This area of darker, more compact cell arrangement is called the **macula densa (5)**. The juxtaglomerular cells (4) in the afferent glomerular arteriole (12) and the macula densa (5) cells in the distal convoluted tubule form the juxtaglomerular apparatus.

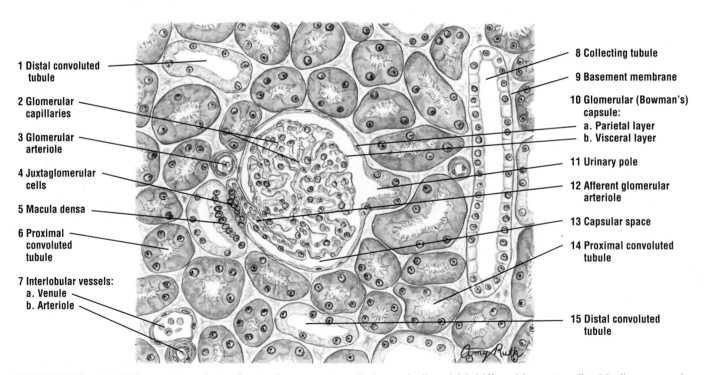

1 Distal convoluted tubule
2 Glomerular capillaries
3 Glomerular arteriole
4 Juxtaglomerular cells
5 Macula densa
6 Proximal convoluted tubule
7 Interlobular vessels:
  a. Venule
  b. Arteriole

8 Collecting tubule
9 Basement membrane
10 Glomerular (Bowman's) capsule:
  a. Parietal layer
  b. Visceral layer
11 Urinary pole
12 Afferent glomerular arteriole
13 Capsular space
14 Proximal convoluted tubule
15 Distal convoluted tubule

FIGURE 16.3 ■ Kidney cortex: juxtaglomerular apparatus. Stain: periodic acid-Schiff and hematoxylin. Medium magnification.

FIGURE 16.4 ■ Kidney: Renal Corpuscle and Juxtaglomerular Apparatus

This high-magnification photomicrograph shows a renal corpuscle with surrounding tubules. The renal corpuscle consists of the **glomerulus (1)** and the **glomerular capsule (2),** with a **parietal layer (2a)** and a **visceral layer (2b).** Between these layers is the **capsular space (3).** At the **vascular pole (5)** of the renal corpuscle, blood vessels enter and leave the renal corpuscle. Adjacent to the vascular pole (5) is the **juxtaglomerular apparatus (6).** The juxtaglomerular apparatus (6) consists of modified smooth muscle cells of the afferent arteriole in the vascular pole (5), the **juxtaglomerular cells (6a),** and the **macula densa (6b)** of the distal convoluted tubule. Surrounding the renal corpuscle are the darker-staining **proximal convoluted tubules (4)** and the **distal convoluted tubules (8).** Between the convoluted tubules are **blood vessels (7).**

FUNCTIONAL CORRELATIONS

Juxtaglomerular Apparatus

Adjacent to the renal corpuscles and distal convoluted tubules lie a special group of cells, called the **juxtaglomerular apparatus.** This apparatus consists of two components, the juxtaglomerular cells and the macula densa.

Juxtaglomerular cells are a group of modified **smooth muscle cells** in the wall of the **afferent arteriole** just before it enters the glomerular capsule to form the glomerulus. The cytoplasm of these cells contains membrane-bound secretory granules of the enzyme **renin.** The **macula densa** is a group of modified distal convoluted tubule cells. The macula densa cells and juxtaglomerular cells are separated by a thin basement membrane. The proximity of juxtaglomerular cells to the macula densa allows integration of their functions.

The main function of the juxtaglomerular apparatus is to maintain normal blood pressure in the kidney for glomerular filtration. The cells of this apparatus act as baroreceptors and chemoreceptors. The juxtaglomerular cells monitor changes in the **systemic blood pressure** by responding to stretching in the wall of the afferent arteriole. The cells in the macula densa probably respond to changes in sodium chloride concentration and the volume of glomerular filtrate as it flows past them in the distal convoluted tubule.

A decrease in systemic blood pressure and/or a decrease in sodium concentration in the filtrate induces the juxtaglomerular cells to release the enzyme renin into the bloodstream. Renin converts the plasma protein **angiotensinogen** to **angiotensin I,** which in turn is converted to **angiotensin II** by another enzyme in the **endothelial cells** of the lung capillaries. Angiotensin II is an active hormone and a powerful **vasoconstrictor** that initially produces arterial constriction, thereby increasing the systemic blood pressure. In addition, angiotensin II stimulates release of the hormone **aldosterone** from the adrenal gland cortex.

Aldosterone acts primarily on the cells of distal convoluted tubules to increase their reabsorption of sodium and chloride ions from the glomerular filtrate. Water follows sodium chloride by osmosis and increases fluid volume in the circulatory system. The combination of these effects raises the systemic blood pressure, increases the glomerular filtration rate in the kidney, and eliminates the need for further release of renin. Aldosterone also facilitates the elimination of potassium and hydrogen ions and is an essential hormone for maintaining electrolyte balance in the body.

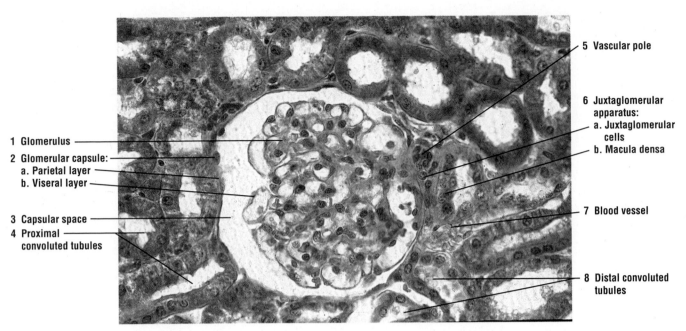

1 **Glomerulus**

2 **Glomerular capsule:**
  a. Parietal layer
  b. Viseral layer

3 **Capsular space**

4 **Proximal**
  convoluted tubules

5 **Vascular pole**

6 **Juxtaglomerular**
  apparatus:
  a. Juxtaglomerular
     cells
  b. Macula densa

7 **Blood vessel**

8 **Distal convoluted**
  tubules

FIGURE 16.4 ■ Kidney: renal corpuscle and juxtaglomerular apparatus. Stain: Mallory's trichrome. 130×

FIGURE 16.5 ■ Kidney Medulla: Papillary Region (Transverse Section)

The papilla in the kidney faces the minor calyx and contains the terminal portions of the collecting tubules, now called the **papillary ducts (3)**. The papillary ducts (3) exhibit large diameters and wide lumina, and they are lined by tall, pale-staining columnar cells. Also in the papillae are the **straight (ascending) segments** of the **distal tubules (7, 10)** and the **straight (descending) segments** of the **proximal tubules (1, 6, 11)**. Note that these straight segments in the medulla are very similar to the corresponding convoluted tubules in the cortex. Interspersed among the ascending (7, 10) and descending (1, 6, 11) straight tubules are transverse sections of the **thin segments** of the **loop of Henle (5, 8)** that resemble the **capillaries (4, 9)** or small **venules (2)**. The capillaries (4, 9) and small venules (2) are distinguished from the thin segments of the loop of Henle (5, 8) by thinner walls and the presence of blood cells in their lumina.

The **connective tissue (12)** surrounding the tubules is more abundant in the papillary region of the kidney, and the papillary ducts (3) are spaced further apart.

FIGURE 16.6 ■ Kidney Medulla: Terminal End of the Papilla (Longitudinal Section)

Several collecting ducts merge in the papilla of the kidney medulla to form large, straight tubules called **papillary ducts (8)**. The openings of numerous papillary ducts (8) at the tip of the papilla produce a sieve-like appearance, called the area cribrosa. The contents from the papillary ducts (8) enter the minor calyx that is adjacent to and surrounds the tip of the each papilla.

In this illustration, the papilla is lined by a stratified **covering epithelium (10)**. At the area cribrosa, the covering epithelium (10) is usually the tall and simple columnar epithelium that is continuous with the papillary ducts (8).

Thin segments of the **loops of Henle (2, 4, 6)** descend deep into the papilla and are identifiable as thin ducts with empty lumina. **Venules (1)** and **capillaries (5)** are usually identified by the presence of blood cells in their lumina. Also visible in the papilla are **straight (ascending) segments** of the **distal tubule (7)** and **connective tissue (3, 9)**.

FUNCTIONAL CORRELATIONS

Collecting Tubules, Collecting Ducts, and Antidiuretic Hormone

Glomerular filtrate flows from the distal convoluted tubules to **collecting tubules** and **collecting ducts**. Under normal conditions, these tubules are not permeable to water. During excessive water loss from the body or dehydration, however, **antidiuretic hormone (ADH)** is released from the posterior lobe (neurohypophysis) of the **pituitary gland** in response to decreased water levels. This hormone causes the epithelium of collecting tubules and collecting ducts to become highly permeable to water. As a result, water leaves the ducts and enters the hypertonic interstitium. Water in the interstitium is collected and returned to the general circulation via the peritubular capillaries, and the glomerular filtrate in the collecting ducts becomes hypertonic (i.e., highly concentrated) urine.

In the absence of circulating ADH, the cells of the collecting tubules remain impermeable to water, and an increased volume of water remains in the collecting ducts. As a result, urine contains an increased volume of water.

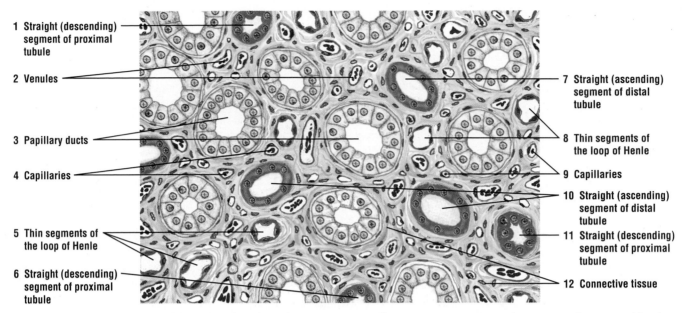

1 Straight (descending) segment of proximal tubule

2 Venules

3 Papillary ducts

4 Capillaries

5 Thin segments of the loop of Henle

6 Straight (descending) segment of proximal tubule

7 Straight (ascending) segment of distal tubule

8 Thin segments of the loop of Henle

9 Capillaries

10 Straight (ascending) segment of distal tubule

11 Straight (descending) segment of proximal tubule

12 Connective tissue

FIGURE 16.5 ■ Kidney medulla: papillary region (transverse section). Stain: hematoxylin and eosin. Medium magnification.

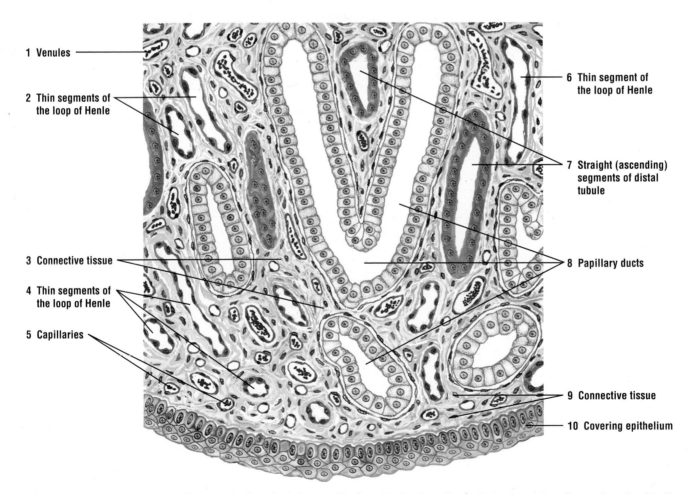

1 Venules

2 Thin segments of the loop of Henle

3 Connective tissue

4 Thin segments of the loop of Henle

5 Capillaries

6 Thin segment of the loop of Henle

7 Straight (ascending) segments of distal tubule

8 Papillary ducts

9 Connective tissue

10 Covering epithelium

FIGURE 16.6 ■ Kidney medulla: terminal end of the papilla (longitudinal section). Stain: hematoxylin and eosin. Medium magnification.

FIGURE 16.7 ■ Kidney: Ducts of Medullary Region (Longitudinal Section)

The medullary region of the kidney consists primarily of various-sized tubules, larger ducts, and blood vessels of the vasa recta. In this photomicrograph, different kidney tubules and blood vessels have been sectioned in a longitudinal plane. The tubules with large, light-staining cuboidal cells are the **collecting tubules (1).** Adjacent to the collecting tubules (1) are tubules with darker-staining, cuboidal cells; these tubules are the **thick segments** of the **loop of Henle (2).** Between the tubules are blood vessels of the **vasa recta (4)** and the **thin segments** of the **loop of Henle (3).** Blood vessels of the vasa recta (4) can be distinguished from the thin segments of the loop of Henle (3) by the presence of blood cells in their lumina.

FIGURE 16.8 ■ Ureter (Transverse Section)

An undistended ureter exhibits an irregular **lumen (4)** that is formed by the longitudinal mucosal folds. The wall of the ureter consists of mucosa, muscularis, and adventitia.

The mucosa consists of **transitional epithelium (9, 10)** and a wide **lamina propria (5).** The transitional epithelium has several cell layers, with the outermost layer being characterized by large cuboidal cells (9). The intermediate cells are polyhedral in shape, whereas the basal cells are low columnar or cuboidal (10). The basal surface of the epithelium is smooth, and no indentations by the connective tissue papillae are found.

The lamina propria (5) contains fibroelastic connective tissue, which is denser and has more fibroblasts under the epithelium and is looser near the muscularis. Diffuse lymphatic tissue and occasional small lymphatic nodules may be observed in the lamina propria.

In the upper ureter, the muscularis consists of an inner **longitudinal smooth muscle layer (3)** and an outer **circular smooth muscle layer (2);** these two layers are not always distinct. An additional outer longitudinal layer of smooth muscle is found in the lower third of the ureter.

The **adventitia (6)** blends with the surrounding fibroelastic **connective tissue** and **adipose tissue (1, 12),** which contain numerous **arteries (8), venules (11),** and small **nerves (7).**

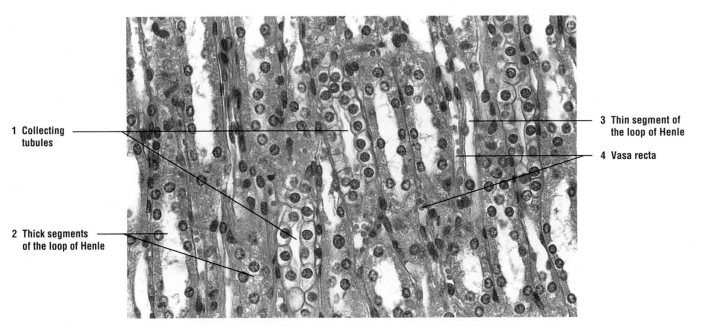

1 Collecting tubules

2 Thick segments of the loop of Henle

3 Thin segment of the loop of Henle

4 Vasa recta

FIGURE 16.7 ■ Kidney: ducts of the medullary region (longitudinal section). Stain: hematoxylin and eosin. 130×

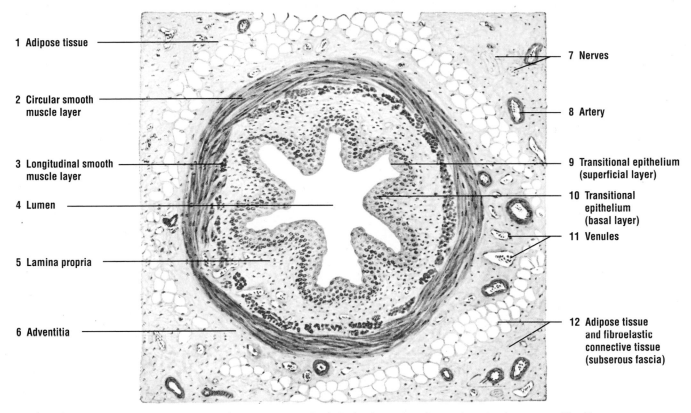

1 Adipose tissue

2 Circular smooth muscle layer

3 Longitudinal smooth muscle layer

4 Lumen

5 Lamina propria

6 Adventitia

7 Nerves

8 Artery

9 Transitional epithelium (superficial layer)

10 Transitional epithelium (basal layer)

11 Venules

12 Adipose tissue and fibroelastic connective tissue (subserous fascia)

FIGURE 16.8 ■ Ureter (transverse section). Stain: hematoxylin and eosin. Low magnification.

FIGURE 16.9 ■ Section of a Ureter Wall (Transverse Section)

This illustration shows a higher magnification of a ureter wall. The **transitional epithelium (7)** in an undistended ureter shows **mucosal folds (6)** and numerous layers with round cells. The superficial cells of the transitional epithelium (7) have a special **surface membrane (5)** that serves as an osmotic barrier between the urine and the underlying tissue.

A thin basement membrane separates the epithelium from the loose **lamina propria (9).**

The muscularis often appears as loosely arranged smooth muscle bundles surrounded by abundant connective tissue. The upper ureter has an inner **longitudinal smooth muscle layer (8)** and a middle **circular smooth muscle layer (2).** A third, longitudinal smooth muscle layer is found in the lower third of the ureter.

The **adventitia (4),** with **adipose cells (3)** and blood vessels (**arteriole and venule [1]**), merges with the connective tissue of the posterior abdominal wall to which the ureter is attached.

FIGURE 16.10 ■ Ureter (Transverse Section)

The ureter is a thick, muscular tube that conveys urine from the kidneys to the bladder. This low-magnification photomicrograph shows a ureter in transverse section. The mucosa of the ureter is highly folded and is lined by a thick **transitional epithelium (1).** Below the transitional epithelium (1) is the connective tissue **lamina propria (2).** The muscularis of the ureter contains two smooth muscle layers, an **inner longitudinal muscle layer (3)** and a **middle circular muscle layer (4).** A third, outer longitudinal muscle layer is added to the wall in the lower third of the ureter. The connective tissue **adventitia (6),** with **blood vessels (5)** and **adipose tissue (7),** surrounds the ureter.

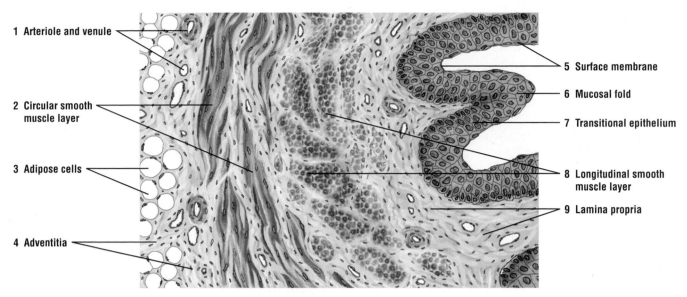

1 Arteriole and venule

2 Circular smooth
  muscle layer

3 Adipose cells

4 Adventitia

5 Surface membrane

6 Mucosal fold

7 Transitional epithelium

8 Longitudinal smooth
  muscle layer

9 Lamina propria

FIGURE 16.9 ■ Section of a ureter wall (transverse section). Stain: hematoxylin and eosin. Medium magnification.

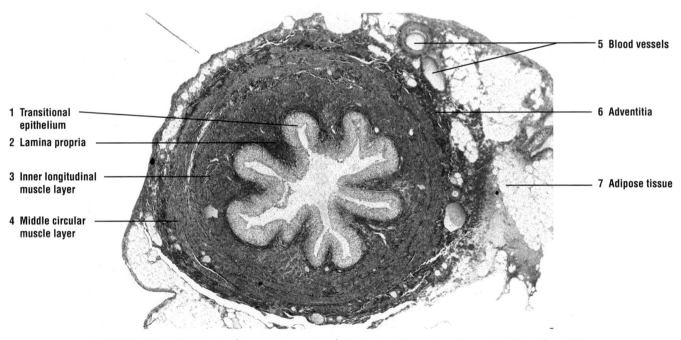

1 Transitional
  epithelium

2 Lamina propria

3 Inner longitudinal
  muscle layer

4 Middle circular
  muscle layer

5 Blood vessels

6 Adventitia

7 Adipose tissue

FIGURE 16.10 ■ Ureter (transverse section). Stain: iron hematoxylin and alcian blue. 10×

FIGURE 16.11 ▪ Urinary Bladder: Wall (Transverse Section)

The **smooth muscle bundles** (1) in the bladder wall are similar to those in the ureters, except for their thickness. The bladder wall consists of a **mucosa** (6, 7, 8), a **muscularis** (1, 9), and a **serosa** (4, 5) on the superior surface of the bladder. The inferior surface of the bladder is covered by adventitia, which merges with the connective tissue of adjacent structures.

An empty bladder exhibits numerous **mucosal folds** (6) that disappear when the bladder is distended. The **transitional epithelium** (7) is thicker and the **lamina propria** (8) wider than in the ureters. The loose connective tissue in the deeper zone contains more elastic fibers.

The muscularis (1, 9) is thick, and the three layers are arranged in anastomosing bundles (1), between which is found **interstitial connective tissue** (2), with blood vessels and **çapillaries** (3). In this illustration, the muscle bundles are sectioned in various planes (1), and the three distinct muscle layers are not distinguishable. The interstitial connective tissue (2) merges with the connective tissue of the serosa (4). **Peritoneal mesothelium** (5) is the outermost layer.

FIGURE 16.12 ▪ Urinary Bladder: Mucosa (Transverse Section)

The mucosa of the bladder wall is illustrated at a higher magnification.

In an empty bladder, the superficial cells of the **transitional epithelium** (4) are low cuboidal or columnar and appear dome-shaped. Also, some superficial cells may be **binucleate cells** (6); in other words, they contain two nuclei. When the bladder wall is stretched, superficial cells appear squamous, and the thickness of the transitional epithelium (4) may be reduced to approximately three layers. The **outer plasma membrane** (5) of the superficial cells in the epithelium is prominent. The deeper cells in the epithelium are round (5), and the basal cells are more columnar (see also Fig. 2-7).

The subepithelial **lamina propria** (3) contains fine connective tissue fibers, numerous fibroblasts, and blood vessels (a **venule** and an **arteriole** [2]). The muscularis consists of three indistinct muscle layers that are visible as **smooth muscle bundles** (1) sectioned here in the longitudinal and transverse planes.

FUNCTIONAL CORRELATIONS

Urinary Bladder

The **urinary bladder** is a hollow organ with a thick, muscular wall. Its main function is to store urine. Because the lumen of the bladder is lined with a **transitional epithelium,** the wall of the organ can stretch or enlarge (change shape) as the bladder fills with urine. When the bladder is empty, the thick transitional epithelium may exhibit five or six layers of cells. The superficial cells in the epithelium are cuboidal, large, and dome-shaped, and they bulge into the lumen. When the bladder fills with urine, however, the transitional epithelium is stretched, and the cells in the epithelium appear thinner and squamous to accommodate the increased volume of urine.

The changes in the appearance and cell shapes in the transitional epithelium result from the unique, thickened regions in the plasma membrane of superficial cells, called **plaques.** The plaques are connected to thinner, shorter, and more flexible **interplaque regions.** These structures act like "hinges," and in an empty bladder, the interplaque regions allow the cell membrane to fold. When the bladder is filled with urine, these folds disappear, and the plaques allow the cells to expand during full stretch.

The exposed cell membrane of superficial cells in the transitional epithelium is also thicker. In addition, **desmosomes** and **occluding junctions** attach the cells to each other. The plaques are impermeable to water, salts, and urine, even when the epithelium is fully stretched. These unique properties of transitional epithelium in the urinary passages provide an effective **osmotic barrier** between urine and the underlying connective tissue.

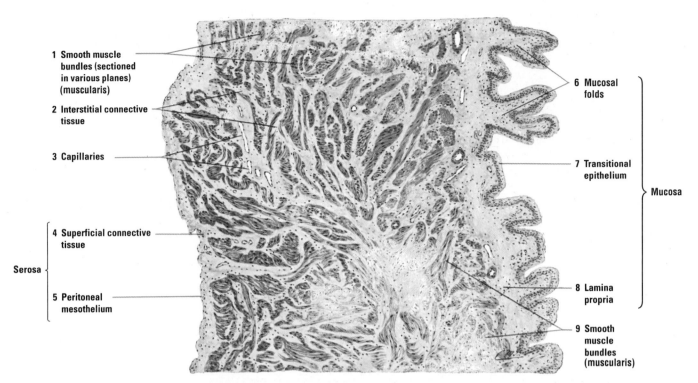

1 Smooth muscle bundles (sectioned in various planes) (muscularis)

2 Interstitial connective tissue

3 Capillaries

6 Mucosal folds

7 Transitional epithelium

Mucosa

Serosa

4 Superficial connective tissue

5 Peritoneal mesothelium

8 Lamina propria

9 Smooth muscle bundles (muscularis)

FIGURE 16.11 ■ Urinary bladder: wall (transverse section). Stain: hematoxylin and eosin. Low magnification.

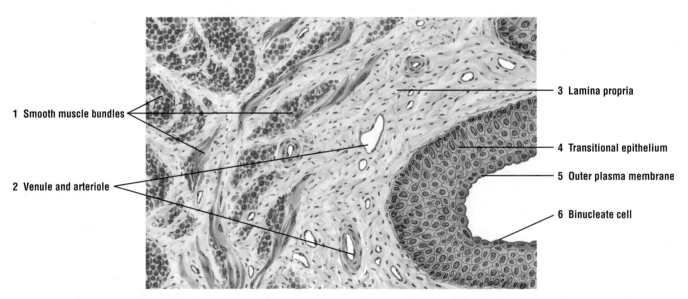

1 Smooth muscle bundles

2 Venule and arteriole

3 Lamina propria

4 Transitional epithelium

5 Outer plasma membrane

6 Binucleate cell

FIGURE 16.12 ■ Urinary bladder: mucosa (transverse section). Stain: hematoxylin and eosin. Medium magnification.

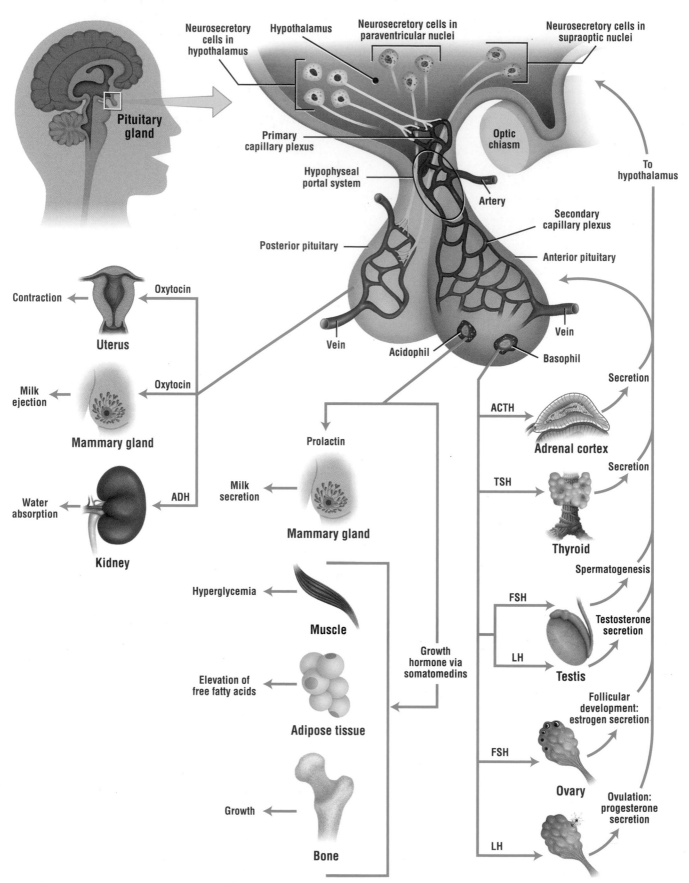

OVERVIEW FIGURE—HYPOTHALAMUS AND HYPOPHYSIS (PITUITARY GLAND) ■ Hypothalamus and hypophysis (pituitary gland). A section of the hypothalamus and hypophysis illustrates the neuronal, axonal, and the vascular connections between these two organs. Also illustrated are the major target cells, tissues, and organs of the hormones that are produced by both the anterior and posterior pituitary gland (hypophysis).

CHAPTER 17

Endocrine System

SECTION 1 ■ Hypophysis (Pituitary Gland)

The endocrine system consists of cells, tissues, and organs that synthesize and secrete **hormones** directly into blood and lymph capillaries. As a result, endocrine glands and organs are **ductless,** because they do not have excretory ducts. Furthermore, the cells in most endocrine tissues and organs are arranged into **cords** and **clumps** and are surrounded by an extensive **capillary network.**

Hormones produced by endocrine cells include peptides, proteins, steroids, amino acid derivatives, and catecholamines. Hormones are released directly into the bloodstream and then transported to distant **target organs.** Here, they influence the structure and function of the target organ cells by binding to specific hormone receptors. **Hormone receptors** can be located on the plasma membrane, cytoplasm, or nucleus of the target cells. Receptors for protein and peptide hormones usually are located on cell surfaces. Other receptors are intracellular and are used by hormones that diffuse through cellular and nuclear membranes.

Numerous organs contain individual endocrine cells or endocrine tissues. Such mixed (endocrine–exocrine) organs are the pancreas, the kidneys, reproductive organs of both sexes, the placenta, and the gastrointestinal tract. Endocrine cells and tissues are discussed with the specific exocrine organs in their respective chapters.

Complete endocrine organs or glands are also found (Overview Figure—Hypothalamus and Hypophysis [pituitary gland]). These include the **hypophysis** or **pituitary gland** (described below), **thyroid gland, adrenal (suprarenal) glands,** and **parathyroid glands** (described in Section 2).

The structure and function of the hypophysis reflect its dual embryological origin. During development, the epithelium of the **pharyngeal roof** (oral cavity) forms an outpocketing, called the **hypophyseal (Rathke's) pouch.** As development proceeds, the hypophyseal pouch detaches from the oral cavity and becomes the cellular or glandular portion of the hypophysis, called the **adenohypophysis (anterior pituitary).** At the same time, the downgrowth from the developing brain (diencephalon) forms the neural portion of the hypophysis, called the **neurohypophysis (posterior pituitary).** The two seperately developed structures then unite to form a single gland, called the **hypophysis.** The hypophysis remains attached to a ventral extension of the brain, called the **hypothalamus.** A short stalk, called the **infundibulum,** is a neural pathway that attaches the hypophysis to the hypothalamus. The neurons in the hypothalamus control the release of hormones from the adenohypophysis and secrete hormones that are stored in and released from the neurohypophysis.

After development, the hypophysis is located in a bony depression of the sphenoid bone of the skull, called the **sella turcica,** that is located inferior to the hypothalamus.

Subdivisions of the Hypophysis

The adenohypophysis has three subdivisions: the pars distalis, pars tuberalis, and pars intermedia. The **pars distalis** is the largest part of the hypophysis. The **pars tuberalis** surrounds the neural stalk. The **pars intermedia** is a thin cell layer between the pars distalis and the neurohypophysis; it represents the remnant of the hypophyseal pouch. The pars intermedia is rudimentary in humans.

The neurohypophysis also consists of three parts: the median eminence, infudibulum, and pars nervosa. The **median eminence** is located at the base of the hypothalamus, from which extends the **infundibulum.** The large portion of the neurohypophysis is the **pars nervosa.**

Vascular and Neural Connections of the Hypophysis

Because the adenohypophysis does not develop from neural tissue, it establishes a rich vascular connection with the **hypothalamus** of the brain via the hypophyseal portal system. **Superior hypophyseal arteries** from the internal carotid artery supply the pars tuberalis, median eminence, and infundibulum of the hypophysis. These arteries form a **primary capillary plexus** in the median eminence of the hypothalamus. Secretory neurons in the hypothalamus synthesize hormones that have a direct influence on cell functions in the adenohypophysis. The axons of these neurons extend to and terminate on the capillaries of the primary capillary plexus, into which they release their hormones.

Small venules drain the primary capillary plexus and deliver blood to a **secondary capillary plexus** in the pars distalis of the adenohypophysis. The venules that connect the primary capillary plexus of the hypothalamus with the secondary capillary plexus in the adenohypophysis form the **hypophyseal portal system.** To ensure efficient transport of hormones, capillaries in the primary and secondary capillary plexuses are **fenestrated** (i.e., contain small pores).

In contrast, the neurohypophysis has a direct neural connection with the brain. As a result, the neurophypophysis does not contain any neurons; it remains connected to the brain by a multitude of unmyelinated axons. The **neurons,** or cell bodies, of these axons are located in the **supraoptic** and **paraventricular nuclei** of the hypothalamus. The unmyelinated axons that extend from the hypothalamus into the neurohypophysis form the **hypothalamohypophyseal tract** and the bulk of the neurohypophysis.

Neurons in the hypothalamus synthesize the hormones that are released from the neurohypophysis. These hormones bind to the carrier glycoprotein **neurophysin** and then are transported from the hypothalamus down the axons to the neurohypophysis. Here, the hormones accumulate and are stored in the distended terminal ends of unmyelinated axons as **Herring bodies.** When needed, hormones from the neurohypophysis are released directly into fenestrated capillaries by nerve impulses from the hypothalamus.

FIGURE 17.1 ■ Hypophysis (Panoramic View, Sagittal Section)

The hypophysis (pituitary gland) consists of two major subdivisions, the adenohypophysis and the neurohypophysis. The adenohypophysis is further subdivided into the **pars distalis (anterior lobe) (5), pars tuberalis (9),** and **pars intermedia (10).** The neurohypophysis is divided into the **pars nervosa (infundibular process) (11), infudibulum (8),** and tuber cinereum of the median eminence (not illustrated). The pars tuberalis (9) surrounds the infundibulum (8) and is visible both above and below the infundibulum (8) in a sagittal section. The infudibulum (8) connects the hypophysis with the hypothalamus at the base of the brain.

The pars distalis (5) contains two main cell types, chromophobe cells (also called **chromophobes) (1)** and chromophil cells. The chromophils are subdivided into **acidophils (alpha cells) (3)** and **basophils (beta cells) (4),** which are illustrated at a higher magnification in Figure 17-2.

The pars intermedia (10) and pars nervosa (11) form the posterior lobe of the hypophysis. The pars nervosa (11) consists primarily of unmyelinated axons and supporting cells' pituicytes. **Connective tissue septa (12)** arise from the surrounding capsule and penetrate the gland.

The pars intermedia (10) is situated between the pars distalis (5) and the pars nervosa (11). The pars intermedia (10) contains follicles and colloid-filled cysts.

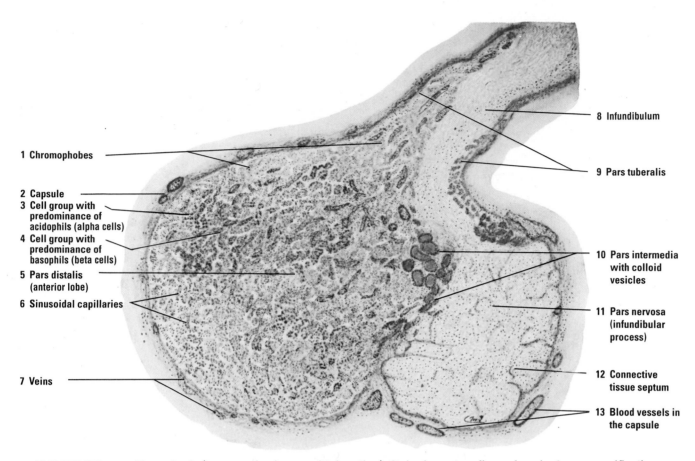

1 Chromophobes

2 Capsule
3 Cell group with
 predominance of
 acidophils (alpha cells)
4 Cell group with
 predominance of
 basophils (beta cells)
5 Pars distalis
 (anterior lobe)
6 Sinusoidal capillaries

7 Veins

8 Infundibulum

9 Pars tuberalis

10 Pars intermedia
 with colloid
 vesicles

11 Pars nervosa
 (infundibular
 process)

12 Connective
 tissue septum

13 Blood vessels in
 the capsule

FIGURE 17.1 ■ Hypophysis (panoramic view, sagittal section). Stain: hematoxylin and eosin. Low magnification.

FIGURE 17.2 ▪ Hypophysis: Sections of Pars Distalis, Pars Intermedia, and Pars Nervosa

With higher magnification, numerous **sinusoidal capillaries (1)** and different cell types are visible in the **pars distalis. Chromophobe cells (2)** have a light-staining, homogeneous cytoplasm and normally are smaller than the chromophils. The cytoplasm of chromophils stains reddish in **acidophils (alpha cells) (3)** and bluish in **basophils (beta cells) (4).**

The **pars intermedia** contains **follicles (6)** and colloid-filled **cystic follicles (7).** Follicles lined with basophils (4) are often present in the pars intermedia.

The **pars nervosa** is characterized by unmyelinated axons and the supportive cells, called **pituicytes (5),** with oval nuclei.

FUNCTIONAL CORRELATIONS

Hypophysis

Hormones produced by neurons in the **hypothalamus** directly influence the synthesis and release of six specific hormones from the adenohypophysis. **Releasing hormones (factors)** are produced by neurons in the hypothalamus for each hormone that is released from the adenohypophysis. For two hormones, growth hormone and prolactin, **inhibitory hormones (factors)** as well as releasing hormones are produced.

The releasing and inhibitory hormones that are secreted from the hypothalamic neurons are carried to the adenohypophysis via the **hypophyseal portal system.** On reaching the adenohypophysis, the hormones bind to specific receptors on cells and either stimulate the cells to secrete and release a specific hormone into the circulation or inhibit this function.

The neurohypophysis stores and releases only two hormones. The neurons in the **supraoptic** and **paraventricular nuclei** of the hypothalamus secrete **vasopressin** (antidiuretic hormone) and **oxytocin,** respectively. These hormones are transported along unmyelinated axons and stored in the axon terminals of the neurohypophysis as **Herring bodies,** from which they are released into the bloodstream as needed.

Cells of the Hypophysis

The cells of the adenohypophysis initially were classified as **chromophobes** and **chromophils** based on the affinity of their cytoplasmic granules for specific stains. The pale-staining chromophobes are believed to be either degranulated chromophils or undifferentiated stem cells. Later, the chromophils were further subdivided into **acidophils** and **basophils** based on their staining properties. Immunocytochemical techniques now identify these cells based on their specific hormones. In the adenohypophysis are two types of acidophils, **somatotrophs** and **mammotrophs,** and three types of basophils, **gonadotrophs, thyrotrophs,** and **corticotrophs.**

The hormones released from these cells are carried in the bloodstream to the target organs, where they bind to specific receptors that influence the structure and function of the target cells. Once the target cells are activated, a **feedback mechanism** (positive or negative) controls further synthesis and release of these hormones by acting directly on cells in the adenohypophysis or neurons in the hypothalamus.

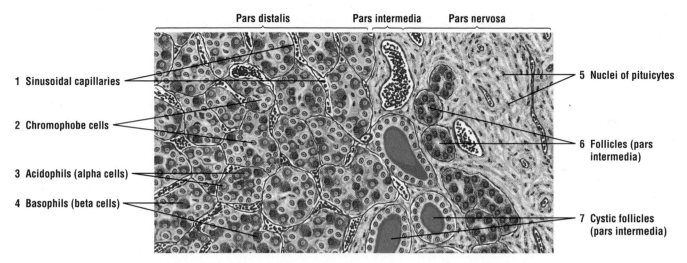

Pars distalis   **Pars intermedia**   **Pars nervosa**

1 Sinusoidal capillaries

2 Chromophobe cells

3 Acidophils (alpha cells)

4 Basophils (beta cells)

5 Nuclei of pituicytes

6 Follicles (pars intermedia)

7 Cystic follicles (pars intermedia)

FIGURE 17.2 ■ Hypophysis: sections of pars distalis, pars intermedia, and pars nervosa. Stain: hematoxylin and eosin. Medium magnification.

FIGURE 17.3 ■ Hypophysis: Pars Distalis (Sectional View)

Cell types in the pars distalis can be identified with special fixation and staining. In this illustration, the hypophysis was fixed with a corrosive sublimate mixture, and the section was stained with azocarmine and differentiated with aniline oil. Phosphotungstic acid was then used to destain the connective tissue; this was followed by cytoplasmic staining with aniline blue and orange G. The cytoplasmic granules stain red, orange, or blue, depending on their respective affinities, and the nuclei of all cells stain orange.

The **chromophobes (3)** usually exhibit pale nuclei and pale-orange cytoplasm with poorly defined cell outlines. The aggregation of chromophobes in groups or clumps is seen in this illustration.

Two types of **acidophils (1, 6)** can be distinguished by their staining. Acidophils (1, 6) with coarse granules stain red (1) with azocarmine stain, and those with smaller granules stain orange with orange G (6).

Basophils (2, 5) contain blue-stained granules. The degree of granularity and the density of the stain vary in different cells.

FIGURE 17.4 ■ Cell Types in the Hypophysis

Groups of different cell types of the hypophysis are illustrated at higher magnification after modified azan staining. The nuclei of all cells are stained orange-red.

The **chromophobes (a)** exhibit a clear and very-light-orange cytoplasm. The clear cytoplasm indicates that the cells do not have granules; as a result, their cell boundaries are indistinct.

The cytoplasmic granules of **acidophils (alpha cells) (b)** stain intensely red, and the cell outlines are distinct. A sinusoid capillary surrounds the acidophils.

The **basophils (beta cells) (c)** exhibit cells that vary in shape and granules that vary in size.

The **pituicytes (d)** of the pars nervosa vary in shape and size. The small, orange-stained cytoplasm is diffuse and barely visible.

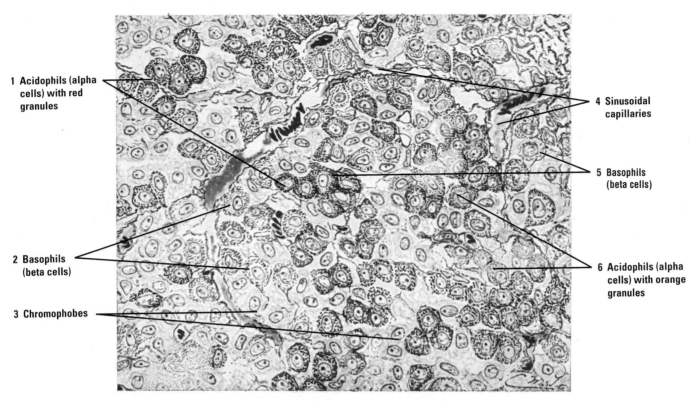

1 Acidophils (alpha cells) with red granules

2 Basophils (beta cells)

3 Chromophobes

4 Sinusoidal capillaries

5 Basophils (beta cells)

6 Acidophils (alpha cells) with orange granules

FIGURE 17.3 ■ Hypophysis: pars distalis (sectional view). Stain: azan (nuclei: orange; cytoplasmic granules of acidophil: red or orange; cytoplasmic organelles of basophils: deep blue; collagen and reticular fibers: blue; erythrocytes: bright red; hemolyzed blood: deep yellow). High magnification.

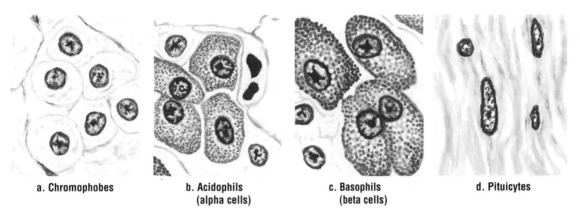

a. Chromophobes

b. Acidophils (alpha cells)

c. Basophils (beta cells)

d. Pituicytes

FIGURE 17.4 ■ Cell types in the hypophysis. Stain: modified azan. Oil immersion.

FIGURE 17.5 ■ Hypophysis: Pars Distalis, Pars Intermedia, and Pars Nervosa (Human)

A higher-power photomicrograph illustrates the cellular pars distalis of the adenohypophysis and pars intermedia and the light-staining pars nervosa of the hypophysis. With this stain, different cell types can be identified in the pars distalis. The red-staining, or eosinophilic, cells are **acidophils (alpha cells) (5).** The cells with bluish cytoplasm are **basophils (beta cells) (4).** The light, unstained cells scattered among the acidophils (5) and basophils (4) are **chromophobes (7).** The pars intermedia exhibits small cysts, or **vesicles (6),** that are filled with colloid.

The pars nervosa is filled with nonmyelinated, light-staining axons of secretory cells, the cell bodies of which are located in the hypothalamus. Most red-staining nuclei in the pars nervosa belong to **pituicytes (2),** the supportive cells. Accumulations of neurosecretory material at the end of the axon terminals in the pars nervosa are the irregularly shaped, red-staining structures called **Herring bodies (3).** Herring bodies (3) are closely associated with capillaries and **blood vessels (1).** Surrounding the secretory cells and axon terminals in the hypophysis are blood vessels (1) and fenestrated capillaries.

FUNCTIONAL CORRELATIONS

Cells and Hormones of the Adenohypophysis

Acidophils

Somatotrophs secrete **somatotropin,** which is also called growth hormone. This hormone stimulates cellular metabolism, general body growth, amino acid uptake, and protein synthesis. Somatotropin also stimulates the liver to produce **somatomedins.** These hormones induce proliferation of cartilage cells in the epiphyseal plates of developing or growing long bones to increase bone length. An increase also occurs in the growth of the skeletal muscle and in the release of fatty acids from the adipose cells for energy production by body cells.

Mammotrophs produce the lactogenic hormone **prolactin,** which stimulates the development of mammary glands during pregnancy. Following parturition (i.e., birth), prolactin maintains milk production in the developed mammary glands during lactation.

Basophils

Thyrotrophs secrete **thyroid-stimulating hormone, or thyrotropin.** Thyrotropin stimulates the synthesis and secretion of the hormones **thyroxine (T_4)** and **triiodothyronine (T_3)** from the thyroid gland.

Gonadotrophs secrete **follicle-stimulating hormone (FSH)** and **luteinizing hormone (LH).** In females, FSH promotes growth and maturation of ovarian follicles and subsequent **estrogen** secretion by developing follicles. In males, FSH promotes **spermatogenesis** in the testes and secretion of **androgen-binding protein** into seminiferous tubules by **Sertoli cells.**

In females, LH, in association with FSH, induces **ovulation,** promotes final maturation of ovarian follicles, and stimulates formation of the **corpus luteum** after ovulation. In addition, LH promotes secretion of estrogen and progesterone from the corpus luteum. In males, LH maintains and stimulates the **interstitial cells** (of Leydig) in the testes to produce the hormone **testosterone.** As a result, LH is sometimes called interstitial cell-stimulating hormone.

Corticotrophs secrete **adrenocorticotropic hormone (ACTH),** which influences the function of the cells in the **adrenal cortex.** In addition, ACTH stimulates the synthesis and release of glucocorticoids from the zona fasciculata and zona reticularis of the adrenal cortex.

Pars Intermedia

In lower vertebrates (amphibians and fishes), the pars intermedia is well developed and produces **melanocyte-stimulating hormone.** This hormone increases skin pigmentation by causing dispersion of melanin granules. In humans and most mammals, the pars intermedia is rudimentary.

Cells and Hormones of the Neurohypophysis

Oxytocin

The main targets of **oxytocin** are the smooth muscles of the pregnant uterus. During labor, the neurohypophysis releases oxytocin to induce strong contractions of smooth muscles in the uterus, resulting in childbirth (i.e., parturition). After parturition, the suckling action of the infant on the nipple activates the **milk-ejection reflex** in the lactating mammary glands. Afferent impulses from the nipple stimulate neurons in the hypothalamus, causing release of oxytocin. Oxytocin then stimulates the contraction of **myoepithelial cells** around the secretory alveoli and ducts in the mammary glands, causing milk ejection into the excretory ducts of the mammary gland and the nipple.

Antidiuretic Hormone or Vasopressin

A sudden decrease of blood pressure is a strong stimulus for the release of **antidiuretic hormone**. Its release into the bloodstream results in strong contraction of the smooth muscle in the walls of small arteries and arterioles. This action constricts their lumina and raises the **blood pressure**. The other main action of antidiuretic hormone is to increase **water permeability** in the **distal convoluted tubules** and **collecting tubules** of the kidney. As a result, more water is resorbed from the filtrate into the interstitium and retained in the body, creating a more concentrated urine.

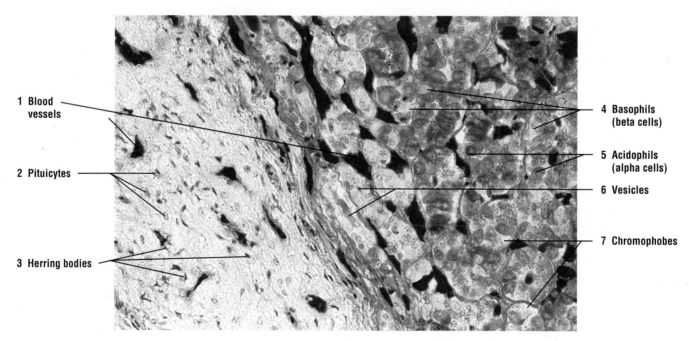

FIGURE 17.5 ■ Hypophysis: pars distalis, pars intermedia, and pars nervosa (human). Stain: mallory-azan and orange G. 80×

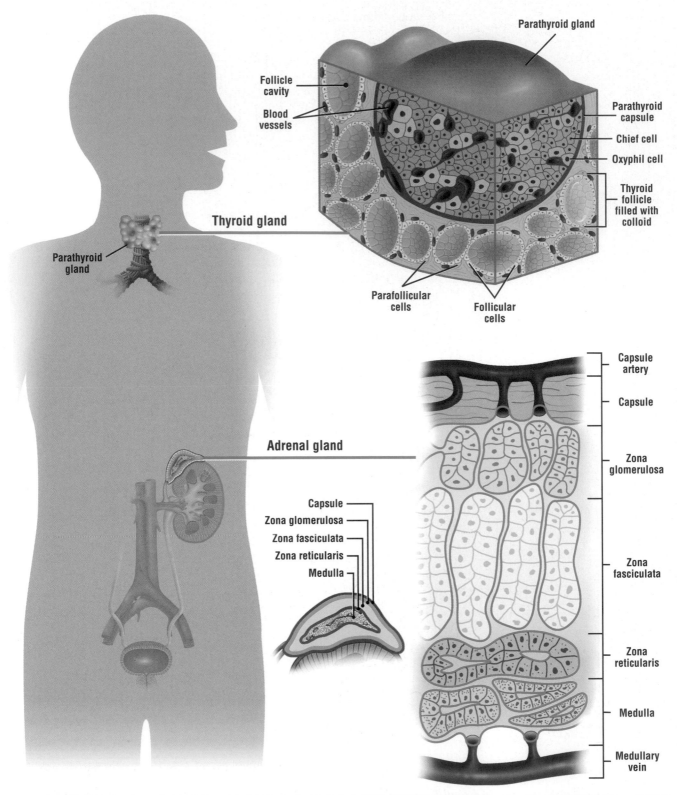

OVERVIEW FIGURE—THYROID GLAND, PARATHYROID GLANDS, AND ADRENAL GLAND ▪ The structural organization and general location in the body of the thyroid gland, parathyroid gland, and adrenal gland are illustrated.

SECTION 2 ▪ Thyroid Gland, Parathyroid Glands, and Adrenal Gland

Thyroid Gland

Located inferior to the larynx, the **thyroid gland** is a single gland that consists of right and left lobes, which are connected in the middle by an isthmus. Most endocrine cells, tisssues, or organs are arranged in cords or clumps, and they store their secretory products within their cytoplasm. The thyroid gland is a unique endocrine organ in that its cells are arranged into spherical structures, called **follicles.** Each follicle is surrounded by reticular fibers and a vascular network of capillaries that allows for easy entrance of thyroid hormones into the bloodstream. The follicular epithelium can be simple squamous, cuboidal, or low columnar, depending on the state of activity of the thyroid gland.

Follicles are the structural and functional units of the thyroid gland. The cells that surround the follicles, the **follicular cells,** also synthesize, release, and store their product outside their cytoplasm (i.e., extracellularly), in the lumen of the follicles, as a gelatinous substance, called **colloid.** Colloid is composed of **thyroglobulin,** which is a glycoprotein containing several iodinated amino acids.

In addition to follicular cells, the thyroid gland also contains larger, pale-staining **parafollicular cells.** These cells are found either peripherally, in the follicular epithelium, or within the follicle. When parafollicular cells are located in a follicle, they are always separated from the follicular lumen by neighboring follicular cells.

Parathyroid Glands

Mammals generally have four **parathyroid glands.** These small glands are situated on the posterior surface of the thyroid gland, but they are separated from the thyroid gland by a thin connective tissue **capsule.** Normally, one parathyroid gland is located on the superior pole and one on the inferior pole of each lobe of the thyroid gland. In contrast to the thyroid gland, cells of the parathyroid glands are arranged into cords or clumps that are surrounded by a rich network of capillaries.

Two types of cells are found in the parathyroid glands, functional **chief cells** and **oxyphil cells.** Oxyphil cells are larger than the chief cells, are found singly or in small groups, and are less numerous than the chief cells. In routine histologic sections, these cells stain deeply acidophilic. On rare occasions, small colloid-filled follicles may be seen in the parathyroid glands.

Adrenal (Suprarenal) Glands

The **adrenal glands** are endocrine organs near the superior pole of each kidney. Each adrenal gland is surrounded by a dense irregular connective tissue capsule and is embedded in adipose tissue around the kidneys. Each adrenal gland consists of an outer **cortex** and an inner **medulla.** These two regions of the adrenal gland are located in one organ and are linked by a common blood supply, but they have distinct embryologic origins, structures, and functions.

Cortex

The adrenal cortex exhibits three concentric zones: the zona glomerulosa, zona fasciculata, and zona reticularis.

The **zona glomerulosa** is a thin zone inferior to the adrenal gland capsule. It consists of cells arranged in small clumps.

The **zona fasciculata** is the intermediate zone. It is also the thickest zone of the adrenal cortex. This zone exhibits vertical columns, with a thickness of one cell, adjacent to straight capillaries.

The **zona reticularis** is the innermost zone and is adjacent to the adrenal medulla. The cells in this zone are arranged in cords or clumps.

In all three zones, the secretory cells are adjacent to fenestrated capillaries. The cells of these zones in the adrenal cortex produce three classes of steroid hormones: **mineralocorticoids, glucocorticoids,** and **sex hormones.**

Medulla

The medulla lies in the center of the adrenal gland. The cells of the adrenal medulla, which are also arranged in small cords, are modified postganglionic sympathetic neurons that synthesize and secrete **catecholamines** (primarily epinephrine and norepinephrine).

The release of epinephrine and norepinephrine from the adrenal medulla is under the direct control of the **autonomic nervous system.** The effects of catecholamines on different organs are similar to those produced by stimulation of the sympathetic division of the autonomic nervous system.

The thyroid gland, parathyroid glands, and adrenal glands are illustrated in Overview Figure 17—Thyroid Gland, Parathyroid Glands, and Adrenal Gland.

FIGURE 17.6 ■ Thyroid Gland: Canine (General View)

The thyroid gland is characterized by variable-sized **follicles (2, 12)** that are filled with an acidophilic **colloid (2, 12).** The follicles usually are lined by a simple cuboidal epithelium consisting of **follicular** (principal cells) **(3, 7).** The **follicles** that are **sectioned tangentially (4)** do not exhibit a lumen. The follicular cells (3, 7) synthesize and secrete the thyroid hormones. In routine histologic preparations, colloid often retracts from the follicular wall (12).

The thyroid gland also contains another cell type, called the **parafollicular cell (1, 8).** These cells occur either alone or in clumps on the periphery of the follicles. The parafollicular cells (1, 8) stain light and are visible in the canine thyroid. Parafollicular cells (1, 8) synthesize and secrete the hormone calcitonin.

Connective tissue septa (5, 9) from the thyroid gland capsule extend into the gland's interior and divide the gland into lobules. Numerous blood vessels, including **arterioles (6), venules (10),** and **capillaries (13),** are seen in the connective tissue septa (5, 9) and around follicles (2, 12). Little **interfollicular connective tissue (11)** is found between individual follicles.

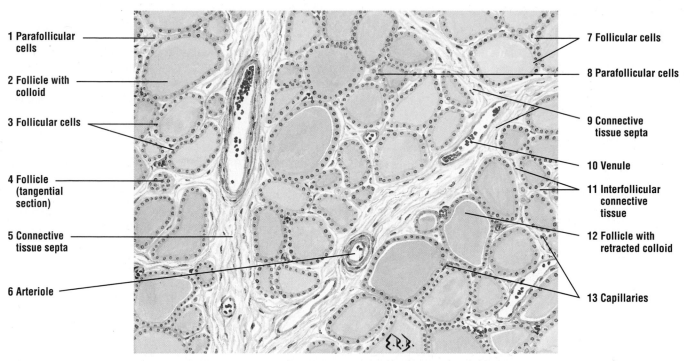

1 Parafollicular cells

2 Follicle with colloid

3 Follicular cells

4 Follicle (tangential section)

5 Connective tissue septa

6 Arteriole

7 Follicular cells

8 Parafollicular cells

9 Connective tissue septa

10 Venule

11 Interfollicular connective tissue

12 Follicle with retracted colloid

13 Capillaries

FIGURE 17.6 ■ Thyroid gland: canine (general view). Stain: hematoxylin and eosin. Low magnification.

FIGURE 17.7 ■ Thyroid Gland Follicles: Canine (Sectional View)

A higher-magnification of the thyroid gland shows details of the thyroid **follicles (2, 9).** The height of the **follicular cells (5, 11)** depends on their function. In highly active follicles, the epithelium is cuboidal (9). In less active follicles, the epithelium appears flat (5). All thyroid follicles (2, 9) are filled with **colloid (2),** some of which show **retraction (12)** from the follicular wall or **distortion (12)** because of slide preparation. A **follicle (7)** that is sectioned at a peripheral or **tangential** angle (7) shows only the follicular cells.

The **parafollicular cells (1, 10)** are located within the follicular epithelium (1) or in small clumps (10) adjacent to the thyroid follicles (2, 9). These cells (1, 10) are larger, oval, or varied in shape, with lighter-staining cytoplasm than that of the follicular cells (5, 11). The parafollicular cells (1, 10) are not directly located on the follicular lumen. Instead, they are separated from the lumen by the processes of neighboring follicular cells (5, 11).

Surrounding the thyroid follicles (2, 9), the follicular cells (5, 11), and the parafollicular cells (1, 10) is a thin **interfollicular connective tissue (3, 8)** with numerous **blood vessels (6)** and **capillaries (4).**

FUNCTIONAL CORRELATIONS

Formation of Thyroid Hormones

The secretory functions of **follicular cells** in the thyroid gland are controlled by **thyroid-stimulating hormone** released from the adenohypophysis. **Iodide** is an essential element for production of the thyroid hormones T_3 and T_4.

In response to thyroid-stimulating hormone from the adenohypophysis, the follicular cells in the thyroid gland take up **iodide** from the circulation via the iodide pump in the follicular basal cell membrane. Iodide is oxidized to iodine in the follicular cells and is transported into the follicular lumen. In the lumen, iodine combines with tyrosine groups to form **iodinated thyroglobulin,** of which the hormones T_3 and T_4, are the principal products. Both T_3 and T_4 remain bound to the iodinated thyroglobulin in thyroid follicles in an inactive form until needed. Released from the adenohypophysis, thyroid-stimulating hormone stimulates the thyroid gland cells to release the thyroid hormones into the bloodstream.

Release of Thyroid Hormones

Release of thyroid hormones involves endocytosis (i.e., take up) of thyroglobulin by follicular cells, hydrolysis of the iodinated thyroglobulin by lysosomes, and release of principal thyroid hormones (T_3 and T_4) at the base of follicular cells into the surrounding capillaries. The presence of thyroid hormones in the general circulation accelerates the metabolic rate of the body and increases cell metabolism, growth, differentiation, and development throughout the body. In addition, thyroid hormones increase the rate of protein, carbohydrate, and fat metabolism.

Parafollicular Cells

The thyroid gland also contains **parafollicular cells.** These cells appear on the periphery of follicular epithelium as single cells or as cell clusters between the follicles. Parafollicular cells are not part of thyroid follicles and are not in contact with colloid.

The parafollicular cells synthesize and secrete the hormone **calcitonin (thyrocalcitonin)** into capillaries. The main function of this hormone is to lower blood calcium levels in the body, which is accomplished primarily by reducing the number of **osteoclasts** in the bones and decreasing their activity. This action reduces bone resorption and calcium release. Calcitonin also promotes increased excretion of calcium and phosphate ions from the kidneys into the urine. The production and release of calcitonin by the parafollicular cells depends only on blood calcium levels and is completely independent of the pituitary gland hormones.

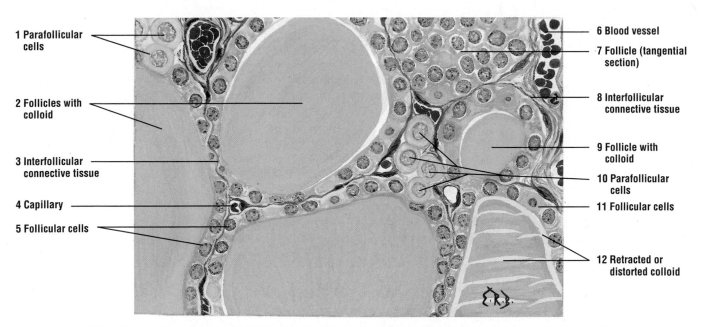

1 Parafollicular cells

2 Follicles with colloid

3 Interfollicular connective tissue

4 Capillary

5 Follicular cells

6 Blood vessel

7 Follicle (tangential section)

8 Interfollicular connective tissue

9 Follicle with colloid

10 Parafollicular cells

11 Follicular cells

12 Retracted or distorted colloid

FIGURE 17.7 ■ Thyroid gland follicles (sectional view). Stain: hematoxylin and eosin. High magnification.

FIGURE 17.8 ■ Thyroid and Parathyroid Glands: Canine (Sectional View)

The **thyroid gland (1)** is closely associated with the **parathyroid gland (3)**. A thin **connective tissue capsule (2)** with **capillaries (9)** and **blood vessels (8)** separates the two glands. **Connective tissue trabeculae (6)** from the surrounding capsule (2) extend into the parathyroid gland (3) and bring larger blood vessels (8) into its interior, where they branch into capillaries (9) around the parathyroid gland cells (3).

The parathyroid gland cells (3) are arranged into anastomosing cords and clumps instead of the **follicles** with **colloid (4)** of the thyroid gland (1). Occasionally, however, an isolated small follicle with colloid material may be observed in the parathyroid gland (3). The parathyroid gland (3) contains two cell types, **chief (principal) cells (7)** and **oxyphil cells (10).** The chief cells (7) are the most numerous cells. They are round and have a pale, slightly acidophilic cytoplasm. The oxyphil cells (10) are larger and less numerous than the chief cells (7), and they exhibit an acidophilic cytoplasm with smaller, darker-staining nuclei (10). The oxyphil cells (10) are found singly or in small clumps. The oxyphil cells (10) increase in number with age.

FIGURE 17.9 ■ Thyroid Gland and Parathyroid Gland

This photomicrograph shows a section of parathyroid gland adjacent to the thyroid gland. A thin **connective tissue septum (3)** separates the two glands. **Follicles** with **colloid (1),** of different size, and lined by **follicular cells (2)** characterize the thyroid gland.

Instead of follicles, the parathyroid gland contains two cell types. The first, **chief cells (4),** are smaller and more numerous, whereas the second, **oxyphil cells (5),** are larger, less numerous, and exhibit a highly eosinophilic cytoplasm. Numerous **blood vessels (6)** surround the secretory cells in both organs.

FUNCTIONAL CORRELATIONS

Parathyroid Glands

The **chief cells** of the parathyroid glands produce **parathyroid hormone (parahormone).** The main function of this hormone is to maintain proper calcium levels in the extracellular body fluids, which is accomplished by raising calcium levels in the blood. This action is opposite, or antagonistic to, that of calcitonin, which is produced by parafollicular cells in the thyroid glands.

Release of parathyroid hormone stimulates the activity and increases the proliferation of **osteoclasts** in bones. This activity results in increased osteolytic activities and release of more calcium into the bloodstream, thereby maintaining normal calcium levels. As the calcium concentration in the bloodstream increases, further production of parathyroid hormone is suppressed.

Parathyroid hormone also targets the kidneys and intestines. The distal convoluted tubules in the kidneys increase both resorption of calcium from the glomerular filtrate and elimination of phosphate, sodium, and potassium ions into urine. Parathyroid hormone also influences the kidneys to form the hormone **calcitriol,** which is the active form of vitamin D. Calcitriol increases calcium absorption from the gastrointestinal tract into the bloodstream.

The secretion and release of parathyroid hormone depends primarily on the calcium levels in the blood, not on pituitary hormones. Because parathyroid hormone maintains optimal levels of calcium in the blood, parathyroid glands are essential to life.

As of this writing, the function of **oxyphil cells** in the parathyroid glands is not known.

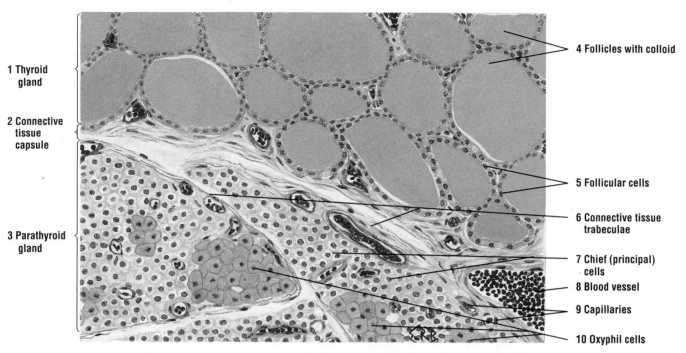

1 Thyroid gland

2 Connective tissue capsule

3 Parathyroid gland

4 Follicles with colloid

5 Follicular cells

6 Connective tissue trabeculae

7 Chief (principal) cells

8 Blood vessel

9 Capillaries

10 Oxyphil cells

FIGURE 17.8 ■ Thyroid and parathyroid glands: canine (sectional view). Stain: hematoxylin and eosin. Low magnification.

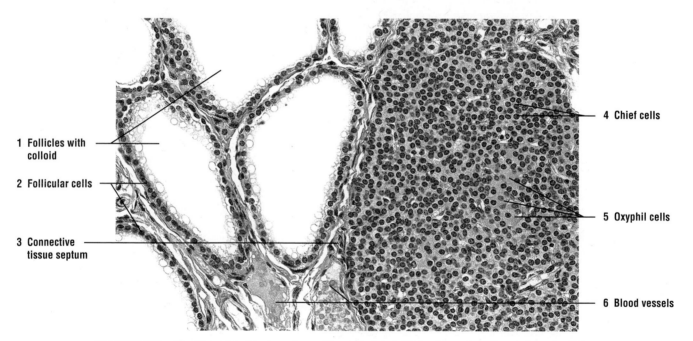

1 Follicles with colloid

2 Follicular cells

3 Connective tissue septum

4 Chief cells

5 Oxyphil cells

6 Blood vessels

FIGURE 17.9 ■ Thyroid gland and parathyroid gland. Stain: hematoxylin and eosin. 80×

FIGURE 17.10 ■ Adrenal (Suprarenal) Gland

The adrenal (suprarenal) gland consists of an outer **cortex (2)** and an inner **medulla (3)** surrounded by a thick connective tissue **capsule (1)** with branches of adrenal arteries, veins, **nerves (5)** (largely unmyelinated), and lymphatics. A **connective tissue septum** with an artery **(4)** passes from the capsule (1) into the cortex. Other septa carry the blood vessels to the medulla (3). The **sinusoidal capillaries (7, 9)** are found throughout the cortex (2) and the medulla (3).

The adrenal cortex (2) is subdivided into three concentric zones. Directly under the connective tissue capsule (1) is the outer **zona glomerulosa (2a).** The **cells** in the zona glomerulosa **(6)** are arranged into ovoid groups. The cytoplasm of these cells (6) contains few lipid droplets.

The middle and widest cell layer is the **zona fasciculata (2b).** The **cells** in the zona fasciculata **(8)** are arranged in columns or radial plates. Because of increased lipid in their cytoplasm, the cells of the zona fasciculata (8) appear vacuolated after normal slide preparation. **Sinusoidal capillaries (9)** between the cell columns follow a similar radial course.

The third and innermost cell layer is the **zona reticularis (2c).** This cell layer borders on the adrenal medulla (3). The **cells** of the zona reticularis **(10, 15)** form anastomosing cords and often contain the dark-staining lipofuscin **pigment (11).** The capillaries in this layer exhibit an irregular arrangement.

The medulla (3) is not sharply demarcated from the cortex. The cytoplasm of the **cells** in the medulla **(14)** appears clear. After tissue fixation in potassium bichromate, called the chromaffin reaction, fine brown granules become visible in the cells of the medulla (14). These granules indicate the presence of the catecholamines epinephrine and norepinephrine.

The medulla also contains **sympathetic ganglion cells (13),** which are seen either singly or in groups. The ganglion cells (13) exhibit a vesicular nucleus, prominent nucleolus, and a small amount of peripheral chromatin.

Sinusoidal capillaries drain the contents of the medulla (3) into the **medullary veins (12).**

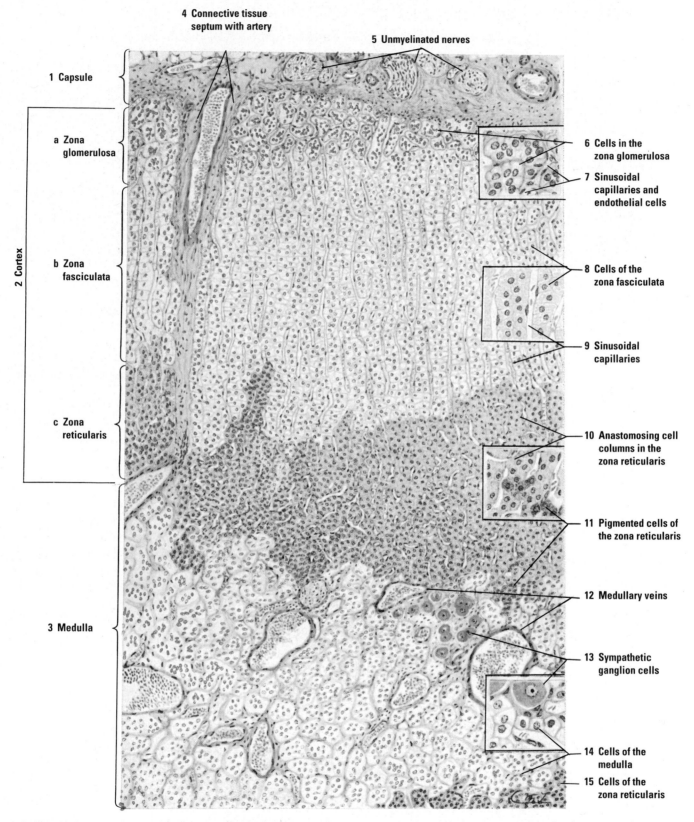

4 Connective tissue septum with artery

5 Unmyelinated nerves

1 Capsule

a Zona glomerulosa

2 Cortex

b Zona fasciculata

c Zona reticularis

3 Medulla

6 Cells in the zona glomerulosa

7 Sinusoidal capillaries and endothelial cells

8 Cells of the zona fasciculata

9 Sinusoidal capillaries

10 Anastomosing cell columns in the zona reticularis

11 Pigmented cells of the zona reticularis

12 Medullary veins

13 Sympathetic ganglion cells

14 Cells of the medulla

15 Cells of the zona reticularis

FIGURE 17.10 ■ Adrenal (suprarenal) gland. Stain: hematoxylin and eosin. Medium magnification (insets: high magnification).

FIGURE 17.11 ■ Adrenal (Suprarenal) Gland: Cortex and Medulla

A lower-magnification photomicrograph illustrates a section of the adrenal gland. The cortex is surrounded by a dense connective tissue **capsule (1)**. Beneath the capsule (1) is the **zona glomerulosa (2),** which contains irregular, ovoid clumps of cells. The intermediate and widest zone is the **zona fasciculata (3)**. Here, the cells are arranged into light-staining, narrow cords, between which are found capillaries and fine connective tissue fibers. The innermost zone of the adrenal cortex is the **zona reticularis (4),** in which the cells are arranged into groups of branching cords and clumps.

The adrenal **medulla (5)** is located adjacent to the zona reticularis (4). In the medulla (5), the cells are larger and also arranged into clumps. Large **blood vessels (6)** (veins) drain the medulla (5).

FUNCTIONAL CORRELATIONS

Adrenal Gland Cortex

The adrenal gland cortex is under the influence of the pituitary gland hormone ACTH. Cells of the adrenal gland cortex synthesize and release three types of steroids: mineralocorticoids, glucocorticoids, and androgens.

The cells of the **zona glomerulosa** produce a potent **mineralocorticoid** hormone, called **aldosterone.** Aldosterone has a major influence on fluid and electrolyte balance in the body. Its primary function is to increase sodium resorption from the glomerular filtrate by cells in the distal convoluted tubules of the kidney and to increase potassium excretion into urine. Because water follows sodium, there is an increase in fluid volume in the circulation. The increased volume increases blood pressure and restores a normal electrolyte balance.

The release of aldosterone from the adrenal gland cortex is initiated via the **renin-angiotensin pathway** in response to decreased arterial blood pressure and low levels of sodium in the plasma. These changes are detected by the **juxtaglomerular apparatus** (juxtaglomerular cells and macula densa) located in the kidney cortex near the renal corpusles.

The cells of the zona fasciculata—and, probably, those of the zona reticularis—secrete **glucocorticoids,** of which **cortisol** and **cortisone** are the most important. Glucocorticoids are released into the circulation in response to stress. These steroids stimulate protein, fat, and carbohydrate metabolism, especially by increasing circulating blood sugar levels. Glucocorticoids also suppress inflammatory responses by reducing the number of circulating lymphocytes from lymphoid tissues and decreasing production of antibodies by lymphocytes. In addition, cortisol suppresses tissue response to injury by decreasing cellular and humoral immunity.

Although the cells of the zona reticularis are believed to produce sex steroids, the steroids are mainly weak androgens and have little physiological significance. Glucocorticoid secretion as well as the secretory functions of the zona fasciculata and zona reticularis are regulated by feedback control from the pituitary gland and ACTH.

Adrenal Gland Medulla

The functions of the adrenal medulla are controlled by the hypothalamus through the sympathetic nervous system. Cells in the adrenal medulla are activated in response to fear or acute emotional stress, causing them to release the catecholamines **epinephrine** and **norepinephrine.** Release of these chemicals prepares the individual for a "fight" or "flight" response, resulting in increased heart rate, increased cardiac output and blood flow, and a surge of glucose into the bloodstream from the liver for added energy.

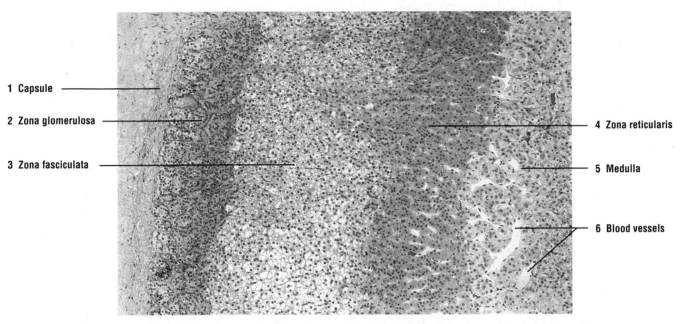

1 Capsule

2 Zona glomerulosa

3 Zona fasciculata

4 Zona reticularis

5 Medulla

6 Blood vessels

FIGURE 17.11 ■ Adrenal (suprarenal) gland: cortex and medulla. Stain: hematoxylin and eosin. 25×

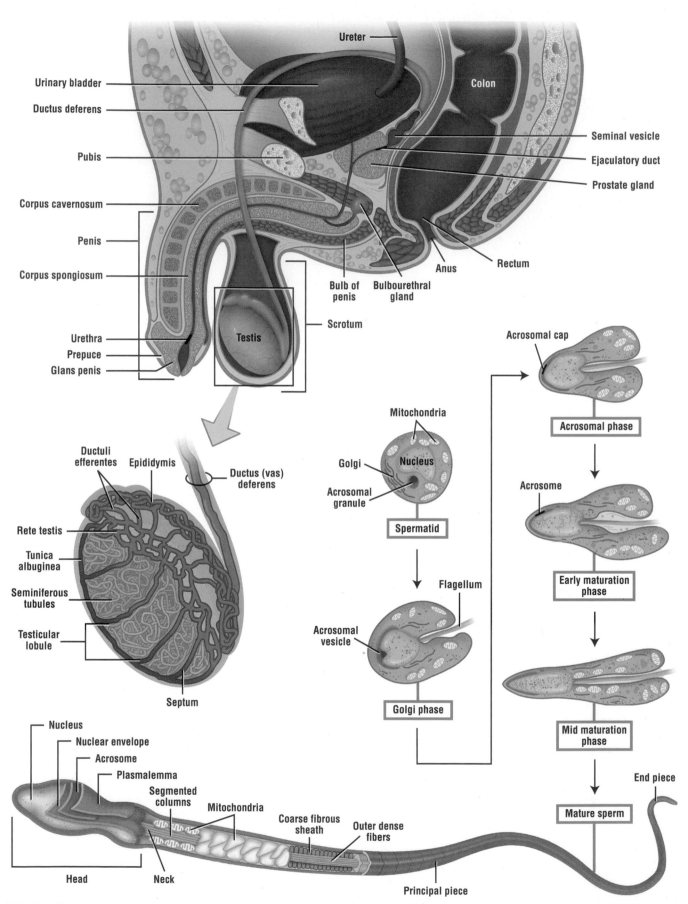

OVERVIEW FIGURE ■ Location of testes and accessory male reproductive organs, with emphasis on the internal organization of the testis, different phases of the spermiogenesis, and structure of a mature sperm.

CHAPTER 18

Male Reproductive System

SECTION 1 ■ Testes, Excurrent Ducts, Ductus Epididymis, and Ductus (Vas) Deferens

The male reproductive system consists of the testes, excurrent ducts, and accessory glands. The **testes** contain **stem cells** that continuously divide and are transformed into **spermatozoa,** or **sperm.** From the testes, the sperm move through excurrent ducts to the **epididymis** for storage and maturation. During sexual excitation, sperm leave the epididymis via the excurrent **ductus (vas) deferens** and exit the reproductive organs through the penile **urethra.**

The **accessory glands** of the male reproductive system are discussed and illustrated in detail in Section 2.

Scrotum

The paired testes are located outside the body cavity in the **scrotum.** In the scrotum, the temperature of the testes is approximately 3° to 4°C lower than normal body temperature. This lower temperature is vital for normal functioning of the testes and **spermatogenesis,** or sperm production. Perspiration and evaporation of sweat from the scrotal surface maintains the testes in a cooler environment.

Equally important in lowering the testicular temperature is the special arrangement of blood vessels that supply the testes. Testicular arteries that descend into the scrotum are surrounded by a complex plexus of veins that ascend from the testes and form the **pampiniform plexus.** Blood returning from the testes in the pampiniform plexus is cooler than the blood in the testicular arteries. By a **countercurrent heat-exchange mechanism,** arterial blood is cooled by venous blood before it enters the testes, which helps to maintain them at a lower temperature.

Testes

A thick connective tissue capsule, called the **tunica albuginea,** surrounds each testis. Posteriorly, the connective tissue of the tunica albuginea extends inward, into each testis, to form the **mediastinum testis.** A thin connective tissue **septum** extends from the mediastinum testis and subdivides each testis into approximately 250 compartments or **testicular lobules,** each containing one to four coiled **seminiferous tubules.** Each seminiferous tubule is lined by stratified **germinal epithelium** containing proliferating **spermatogenic (germ) cells** and nonproliferating **supporting (sustentacular)** or **Sertoli cells.** In the seminiferous tubules, spermatogenic cells divide and are transformed into sperm (see overview figure).

Surrounding each seminiferous tubule are fibroblasts, muscle-like cells, nerves, blood vessels, and lymphatic vessels. In addition, between the seminiferous tubules are clusters of epithelioid cells, called the **interstitial cells (of Leydig).** These cells are secretory and produce the male sex hormone **testosterone.**

Formation of Sperm (Spermiogenesis)

The spermatogenic cells divide mitotically to produce a progeny of cells, including the **primary spermatocytes** and the **secondary spermatocytes.** These spermatocytes undergo meiotic divisions and produce cells, called **spermatids,** with a haploid number (23) of chromosomes. Spermatids do not undergo further divisions.

Spermiogenesis is a complex morphological process by which the spherical spermatids are transformed into elongated sperm cells. During spermiogenesis, the cell size and shape of the spermatids are altered, and the nuclear chromatin condenses. In the **Golgi phase,** small granules accumulate in the Golgi apparatus of the spermatid and form an **acrosomal granule** within a membrane-bound **acrosomal vesicle.** During the **acrosomal phase,** both the acrosomal vesicle and the acrosomal granule spread over the condensing spermatid nucleus at the anterior tip of the spermatid as an **acrosome.** The acrosome functions as a specialized type of lysosome and contains several hydrolytic enzymes that assist the sperm in penetrating the cells (corona radiata) and the membrane (zona pellucida) that surround the ovulated oocyte. During the **maturation phases,** the plasma membrane moves posteriorly from the nucleus to cover the developing **flagellum** (i.e., the sperm tail). The mitochondria migrate both to and from a tight sheath around the middle piece of the flagellum. The final maturation phase is characterized by shedding of the excess or residual cytoplasm of the spermatid and release of the sperm cell into the lumen of the seminiferous tubule. Sertoli cells then phagocytose the residual cytoplasm.

The mature sperm cell is composed of a **head** and an acrosome that surrounds the anterior portion of the nucleus, a **neck,** a **middle piece** that is characterized by the presence of a compact mitochondrial sheath, and a main or **principal piece** (see overview figure).

Excurrent Ducts

Sperm from the seminiferous tubules pass into the intertesticular excurrent ducts that connect each testis with the overlying epididymis. The excurrent ducts consist of the **straight tubules** (tubuli recti) and the **rete testis,** the epithelial-lined spaces in the mediastinum testis. From the rete testis, the sperm enter approximately 12 short tubules, called the **ductuli efferentes** (efferent ducts), that conduct sperm from the rete testis to the initial segment or head of the **epididymis.**

The extratesticular duct that conducts the sperm to the penile urethra is the **ductus epididymis.** This duct continues with the **ductus (vas) deferens** and **ejaculatory ducts** in the prostate gland. During sexual excitation and ejaculation, strong contractions of the **smooth muscle** that surrounds the **ductus epididymis** expel the sperm (see overview figure).

FUNCTIONAL CORRELATIONS

Spermatogonia

The testes produce both sperm and testosterone. Testosterone is a hormone essential for development and maintenance of male sexual characteristics and normal functioning of the accessory reproductive glands.

The spermatogenic cells in the seminiferous tubules divide, differentiate, and produce sperm by a process called **spermatogenesis.** This process involves three phases:
1. Mitotic divisions of spermatogonia that form **primary** and **secondary spermatocytes.**
2. Two successive **meiotic divisions** of spermatocytes that reduce the somatic chromosome numbers by half. This process results in the production of **spermatids,** which are germ cells that contain only 23 single chromosomes (22 + X, or 22 + Y).
3. **Spermiogenesis,** which is a morphological process that transforms spermatids into sperm.

Sertoli Cells

Sertoli cells are the supportive cells of the testes and are located among the spermatogenic cells in the seminiferous tubules. They perform numerous important functions in the testes, including:
- Physical support, protection, and nutrition of the developing sperm (spermatids).
- Phagocytosis of excess cytoplasm (residual bodies) from the developing spermatids.
- Release of mature sperm, called spermiation, into the lumen of seminiferous tubules.
- Secretion of fructose-rich testicular fluid for nourishment and transport of sperm to the excurrent ducts.
- Production and release of androgen-binding protein (ABP), which binds to and increases the concentration of testosterone in the lumen of the seminiferous tubules.
- Secretion of the hormone inhibin, which is a peptide that suppresses the release of follicle-stimulating hormone (FSH) from the hypophysis (pituitary gland).
- Production and release of the antimullerian hormone, also called mullerian-inhibiting hormone, which is a glycoprotein that suppresses the development of mullerian ducts in the male and the development of female reproductive organs.

Blood-Testis Barrier

The adjacent cytoplasm of Sertoli cells are joined by occluding **tight junctions,** producing a **blood-testis barrier** that subdivides each seminiferous tubule into a **basal compartment** and an **adluminal compartment.** This important barrier isolates and protects the more advanced progeny of spematogonia in the adluminal compartment from the immune system, restricting the passage of membrane **antigens** from developing sperm into the bloodstream. Thus, the blood-testis barrier prevents an autoimmune response to the individual's own sperm, antibody formation, and eventual induction of sterility. The blood-testis barrier also keeps harmful substances in the blood from entering the germinal epithelium.

FIGURE 18.1 ■ Testis (Sectional View)

Each testis is enclosed in a thick connective tissue capsule, called the **tunica albuginea (1)**, internal to which is a vascular layer of loose connective tissue, called the **tunica vasculosa (2, 8)**. The connective tissue extends inward from the tunica vasculosa (2, 8) into the testis to form the **interstitial connective tissue (3, 12)**. The interstitial connective tissue (3, 12) surrounds, binds, and supports the **seminiferous tubules (4, 6, 9)**. Extending from the mediastinum testis toward the tunica albuginea (1) are thin fibrous **septa (7, 10)** that divide the testis into compartments, called lobules. Within each lobule are one to four seminiferous tubules (4, 6, 9). The septa (7, 10) are not solid, and there is intercommunication between lobules.

Located in the interstitial connective tissue (3, 12) around the seminiferous tubules (4, 6, 9) are **blood vessels (13)**, loose connective tissue cells, and clusters of epithelial **interstitial cells (of Leydig) (5, 11)**. The interstitial cells (5, 11) are the endocrine cells of the testis, and they secrete the male sex hormone testosterone into the bloodstream.

The seminiferous tubules (4, 6, 9) are long, convoluted tubules in the testis that normally are observed cut in transverse (4), longitudinal (6), or tangential (9) planes of section. The seminiferous tubules (4, 6, 9) are lined with a stratified epithelium, called the **germinal epithelium (14)**. The germinal epithelium (14) contains two cell types, the spermatogenic cells that produce sperm and the supportive Sertoli cells that nourish the developing sperm. The germinal epithelium (14) rests on the basement membrane of the seminiferous tubules (4, 6, 9); its cells are illustrated in greater detail in Figures 18-3, 18-4, and 18-5.

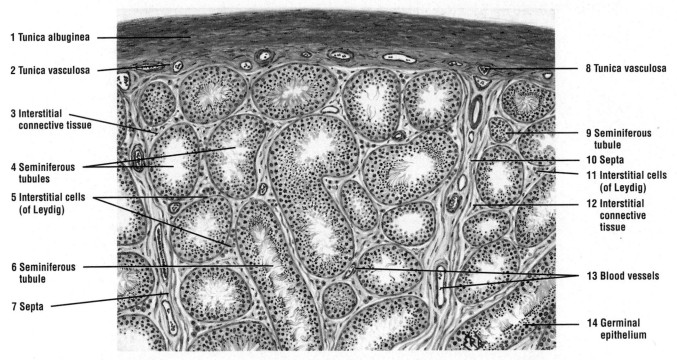

1 Tunica albuginea

2 Tunica vasculosa

3 Interstitial connective tissue

4 Seminiferous tubules

5 Interstitial cells (of Leydig)

6 Seminiferous tubule

7 Septa

8 Tunica vasculosa

9 Seminiferous tubule

10 Septa

11 Interstitial cells (of Leydig)

12 Interstitial connective tissue

13 Blood vessels

14 Germinal epithelium

FIGURE 18.1 ■ Testis (sectional view). Stain: hematoxylin and eosin. Low magnification.

FIGURE 18.2 ■ Seminiferous Tubules, Straight Tubules, Rete Testis, and Ductuli Efferentes
(Efferent Ductules)

In the posterior region of the testis, the tunica albuginea extends into the testis interior as the **mediastinum testis (10, 16).** In this illustration, the plane of section passes through the **seminiferous tubules (3, 5),** the connective tissue and blood vessels of the mediastinum testis (10, 16), and the excretory ducts, called the **ductuli efferentes** (efferent ductules) **(9, 13).**

A few seminiferous tubules (3, 5) are visible on the left. The seminiferous tubules (3, 5) are lined with spermatogenic epithelium and sustentacular (Sertoli) cells. The **interstitial connective tissue (4)** is continuous with the mediastinum testis (10, 16) and contains the steroid- (testosterone-) producing **interstitial cells (of Leydig) (1).** In the mediastinum testis (10, 16), the seminiferous tubules (3, 5) terminate in the **straight tubules (2, 6).** The straight tubules (2, 6) are short, narrow ducts lined with cuboidal or low columnar epithelium that are devoid of spermatogenic cells.

The straight tubules (2, 6) continue into the **rete testis (7, 8, 12)** of the mediastinum testis (10, 16). The rete testis (7, 8, 12) is an irregular, anastomosing network of tubules with wide lumina that are lined by a simple squamous to low cuboidal or low columnar epithelium. The rete testis (7, 8, 12) becomes wider near the ductuli efferentes (9, 13), into which the rete testis empties. The ductuli efferentes (9, 13) are generally straight, but they become highly convoluted in the head of the ductus epididymis. The ductuli efferentes (9, 13) connect the rete testis (7, 8, 12) with the epididymis (see Fig. 18-6). Some tubules in the rete testis (12) and ductuli efferentes (9, 13) contain accumulations of **sperm (11, 14).**

The epithelium of the ductuli efferentes (9, 13) consists of groups of tall columnar cells that alternate with groups of shorter cuboidal cells. Because of the alternating cell heights, the lumina of the ductuli efferentes are uneven. The tall cells in the ductuli efferentes (9, 13) exhibit **cilia (15),** and the cuboidal cells exhibit microvilli.

FUNCTIONAL CORRELATIONS

Hormones of Male Reproductive Organs

Normal spermatogenesis is dependent on the action of **luteinizing hormone (LH)** and **FSH** produced by **gonadotrophs** in the **adenohypophysis** of the pituitary gland. The LH binds to receptors on **interstitial cells (of Leydig)** and stimulates them to synthesize the hormone **testosterone.** The FSH stimulates **Sertoli cells** to synthesize and release **ABP** into the seminiferous tubules. The ABP combines with testosterone and increases its concentration in the seminiferous tubules, which then stimulates spermatogenesis. An increased concentration of testosterone in the seminiferous tubules is essential for proper **spermatogenesis.** In addition, the structure and function of the accessory reproductive glands, as well as the development and maintenance of male secondary sexual characteristics, are dependent on proper testosterone levels.

The hormone **inhibin,** which is also secreted by the Sertoli cells, has an inhibitory effect on the pituitary gland. Inhibin suppresses or inhibits additional production of FSH.

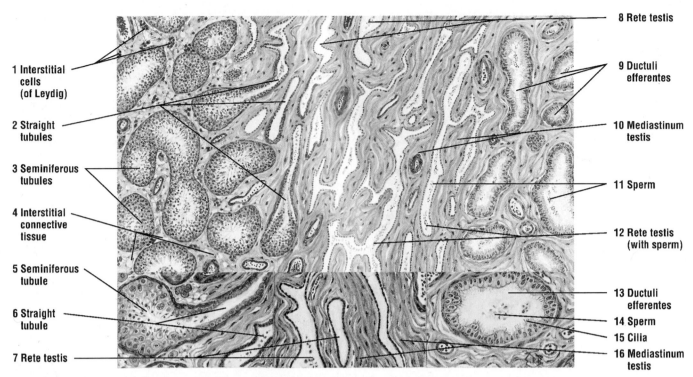

1 Interstitial cells (of Leydig)

2 Straight tubules

3 Seminiferous tubules

4 Interstitial connective tissue

5 Seminiferous tubule

6 Straight tubule

7 Rete testis

8 Rete testis

9 Ductuli efferentes

10 Mediastinum testis

11 Sperm

12 Rete testis (with sperm)

13 Ductuli efferentes

14 Sperm

15 Cilia

16 Mediastinum testis

FIGURE 18.2 ■ Seminiferous tubules, straight tubules, rete testis, and ductuli efferentes (efferent ductules). Stain: hematoxylin and eosin. Low magnification (inset: high magnification).

FIGURE 18.3 ■ Primate Testis: Spermatogenesis in Seminiferous Tubules (Transverse Section)

Different stages of spermatogenesis are illustrated in a **seminiferous tubule (3).** Each seminiferous tubule (3) is surrounded by an outer layer of connective tissue with **fibroblasts (1)** and an inner **basement membrane (2).** Between the seminiferous tubules (3) is the interstitial tissue with **fibroblasts (1, 18), blood vessels (10),** nerves, lymphatics, and the **interstitial cells (of Leydig) (11, 15).**

The stratified germinal epithelium of the seminiferous tubule (3) consists of supporting or **Sertoli cells (6, 7, 14)** and spermatogenic cells, such as **primary spermatocytes (5), spermatids (9),** and **spermatogonia (12).** Sertoli cells (6, 7, 14) are slender, elongated cells with irregular outlines that extend from the basement membrane (2) to the lumen of the seminiferous tubule (3). The nuclei of Sertoli cells (6, 7, 14) are ovoid or elongated and contain fine, sparse chromatin. A distinct nucleolus distinguishes Sertoli cells (6, 7, 14) from the spermatogenic cells (5, 9, 12) that surround the Sertoli cells (6, 7, 14).

The immature spermatogenic cells, called the spermatogonia (12), are adjacent to the basement membrane (2) of the seminiferous tubules (3). The spermatogonia (12) divide mitotically to produce several generations of cells. Three types of spermatogonia are recognized. The **pale type A** spermatogonia (12a) have a light-staining cytoplasm and a round or ovoid nucleus with pale, finely granular chromatin. The **dark type A** spermatogonia (12b) appear similar, but with darker chromatin.

Dark type A spermatogonia (12a) serve as stem cells for the germinal epithelium and give rise to other type A and type B spermatogonia. The final mitotic division of type B spermatogonia produces **primary spermatocytes (5, 16).**

The primary spermatocytes (5, 16) are the largest germ cells in the seminiferous tubules (3) and occupy the middle region of the germinal epithelium. Their cytoplasm contains large nuclei with coarse clumps or thin threads of chromatin. The first meiotic division of the primary spermatocytes (Fig. 18-4, labels I, 5) produces smaller secondary spermatocytes with less dense nuclear chromatin (Fig. 18-4, labels I, 3). The secondary spermatocytes (Fig. 18-4, labels I, 3) undergo a second meiotic division shortly after their formation and are not frequently seen in the seminiferous tubules (3).

The second meiotic division produces **spermatids (4, 8, 9, 13, 17),** which are smaller cells in comparison to the primary or secondary spermatocytes (Fig. 18-4, labels I, 2, 3, 5). The spermatids (4, 8, 9, 13, 17) are grouped in the adluminal compartment of the seminiferous tubule (3) and are closely associated with Sertoli cells (6, 13, 14). Here, the spermatids (4, 8, 9, 13, 17) differentiate into sperm by a process called spermiogenesis. The small, dark-staining heads of the maturing spermatids (4, 8) are embedded in the cytoplasm of Sertoli cells (6, 7, 14), with their tails extending into the lumen of the seminiferous tubule (3).

FIGURE 18.4 ■ Primate Testis: Stages of Spermatogenesis

Three stages of spermatogenesis are illustrated. In the left illustration (**I**), the **primary spermatocytes (in meiosis) (5)** form the **secondary spermatocytes (3),** which undergo rapid meiotic division to form the **spermatids (1, 2)** that become embedded deep in the **Sertoli cell (4)** cytoplasm. Adjacent to the basement membrane are the **type A spermatogonia (6).**

In the middle illustration (**II**), the **spermatids (7)** are near the lumen of the seminiferous tubule before their release. Also visible are round **spermatids (8)** and **primary spermatocytes (9)** close to **Sertoli cells (10).** Near the base of the seminiferous tubule are the **spermatogonia (11).**

In the right illustration (**III**), the mature sperm have been released (spermiation) into the seminiferous tubule, and the germinal epithelium contains only **spermatids (8), primary spermatocytes (9), spermatogonia (11),** and the supporting **Sertoli cells (10).**

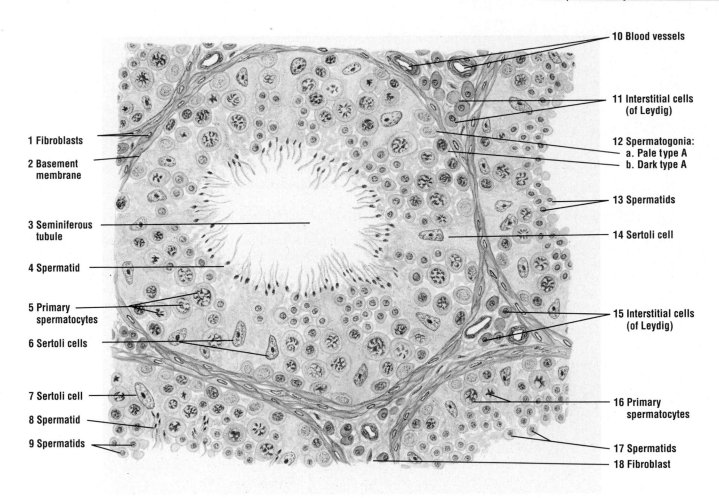

10 Blood vessels

11 Interstitial cells (of Leydig)

12 Spermatogonia:
a. Pale type A
b. Dark type A

13 Spermatids

14 Sertoli cell

15 Interstitial cells (of Leydig)

16 Primary spermatocytes

17 Spermatids
18 Fibroblast

1 Fibroblasts

2 Basement membrane

3 Seminiferous tubule

4 Spermatid

5 Primary spermatocytes

6 Sertoli cells

7 Sertoli cell

8 Spermatid

9 Spermatids

FIGURE 18.3 ■ Primate testis: spermatogenesis in seminiferous tubules (transverse section). Stain: hematoxylin and eosin. Medium magnification.

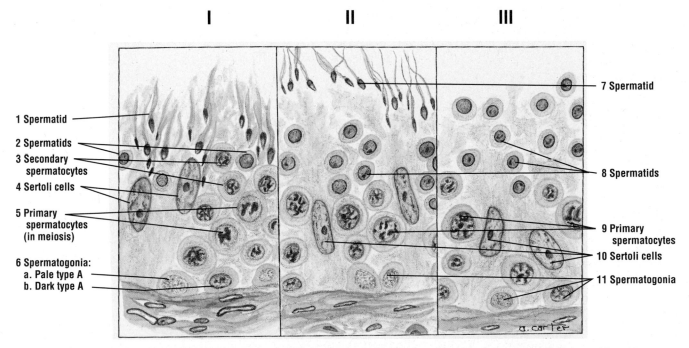

I   II   III

1 Spermatid

2 Spermatids
3 Secondary spermatocytes

4 Sertoli cells

5 Primary spermatocytes (in meiosis)

6 Spermatogonia:
a. Pale type A
b. Dark type A

7 Spermatid

8 Spermatids

9 Primary spermatocytes
10 Sertoli cells

11 Spermatogonia

a. carter

FIGURE 18.4 ■ Primate testis: stages of spermatogenesis. Stain: hematoxylin and eosin. High magnification.

FIGURE 18.5 ■ Testis: Seminiferous tubules (Transverse Section)

This photomicrograph illustrates a **seminiferous tubule (5)** and parts of adjacent seminiferous tubules. A thick germinal epithelium lines each seminiferous tubule (5).

The **dark type A (1a)** and the **pale type B (1b) spermatogonia (1)** are in the base of the tubule. The **primary spermatocytes (2)** and **spermatids (7)** at different stages of maturation are embedded in the germinal epithelium closer to the lumen. The tails of the spermatids (7) protrude into the lumen of the seminiferous tubules (5). The supportive **Sertoli cells (6)** are located throughout the germinal epithelium.

Each seminiferous tubule (5) is surrounded by a fibromuscular interstitial **connective tissue (3)**. Here, the testosterone-secreting **interstitial cells (4)** are found.

FIGURE 18.6 ■ Ductuli Efferentes and Tubules of Ductus Epididymis

The **ductuli efferentes (1)**, or efferent ductules, emerge from the mediastinum on the posterior–superior surface of the testis and connect the rete testis with the ductus epididymis. The ductuli efferentes are located in the **connective tissue (2, 12)** and form a portion of the head of the epididymis.

The lumen of the ductuli efferentes (1) exhibits an irregular contour, because the lining epithelium consists of simple alternating groups of tall ciliated and shorter nonciliated cells. The basal surface of the tubules has a smooth contour. Located under the basement membrane is a thin layer of connective tissue (2) containing a thin **smooth muscle layer (5, 11)**. As the ductuli efferentes (1) terminate in the ductus epididymis, the lumina are lined with **pseudostratified columnar epithelium (6, 8)** of the ductus epididymis (3, 4).

The **ductus epididymis (3, 4)** is a long, convoluted tubule that is surrounded by connective tissue (2) and a thin smooth muscle layer (5, 11). A section through the ductus epididymis shows both **cross-sections (3)** and **longitudinal sections (4)**. Some parts of the ductus contain mature **sperm (7)**.

The pseudostratified columnar epithelium (6, 8) consists of tall columnar **principal cells (9)** with long, nonmotile **stereocilia (8)** and small **basal cells (10)**.

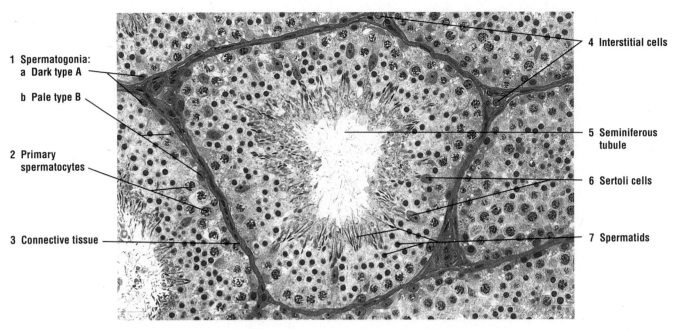

1 Spermatogonia:
 a Dark type A

 b Pale type B

2 Primary
 spermatocytes

3 Connective tissue

4 Interstitial cells

5 Seminiferous
 tubule

6 Sertoli cells

7 Spermatids

FIGURE 18.5 ■ Testis: seminiferous tubules (transverse section). Stain: hematoxylin and eosin (plastic section). 80×

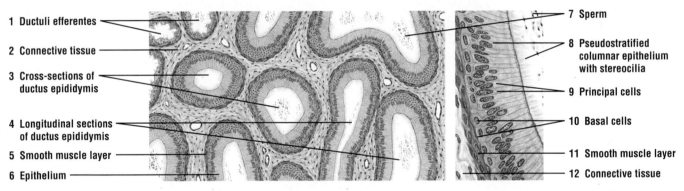

1 Ductuli efferentes

2 Connective tissue

3 Cross-sections of
 ductus epididymis

4 Longitudinal sections
 of ductus epididymis

5 Smooth muscle layer

6 Epithelium

7 Sperm

8 Pseudostratified
 columnar epithelium
 with stereocilia

9 Principal cells

10 Basal cells

11 Smooth muscle layer

12 Connective tissue

FIGURE 18.6 ■ Ductuli efferentes and tubules of the ductus epididymis. Stain: hematoxylin and eosin. Left side: low magnification; right side: high magnification.

FIGURE 18.7 ■ Tubules of the Ductus Epididymis (Transverse Section)

This photomicrograph illustrates the tubules of the ductus epididymis, some of which are filled with **sperm (1)**. The tubules of the ductus are lined with **pseudostratified epithelium (2)**. The **principal cells (2a)** are tall columnar and are lined with **stereocilia (5)**, the long, branching microvilli. The **basal cells (2b)** are small and spherical and are situated near the base of the epithelium. A thin layer of **smooth muscle (3)** surrounds each tubule. Adjacent to the smooth muscle layer (3) are cells and fibers of the **connective tissue (4)**.

FIGURE 18.8 ■ Ductus (Vas) Deferens (Transverse Section)

The ductus (vas) deferens exhibits a narrow and irregular lumen with **longitudinal mucosal folds (6)**, a thin mucosa, a thick muscularis, and an adventitia.

The lumen of the ductus deferens is lined by **pseudostratified columnar epithelium (8)** with stereocilia. The epithelium of the ductus deferens is somewhat lower than in the ductus epididymis. The underlying thin **lamina propria (7)** consists of compact collagen fibers and a fine network of elastic fibers.

The thick muscularis consists of three smooth muscle layers: a thinner **inner longitudinal muscle layer (1)**, a thick **middle circular muscle layer (2)**, and a thinner **outer longitudinal muscle layer (3)**. The muscularis is surrounded by **adventitia (5)**, in which abundant **blood vessels (venule** and **arteriole) (4)** and nerves are found. The adventitia (5) of the ductus deferens merges with the connective tissue of the spermatic cord.

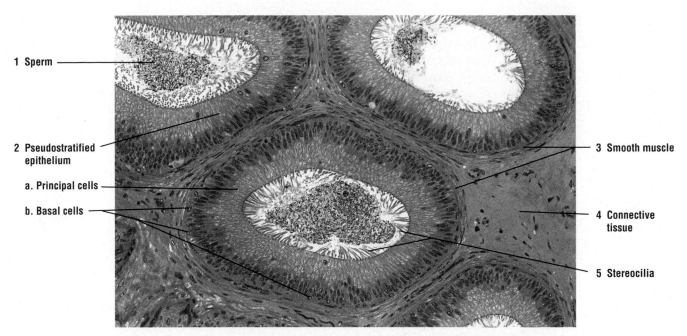

1 Sperm

2 Pseudostratified epithelium

a. Principal cells

b. Basal cells

3 Smooth muscle

4 Connective tissue

5 Stereocilia

FIGURE 18.7 ■ Tubules of the ductus epididymis (transverse section). Stain: hematoxylin and eosin (plastic section). 50×

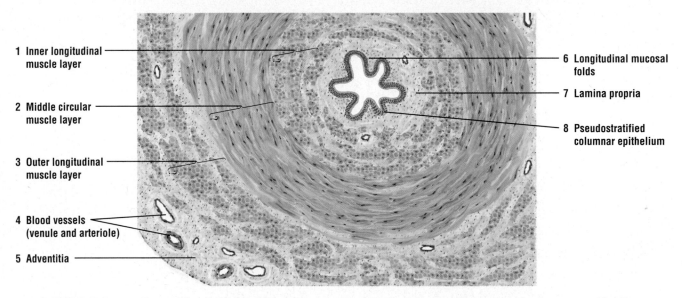

1 Inner longitudinal muscle layer

2 Middle circular muscle layer

3 Outer longitudinal muscle layer

4 Blood vessels (venule and arteriole)

5 Adventitia

6 Longitudinal mucosal folds

7 Lamina propria

8 Pseudostratified columnar epithelium

FIGURE 18.8 ■ Ductus (vas) deferens (transverse section). Stain: hematoxylin and eosin. Low magnification.

FIGURE 18.9 ■ Ampulla of the Ductus (Vas) Deferens (Transverse Section)

The terminal portion of the ductus deferens enlarges into an ampulla. The ampulla differs from the ductus deferens mainly in the structure of its mucosa.

The **lumen (3)** of the ampulla is larger than that of the ductus deferens. The mucosa also exhibits numerous irregular, branching **mucosal folds (4)** and deep **glandular diverticula** or **crypts (1)** between the folds that extend to the surrounding muscle layer. The secretory epithelium that lines the lumen (3) and the glandular diverticula (1) is simple columnar or cuboidal. Below the epithelium is the **lamina propria (6)**.

The smooth muscle layers in the muscularis are similar to those in the ductus deferens. These consist of a thin **inner longitudinal muscle layer (7)**, a thick **middle circular muscle layer (8)**, and a thin **outer longitudinal muscle layer (9)**. Surrounding the ampulla is the connective tissue **adventitia (5)**.

FUNCTIONAL CORRELATIONS

Excurrent Ducts

The motility of cilia in the **ductuli efferentes** creates a current that assists in transporting fluid and sperm from the seminiferous tubules to the **ductus epididymis.** The nonciliated cuboidal cells in the ductuli efferentes absorb some of the testicular fluid that was produced in the seminiferous tubules by Sertoli cells.

The highly coiled ductus epididymis is the site for **accumulation, storage,** and **maturation** of sperm. When sperm enter the epididymis, they are nonmotile and incapable of fertilizing an oocyte. Approximately a week later, however, in transit through the ductus epididymis, the sperm acquire motility. The **principal cells** in the ductus epididymis are lined with long, branching microvilii, or **stereocilia,** that continue to absorb testicular fluid that was not absorbed in the ductuli efferentes during the passage of sperm from the testes. The principal cells in the epididymis also phagocytose the remaining residual bodies that were not removed by the Sertoli cells in the seminiferous tubules as well as any abnormal or degenerating sperm cells. These cells also produce a glycoprotein that **inhibits capacitation,** or the fertilizing ability of the sperm, until they are deposited in the female reproductive tract.

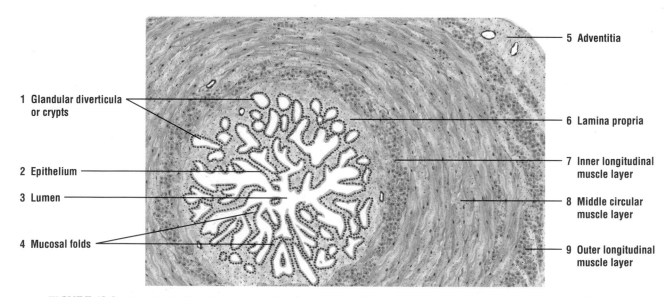

FIGURE 18.9 ■ Ampulla of the ductus (vas) deferens. Stain: hematoxylin and eosin. Low magnification.

SECTION 2 ■ Accessory Reproductive Glands: Seminal Vesicles, Prostate Gland, Bulbourethral Glands, and Penis

The accessory glands of the male reproductive system consist of paired **seminal vesicles,** paired **bulbourethral glands,** and a single **prostate gland.** These structures are directly associated with the male reproductive tract and produce numerous secretory products that mix with sperm to produce a fluid, called **semen.** The penis serves as the copulatory organ; the penile urethra serves as a common passageway for urine or semen.

The seminal vesicles are posterior to the bladder and superior to the prostate gland. The excretory duct of each seminal vesicle joins the dilated terminal part of each ductus (vas) deferens, the **ampulla,** to form the **ejaculatory ducts.** The ejaculatory ducts enter and continue through the prostate gland to open into the **prostatic urethra.**

The prostate gland is inferior to the neck of the bladder. The **urethra** exits the bladder and passes through the prostate gland as the **prostatic urethra.** In addition to the ejaculatory ducts, numerous excretory ducts from prostatic glands open into the prostatic urethra.

The bulbourethral glands are small, pea-sized glands that are located at the root of the **penis** and embedded in the skeletal muscles of the urogenital diaphragm. Their excretory ducts terminate in the proximal portion of the **penile urethra.**

The **penis** consists of **erectile tissues,** the paired dorsal **corpora cavernosa** and a single ventral **corpus spongiosum** that expands distally into the **glans penis.** Because the penile urethra extends through the entire length of the corpus spongiosum, this portion of the penis is also called **corpus cavernosum urethrae.** Each erectile body in the penis is surrounded by the connective tissue layer **tunica albuginea.**

The erectile tissues in the penis consist of irregular vascular spaces lined by vascular endothelium. The trabeculae between these spaces contain collagen and elastic fibers and smooth muscles. Blood enters the vascular spaces from the branches of the **dorsal artery** and **deep arteries of the penis** and is drained by peripheral veins.

FIGURE 18.10 ■ Prostate Gland and Prostatic Urethra

The prostate gland is an encapsulated organ inferior to the neck of the bladder. The urethra that leaves the bladder and passes through the prostate gland is called the **prostatic urethra (1).** A **transitional epithelium (6)** lines the lumen of the crescent-shaped prostatic urethra (1). Most of the prostate gland consists of small, branched tubuloacinar **prostatic glands (5, 11).** Some prostatic glands (5, 11) contain solid secretory aggregations, called prostatic **concretions (11),** in their acini. The prostatic concretions (11) appear as small, red dots in this illustration. A characteristic **fibromuscular stroma (10)** with **smooth muscle bundles (4),** mixed with collagen and elastic fibers, surrounds the prostatic glands (5, 11) and the prostatic urethra (1).

A longitudinal urethral crest of dense fibromuscular stroma without glands widens in the prostatic urethra (1) to form a smooth, dome-like structure, called the **colliculus seminalis (7).** The colliculus seminalis (7) protrudes into and gives the prostatic urethra (1) a crescent shape. On each side of the colliculus seminalis (7) are the **prostatic sinuses (2).** Most excretory **ducts** of **prostatic glands (9)** open into the prostatic sinuses (2).

In the middle of the colliculus seminalis (7) is a cul de sac, called the **utricle (8).** The utricle (8) often shows dilation at its distal end before it opens into the prostatic urethra (1). The thin mucous membrane of the utricle (8) typically is folded, and the epithelium usually is of the simple secretory or pseudostratified columnar type. Also, two **ejaculatory ducts (3)** open at the colliculus, one on each side of the utricle (8).

FIGURE 18.11 ■ Prostate Gland: Glandular Acini and Prostatic Concretions

A small section of the prostate gland from Figure 18-10 is illustrated at a higher magnification.

The size of the **glandular acini (1)** in the prostate gland is highly variable. The lumina of the acini are normally wide and typically irregular because of the protrusion of the epithelium-covered **connective tissue folds (10).** Some of the glandular acini (1) contain proteinaceous **prostatic secretions (9).** Other glandular acini (1) contain spherical **prostatic concretions (4, 6, 8)** that are formed by concentric layers of condensed prostatic secretions. The prostatic concretions (4, 6, 8) are characteristic features of the prostate gland acini. The number of prostatic concretions (4, 6, 8) increases with the age of the individual, and they may become calcified.

Although the **glandular epithelium (5)** is usually simple columnar or pseudostratified and the cells are light-staining, considerable variation is found. In some regions, the epithelium may be squamous or cuboidal.

The **excretory ducts** of the **prostatic glands (2)** often may resemble the glandular acini (1). In the terminal portions of the ducts (2), the epithelium usually is columnar and stains darker before entering the urethra.

The **fibromuscular stroma (7)** is another characteristic feature of the prostate gland. **Smooth muscle bundles (3)** and the connective tissue fibers blend together in the stroma (7) and are distributed throughout the gland.

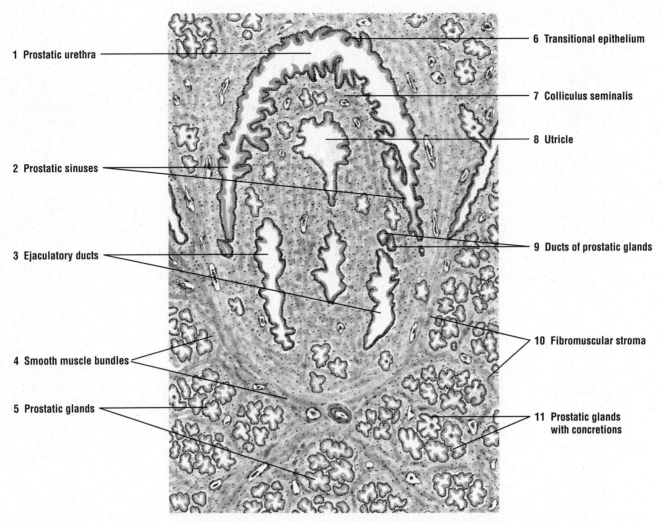

1 Prostatic urethra

2 Prostatic sinuses

3 Ejaculatory ducts

4 Smooth muscle bundles

5 Prostatic glands

6 Transitional epithelium

7 Colliculus seminalis

8 Utricle

9 Ducts of prostatic glands

10 Fibromuscular stroma

11 Prostatic glands with concretions

FIGURE 18.10 ■ Prostate gland and prostatic urethra. Stain: hematoxylin and eosin. Low magnification.

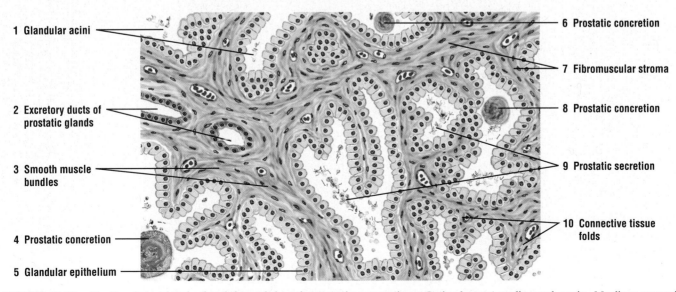

1 Glandular acini

2 Excretory ducts of prostatic glands

3 Smooth muscle bundles

4 Prostatic concretion

5 Glandular epithelium

6 Prostatic concretion

7 Fibromuscular stroma

8 Prostatic concretion

9 Prostatic secretion

10 Connective tissue folds

FIGURE 18.11 ■ Prostate gland: glandular acini and prostatic concretions. Stain: hematoxylin and eosin. Medium magnification.

FIGURE 18.12   ■   Prostate Gland: Prostatic Glands with Prostatic Concretions

The parenchyma of the prostate gland consists of individual **prostatic glands** (3) that vary in size and shape. The glandular epithelium also varies from simple cuboidal or **columnar epithelium** (2) to pseudostratified epithelium. In older individuals, the secretory material of the prostatic glands (3) precipitates to form the characteristic, dense-staining **prostatic concretions** (1, 5). The prostate gland is also characterized by the **fibromuscular stroma** (4). In this photomicrograph, the **smooth muscle fibers** (4a) in the fibromuscular stroma (4) are stained red, and the **connective tissue fibers** (4b) are stained blue.

FIGURE 18.13   ■   Seminal Vesicle

The paired seminal vesicles are elongated glands on the posterior side of the bladder. The excretory duct from each seminal vesicle joins the ampulla of each ductus deferens to form the ejaculatory duct, which then runs through the prostate gland to open into the prostatic urethra.

The seminal vesicle exhibits highly convoluted and irregular lumina. A cross-section through the gland illustrates the complexity of the **primary mucosal folds** (1). These folds branch into numerous **secondary mucosal folds** (2), which frequently anastomose and form irregular cavities, chambers, or **mucosal crypts** (7). The **lamina propria** (6) projects into and forms the core of the larger primary folds (1) and the smaller secondary folds (2). The folds extend far into the lumen of the seminal vesicle.

The glandular **epithelium** (5) of the seminal vesicles varies in appearance. Usually, however, it is low pseudostratified and low columnar or cuboidal.

The muscularis consists of an **inner circular muscle layer** (3) and an **outer longitudinal muscle layer** (4). This arrangement of the smooth muscles often is difficult to observe because of the complex folding of the mucosa. The **adventitia** (8) surrounds the muscularis and blends with the connective tissue.

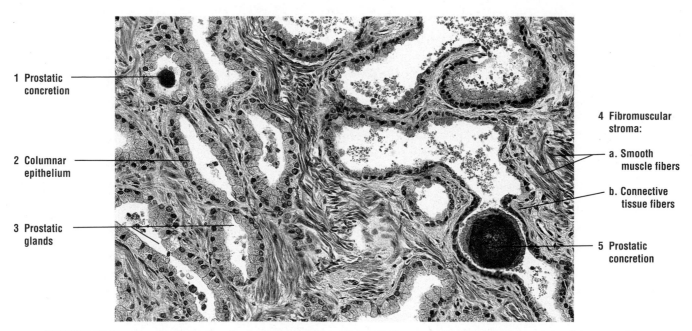

1 Prostatic concretion

2 Columnar epithelium

3 Prostatic glands

4 Fibromuscular stroma:

a. Smooth muscle fibers

b. Connective tissue fibers

5 Prostatic concretion

FIGURE 18.12 ■ Prostate gland: prostatic glands with prostatic concretions. Stain: Masson's trichrome. 64×

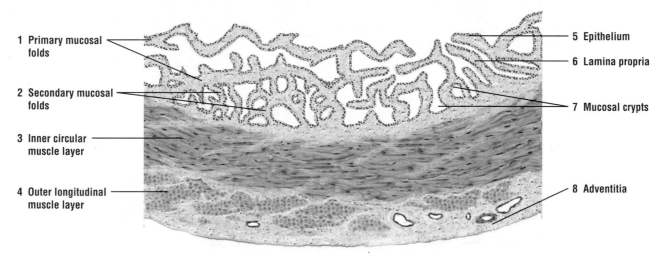

1 Primary mucosal folds

2 Secondary mucosal folds

3 Inner circular muscle layer

4 Outer longitudinal muscle layer

5 Epithelium

6 Lamina propria

7 Mucosal crypts

8 Adventitia

FIGURE 18.13 ■ Seminal vesicle: Stain: hematoxylin and eosin. Low magnification.

FIGURE 18.14 ■ Bulbourethral Gland

The paired bulbourethral glands are compound tubuloacinar glands. The fibroelastic capsule that surrounds these glands contains **connective tissue (3)**, smooth muscle fibers, and **skeletal muscle fibers (2, 7)** in the interlobular **connective tissue septum (5).** Because the bulbourethral glands are located in the urogenital diaphragm, the skeletal muscles fibers (2, 7) from the diaphragm are present in the glands. Connective tissue septa (5) from the capsule (3) divide the gland into several lobules.

The secretory units vary in structure and size, and they resemble mucous glands. The glands exhibit either **acinar secretory units (6)** or **tubular secretory units (1).** The secretory cells are cuboidal, low columnar, or squamous, and they are light-staining. The height of the epithelial cells depends on the functional state of the gland. The secretory product of the bulbourethral glands is primarily mucus.

Smaller **excretory ducts (4)** from the secretory units may be lined with secretory cells. The larger excretory ducts exhibit pseudostratified or stratified columnar epithelium.

FUNCTIONAL CORRELATIONS

Accessory Reproductive Glands

The secretory products from the seminal vesicles, prostate gland, and bulbourethral glands mix with sperm and form **semen.** Semen provides the sperm with a liquid transport medium as well as nutrients. It also neutralizes the acidity of the male urethra and vaginal canal and activates the sperm after ejaculation.

The **seminal vesicles** produce a yellowish, viscous fluid that contains a high concentration of **fructose,** which is the main carbohydrate component of semen. Fructose is metabolized by sperm and servers as the main **energy** source for sperm motility. Seminal vesicles produce most of the fluid found in semen.

The **prostate gland** produces a thin, watery, slightly acidic fluid that is rich in citric acid, acid phosphatase, and amylase. The enzyme fibrinolysin in the fluid liquefies the congealed semen after ejaculation.

The **bulbourethral glands** produce a clear, viscid, mucus-like secretion that, during erotic stimulation, is released and serves as a lubricant for the penile urethra. During ejaculation, secretions from bulbourethral glands precede other components of the semen.

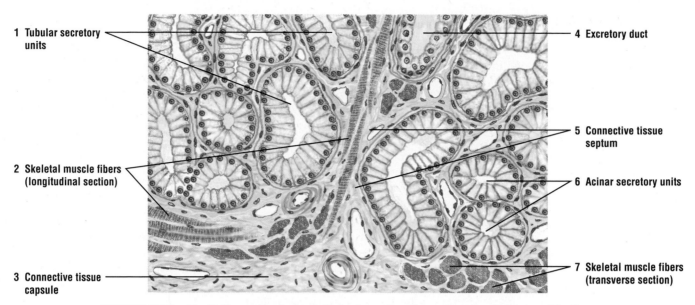

1 Tubular secretory units

2 Skeletal muscle fibers (longitudinal section)

3 Connective tissue capsule

4 Excretory duct

5 Connective tissue septum

6 Acinar secretory units

7 Skeletal muscle fibers (transverse section)

FIGURE 18.14 ■ Bulbourethral gland. Stain: hematoxylin and eosin. High magnification.

FIGURE 18.15 ■ Human Penis (Transverse Section)

A cross-section of the human penis illustrates the two dorsal **corpora cavernosa (15)** (singular, corpus cavernosum) and a single ventral **corpus spongiosum (21)** that form the body of the organ. The **urethra (9)** passes through the entire length of the penis in the corpus spongiosum (21). A thick connective tissue capsule, called the **tunica albuginea (4)**, surrounds the corpora cavernosa (15) and forms a **median septum (17)** between the two bodies. A thinner **tunica albuginea (8)**, with smooth muscle fibers and elastic fibers, surrounds the corpus spongiosum (21).

All three cavernous bodies (15, 21) are surrounded by loose connective tissue, called the **deep penile (Buck's) fascia (5, 16)**, which in turn is surrounded by the connective tissue of the **dermis (10)** below the stratified squamous keratinized epithelium of the **epidermis (11)**. Strands of smooth muscle of the **dartos tunic (7), nerves (2), sebaceous glands (20)**, and peripheral blood vessels are located in the dermis (10).

Trabeculae (19) with collagenous, elastic, nerve, and smooth muscle fibers surround and form the core of the **cavernous sinuses** (veins) **(18, 22)** in the corpora cavernosa (15) and corpus spongiosum (21). The cavernous sinuses (18) of the corpora cavernosa (15) are lined with endothelium and receive the blood from the **dorsal arteries (1, 14)** and **deep arteries (3)** of the penis. The deep arteries (3) branch in the corpora cavernosa (15) and form the **helicine arteries (6)**, which empty directly into the cavernous sinuses (18). The cavernous sinuses (22) in the corpus spongiosum (21) receive their blood from the bulbourethral artery, which is a branch of the internal pudendal artery. Blood leaving the cavernous sinuses (18, 22) exits mainly through the **superficial dorsal vein (12)** and the **deep dorsal vein (13)**.

As the urethra (9) passes the base of the penis, it is lined with pseudostratified or stratified columnar epithelium. As the urethra (9) exits the penis, the epithelium changes to stratified squamous. The urethra (9) also shows invaginations called urethral lacunae (of Morgagni) with mucous cells. Branched tubular urethral glands (of Littre) below the epithelium open into these recesses. These glands are shown at higher magnification in Fig. 18-16.

FIGURE 18.16 ■ Penile Urethra (Transverse Section)

The penile urethra extends the entire length of the penis and is surrounded by the **corpus spongiosum (9)**. This illustration shows a transverse section through the **lumen** of the **penile urethra (3)** and the surrounding corpus spongiosum (9). The lining of this portion of the urethra is a pseudostratified or stratified **columnar epithelium (2)**. A thin, underlying **lamina propria (5)** merges with the surrounding connective tissue of the corpus spongiosum (9).

Numerous irregular outpockets or **urethral lacunae (4)** with mucous cells are found in the lumen of the penile urethra (3). The urethral lacunae (4) are connected with the branched mucous **urethral glands (of Littre) (6, 7)** in the surrounding connective tissue of the corpus spongiosum (9) and are found throughout the length of the penile urethra. The **ducts** from the urethral glands (6) open into the lumen of the penile urethra (3).

The corpus spongiosum (9) consists of **cavernous sinuses (1, 10)** that are lined by endothelial cells and separated by connective tissue **trabeculae (8)** that contain smooth muscle fibers and collagen fibers. Numerous **blood vessels (arteriole and venule) (11)** supply the corpus spongiosum (9). The internal structure of the corpus spongiosum (9) is similar to that of the corpora cavernosa described in Figure 18-15.

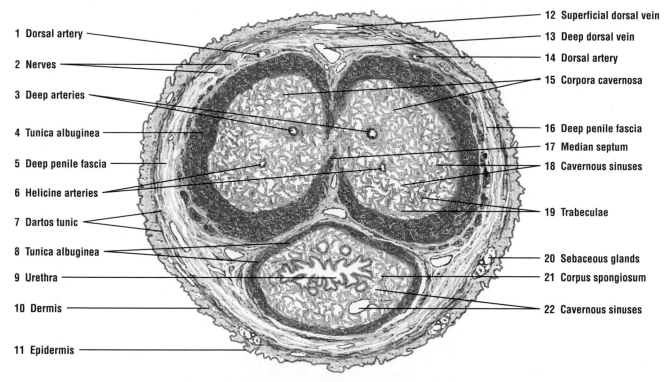

1 Dorsal artery

2 Nerves

3 Deep arteries

4 Tunica albuginea

5 Deep penile fascia

6 Helicine arteries

7 Dartos tunic

8 Tunica albuginea

9 Urethra

10 Dermis

11 Epidermis

12 Superficial dorsal vein

13 Deep dorsal vein

14 Dorsal artery

15 Corpora cavernosa

16 Deep penile fascia

17 Median septum

18 Cavernous sinuses

19 Trabeculae

20 Sebaceous glands

21 Corpus spongiosum

22 Cavernous sinuses

FIGURE 18.15 ■ Human penis (transverse section). Stain: hematoxylin and eosin. Low magnification.

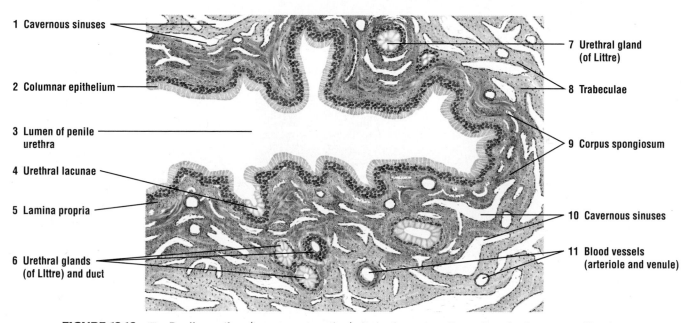

1 Cavernous sinuses

2 Columnar epithelium

3 Lumen of penile urethra

4 Urethral lacunae

5 Lamina propria

6 Urethral glands (of LIttre) and duct

7 Urethral gland (of Littre)

8 Trabeculae

9 Corpus spongiosum

10 Cavernous sinuses

11 Blood vessels (arteriole and venule)

FIGURE 18.16 ■ Penile urethra (transverse section). Stain: hematoxylin and eosin. Low magnification.

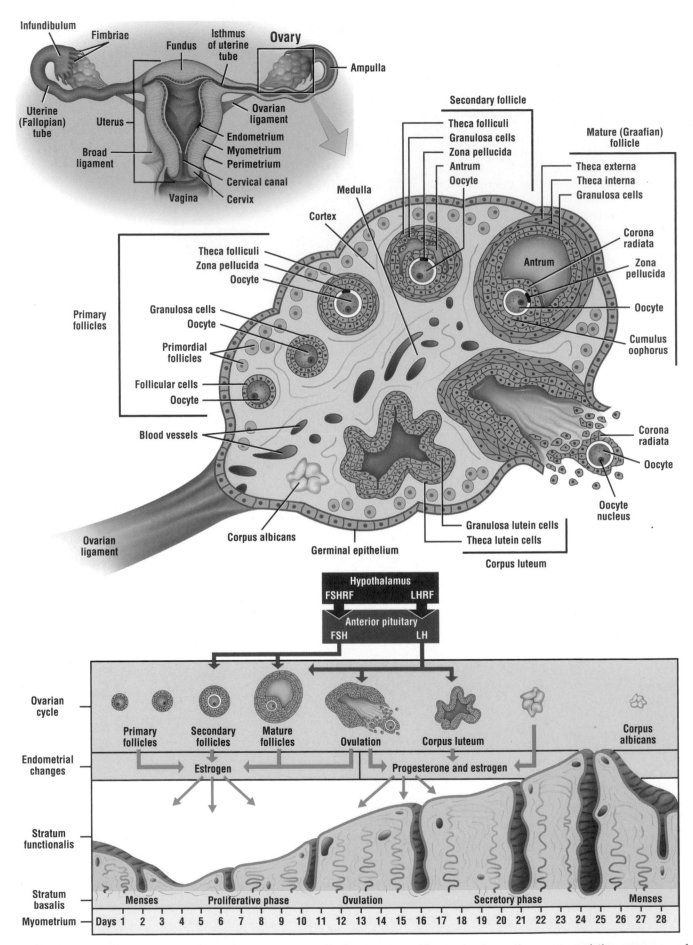

OVERVIEW FIGURE ■ Anatomy of the female reproductive organs, with emphasis on the ovary and the sequence of changes during follicular development, culminating in ovulation and corpus luteum formation. Changes in the uterine wall during the menstrual cycle are correlated with pituitary hormones and ovarian functions.

CHAPTER 19

Female Reproductive System

SECTION 1 ■ Ovaries, Uterine Tubes, and Uterus

The human female reproductive system consists of paired internal **ovaries,** paired **uterine tubes** (**oviducts**)**,** and a single **uterus.** Inferior to the uterus and separated by the **cervix** is the **vagina.** Because **mammary glands** are associated with the female reproductive system, their histologic structure and function are included in this chapter.

During reproductive life, the female reproductive organs exhibit cyclic, monthly changes in both structure and function. In humans, these changes comprise the **menstrual cycle.** The menstrual cycle is primarily controlled by two hormones that are secreted by the adenohypophysis of the pituitary gland, **follicle-stimulating hormone (FSH)** and **luteinizing hormone (LH),** and by two ovarian hormones, **estrogen** and **progesterone.** Release of FSH and LH from the pituitary gland is controlled by releasing factors that are secreted by the neurons in the hypothalamus, **FSH-releasing factor** and **LH-releasing factor** (see overview figure).

The individual organs of the female reproductive system perform numerous important functions, including secretion of female sex hormones (estrogen and progesterone), production of oocytes for fertilization by sperm, provision of a suitable environment for fertilization of the oocytes, transportation of the embryo to the uterus, implantation of the embryo, development of the fetus during pregnancy, and nutrition of the newborn.

In humans, a mature ovarian follicle releases an immature egg, called the oocyte, into the uterine tube approximately every 28 days. The oocyte remains in the female reproductive tract until it degenerates or is fertilized. The transformation or maturation of the immature oocyte into the mature egg or ovum occurs at the time of fertilization, when the sperm penetrates the oocyte.

Ovaries

Each ovary is a flattened, ovoid structure deep in the pelvic cavity. One section of the ovary is attached to the **broad ligament** by a peritoneal fold, called the **mesovarium,** and another section is attached to the uterine wall by an **ovarian ligament.** The ovarian surface is covered by a single layer of cells, called the **germinal epithelium,** that overlies the dense irregular connective tissue **tunica albuginea.** Located below the tunica albuginea is the **cortex** of the ovary. Deep to the cortex is the highly vascularized connective tissue core of the ovary, called the **medulla.** No distinct boundary line exists between the cortex and the medulla; these two regions blend together.

Normally, the cortex is filled with numerous **ovarian follicles** at various stages of development, including the large, **mature follicles** that extend deep into the medulla. In addition, the ovary may contain a large **corpus luteum** of an ovulated follicle, the **corpus albicans** of a degenerated corpus luteum, and **atretic follicles** at various stages of degeneration.

Uterine Tubes (Oviducts)

Each uterine tube is approximately 12 cm in length and extends from the ovaries to the uterus. One end of the uterine tube opens into the uterus; the other end opens into the peritoneal cavity near the ovary. Normally, the uterine tubes are divided into four continuous regions. The region closest to the ovary is the funnel-shaped **infundibulum.** Extending from the infundibulum are slender, finger-like processes, called **fimbriae** (singular, fimbria), that are located close to the ovary. Continuous with the infundibulum is the second region, called the **ampulla,** which is the widest and longest portion. The **isthmus** is short and narrow, and it joins each uterine tube to the uterus. The last portion of the uterine tube is the **interstitial (intramural) region,** which passes through the thick uterine wall to open into the uterine cavity.

Uterus

The human uterus is a pear-shaped organ with a thick muscular wall. The **body** or **corpus** forms the major portion of the uterus. The rounded upper portion of the uterus above the entrance of uterine tubes is called the **fundus.** The lower, narrower, and terminal portion of the uterus below the body or corpus is called the **cervix.** The cervix protrudes and opens into the vagina.

The wall of the uterus is composed of three layers: an outer **perimetrium** lined by serosa or adventitia; a thick smooth muscle layer, called the **myometrium;** and an inner **endometrium.** The endometrium is lined by simple epithelium that descends into a lamina propria to form numerous **uterine glands.**

Normally, the endometrium is subdivided into two functional layers, the luminal **stratum functionalis** and the basal **stratum basalis.** In a nonpregnant female, the superficial functionalis layer with the uterine glands is sloughed off, or shed, during **menstruation,** leaving intact the deeper basalis layer with the basal remnants of the uterine glands—the source of cells for regeneration of a new functionalis layer. The arterial supply to the endometrium plays an important role during the menstrual phase of the menstrual cycle.

Uterine arteries in the broad ligament give rise to the **arcuate arteries.** These arteries penetrate and assume a circumferential course in the myometrium of the uterus. Arcuate vessels divide into **straight** and **spiral arteries** that supply blood to the endometrium. The straight arteries are short and supply the basalis layer of the endometrium, whereas the spiral arteries are long and coiled and supply the surface or functionalis layer of endometrium. In contrast to the straight arteries, spiral arteries are highly sensitive to hormonal levels in the blood. Decreased blood levels of the ovarian hormones estrogen and progesterone during the menstrual cycle result in the shedding of stratum functionalis and menstruation.

FIGURE 19.1 ■ Ovary: Dog (Panoramic View)

The ovarian surface is covered by a single layer of low cuboidal or squamous cells, called the **germinal epithelium (1, 12),** that is continuous with the **mesothelium (14)** of the visceral peritoneum. Beneath the germinal epithelium (1, 12) is a dense connective tissue layer, called the **tunica albuginea (2).**

The ovary has a peripheral **cortex (8)** and a central **medulla (24).** The cortex (8) occupies most of the ovary and contains fibrocytes with collagen and reticular fibers. The medulla (24) is a typical dense irregular connective tissue that is continuous with the ligament **mesovarium (13).** Larger **blood vessels** in the **medulla (10)** distribute smaller vessels to all parts of the cortex. The mesovarium (13) is covered by the germinal epithelium (12) and the peritoneal mesothelium (14).

Numerous **ovarian follicles (3, 4, 6, 9, 16, 17, 18, 19, 20, 22, 25, 28, 29)** at various stages of development are located in the stroma of the cortex (8). The most numerous are the **primordial follicles (3, 29 [lower leader]),** which are located in the periphery of the cortex (8) and under the tunica albuginea (2). These follicles are the smallest and the simplest in structure. The primordial follicles (3, 29 [lower leader]) are surrounded by a squamous layer of follicular cells. In the primordial follicles, the immature primary oocyte is small but gradually increases in size in the primary, growing, and mature follicles.

The smaller follicles with cuboidal, columnar, or stratified cuboidal cells surrounding the oocyte are the **primary follicles (4).** The larger follicles with antral cavities are called **secondary (antral) follicles (6, 7, 9, 28)** and are situated deeper in the cortex. Secondary follicles (7, 6, 9, 28) are surrounded by modified stromal cells, called the **theca folliculi (6).** Theca folliculi (6) cells differentiate into an inner secretory layer, called the **theca interna (16 [upper leader])** and an outer connective tissue layer, called the **theca externa (16 [lower leader]).** All follicles contain an immature primary **oocyte (20, 28)** with a nucleus.

The largest ovarian follicle is the **mature follicle (16–20).** Mature follicles (16-20) consist of the theca interna and theca externa (16), **granulosa cells (17),** a large **antrum (18)** with liquor folliculi (follicular fluid), and the **cumulus oophorus (19)** that contains the primary oocyte (20).

Most follicles do not attain maturity. Instead, they undergo degeneration (i.e., atresia) at various stages of growth and become **atretic follicles (11, 21, 26, 30).** Atretic follicles are replaced by the connective tissue.

Another regressing structure in the illustrated ovary is the **corpus luteum (23, 27).** After ovulation, the follicle transforms into a corpus luteum. If fertilization and implantation do not occur, the corpus luteum regresses, degenerates, and ultimately, turns into a scar tissue, called the **corpus albicans (5).**

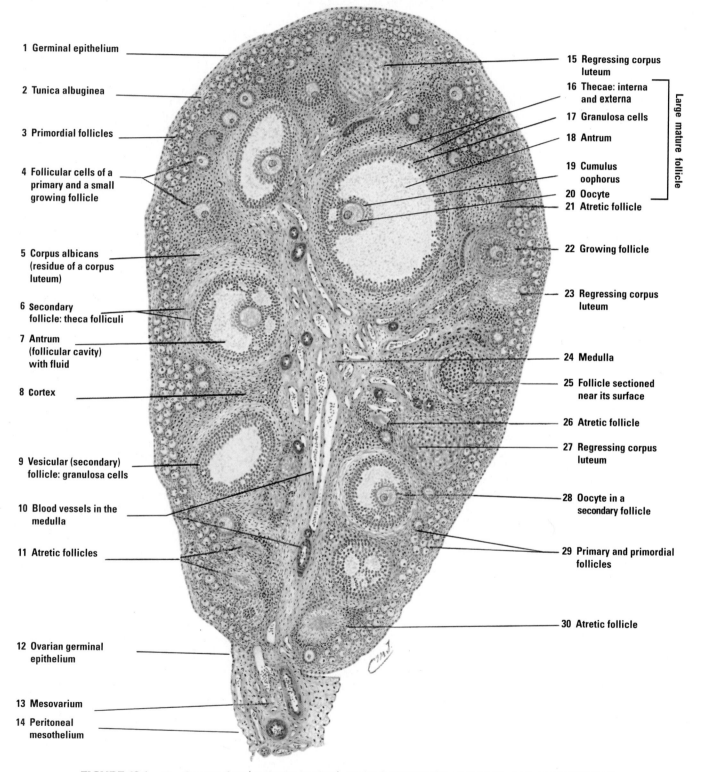

1 Germinal epithelium

2 Tunica albuginea

3 Primordial follicles

4 Follicular cells of a primary and a small growing follicle

5 Corpus albicans (residue of a corpus luteum)

6 Secondary follicle: theca folliculi

7 Antrum (follicular cavity) with fluid

8 Cortex

9 Vesicular (secondary) follicle: granulosa cells

10 Blood vessels in the medulla

11 Atretic follicles

12 Ovarian germinal epithelium

13 Mesovarium

14 Peritoneal mesothelium

15 Regressing corpus luteum

16 Thecae: interna and externa

17 Granulosa cells

18 Antrum

19 Cumulus oophorus

20 Oocyte

21 Atretic follicle

Large mature follicle

22 Growing follicle

23 Regressing corpus luteum

24 Medulla

25 Follicle sectioned near its surface

26 Atretic follicle

27 Regressing corpus luteum

28 Oocyte in a secondary follicle

29 Primary and primordial follicles

30 Atretic follicle

FIGURE 19.1 ■ Ovary: dog (panoramic view). Stain: hematoxylin and eosin. Low magnification.

FUNCTIONAL CORRELATIONS

Ovaries

During the reproductive years, ovaries exhibit structural and functional changes during each menstrual cycle, which lasts an average of 28 days. These changes involve the growth of different follicles; maturation of follicles; ovulation from a mature, dominant follicle; and formation and degeneration of the corpus luteum. The pituitary hormones FSH and LH are primarily responsible for the development, maturation, and ovulation of ovarian follicles and for the production of estrogen and progesterone.

The first half of the menstrual cycle lasts approximately 14 days and involves the growth of ovarian follicles. During follicular growth, the follicular cells possess FSH receptors. At this time, FSH is the principal circulating gonadotrophic hormone. It controls the growth and maturation of ovarian follicles, and initially, it stimulates the **theca interna cells** around the follicles to produce **androgenic steroid precursors.** These precursors diffuse into the follicle, where the **granulosa cells** of the follicles convert them into estrogen. As the follicles develop and mature, the circulating levels of estrogen in the blood rise. High estrogen levels inhibit the release of FSH-releasing factor from the hypothalamus and the release of FSH from the pituitary gland. In addition, a hormone called **inhibin,** which is produced by granulosa cells in ovarian follicles, further inhibits the release of FSH from the pituitary gland.

At midcycle or shortly before ovulation, estrogen levels peak. This peak causes a surge of LH from the adenohypophysis of the pituitary gland. At this time, theca cells and granulosa cells in the follicles have LH receptors. A concomitant, smaller release of FSH also occurs. Increased blood levels of both LH and FSH cause:

- Final **maturation** of a mature ovarian follicle, and **ovulation** (i.e., rupture) at approximately the 14th day of the cycle.
- Completion of the **first meiotic division,** and liberation of a **secondary oocyte** into the uterine tube.
- Collapse of the ovulated follicle, and its luteinization or modification of the granulosa cells and theca lutein cells that surrounded the oocyte.
- Transformation of the postovulatory mature follicle into the corpus luteum, a temporary endocrine organ.

Final maturation of the secondary oocyte occurs only when it is fertilized by a sperm. The liberated oocyte remains viable in the female reproductive tract for approximately 24 hours before it begins to degenerate.

FIGURE 19.2 ■ Ovary: Ovarian Cortex and Primary and Primordial Follicles

The ovarian surface is covered by a cuboidal **germinal epithelium (10).** Located directly beneath the germinal epithelium (10) is a layer of dense connective tissue, called the **tunica albuginea (16).** Numerous **primordial follicles (14, 17)** are located in the cortex below the tunica albuginea (16). Each primordial follicle (14, 17) is surrounded by a single layer of squamous **follicular cells (17).** As the follicles grow larger, the follicular cells (17) of the primordial follicles (14, 17) change to cuboidal or low columnar, and at this point, the follicles are called **primary follicles (4, 11).** The developing oocytes (4, 13) also have a large, eccentric **nucleus (7, 13)** with a conspicuous nucleolus.

In the growing or primary follicles (4, 11), the follicular cells proliferate by **mitosis (3)** and form layers of cuboidal cells, called the **granulosa cells (8, 12),** that surround the primary oocytes (4, 13). A single layer of the granulosa cells that surround the oocyte form the **corona radiata (5).**

Between the corona radiata (5) and the oocyte is the noncellular glycoprotein layer, called the **zona pellucida (6).** The stromal cells that surround the follicular cells now differentiate into the **theca interna (9)** layer that is adjacent to the granulosa cells (8, 12). A thin basement membrane (not shown) separates the granulosa cells (8, 12) from the theca interna (9) cells.

Many primordial, developing, or mature follicles exhibit degeneration, die, and are lost through a process called atresia. A degenerating **atretic follicle (1)** is illustrated in the upper left corner of the illustration. Numerous blood vessels, such as a **capillary (2),** surround the developing follicles and the **connective tissue (15)** of the **cortex (15).**

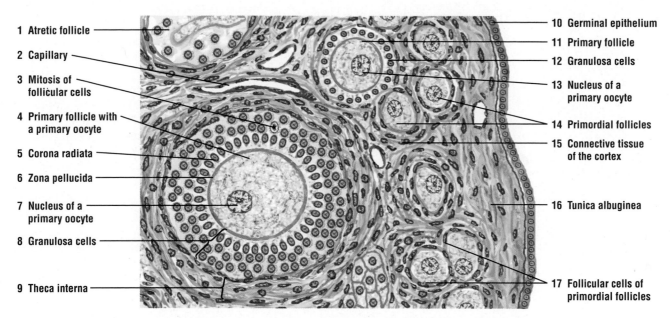

1 Atretic follicle

2 Capillary

3 Mitosis of follicular cells

4 Primary follicle with a primary oocyte

5 Corona radiata

6 Zona pellucida

7 Nucleus of a primary oocyte

8 Granulosa cells

9 Theca interna

10 Germinal epithelium

11 Primary follicle

12 Granulosa cells

13 Nucleus of a primary oocyte

14 Primordial follicles

15 Connective tissue of the cortex

16 Tunica albuginea

17 Follicular cells of primordial follicles

FIGURE 19.2 ■ Ovary: ovarian cortex and primary and primordial follicles. Stain: hematoxylin and eosin. Low magnification.

FIGURE 19.3 ■ Ovary: Primary Oocyte and Wall of a Mature Follicle

During the growth of the follicles, fluid begins to accumulate between the granulosa cells that surround the oocyte, forming a fluid-filled cavity, called the antrum. When the antrum is present, the follicle is called a secondary follicle.

This figure illustrates the **cytoplasm** and **nucleus** of **primary oocyte (3)** and the wall of a fluid-filled, mature follicle. A local thickening of the **granulosa cells (5)** on one side of the follicle surrounds the primary oocyte (3) and projects into the **antrum (4, 7)** of the follicle. Here, the granulosa cells form a hillock or mound, called the **cumulus oophorus (8).** The single layer of granulosa cells (5) immediately adjacent to the primary oocyte (3) forms the **corona radiata (1).** Between the corona radiata (1) and the cytoplasm of the primary oocyte (3) is a prominent, acidophilic-staining glycoprotein, called the **zona pellucida (2).**

The granulosa cells (5) surround the antrum (4, 7) and secrete follicular fluid that fills the antral cavity. Smaller, isolated accumulations of the fluid also occur among the granulosa cells (5) as **intercellular follicular fluid (6, 9).**

The basal row of granulosa cells (5) rests on a thin **basement membrane (10)** that separates the granulosa cells (5) from the cells of the **theca interna (11),** which is an inner layer of vascularized, secretory cells of the follicle. Surrounding the cells of the theca interna (11) is the **theca externa (12)** layer, which blends with the **connective tissue (13)** of the ovarian cortex.

FIGURE 19.4 ■ Ovary: Primordial and Primary Follicles

This photomicrograph shows different types of follicles in the cortex of an ovary. The immature **primordial follicles (2)** consist of a primary **oocyte (3)** that is surrounded by a layer of simple squamous **follicular cells (1, 7).** As the primordial follicles (2) grow to become **primary follicles (4),** the layer of simple squamous follicular cells around the oocyte changes to a cuboidal layer. In a larger **primary follicle (8),** the follicular cells have proliferated into a stratified layer around the oocyte, called the **granulosa cells (11).** A prominent layer of glycoprotein, called the **zona pellucida (10),** develops between the granulosa cells (11) and the immature **oocyte (9).**

The cells around the developing follicles also organize into two distinct cell layers, the inner, hormone-secreting **theca interna (12)** and the outer, connective tissue layer **theca externa (13).** The theca interna (12) and theca externa (13) are separated from the granulosa cells (11) by a thin **basement membrane (6).** Surrounding the follicles in the cortex are cells and fibers of the **connective tissue (5).**

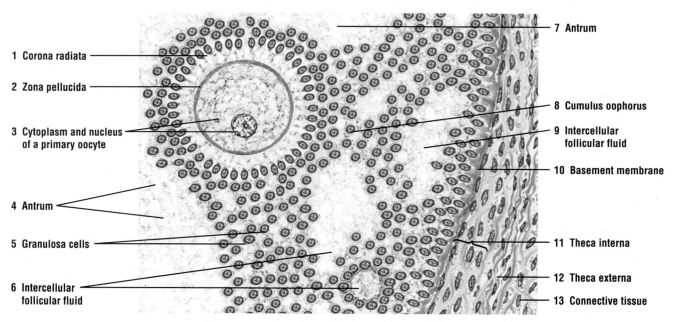

1 Corona radiata

2 Zona pellucida

3 Cytoplasm and nucleus of a primary oocyte

4 Antrum

5 Granulosa cells

6 Intercellular follicular fluid

7 Antrum

8 Cumulus oophorus

9 Intercellular follicular fluid

10 Basement membrane

11 Theca interna

12 Theca externa

13 Connective tissue

FIGURE 19.3 ■ Ovary: primary oocyte and wall of a mature follicle. Stain: hematoxylin and eosin. High magnification.

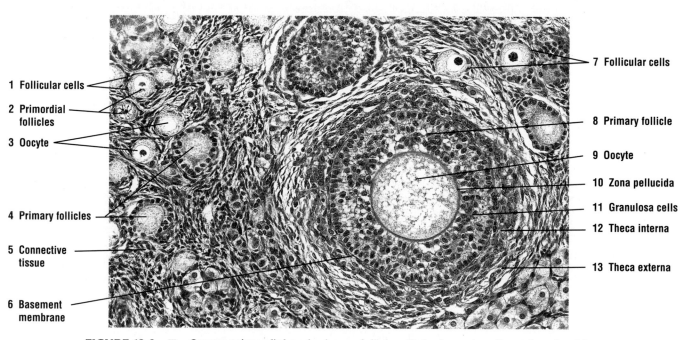

1 Follicular cells

2 Primordial follicles

3 Oocyte

4 Primary follicles

5 Connective tissue

6 Basement membrane

7 Follicular cells

8 Primary follicle

9 Oocyte

10 Zona pellucida

11 Granulosa cells

12 Theca interna

13 Theca externa

FIGURE 19.4 ■ Ovary: primordial and primary follicles. Stain: hematoxylin and eosin. 64×

FIGURE 19.5 ■ Human Ovary: Corpora Lutea and Atretic Follicles

This figure illustrates the newly formed corpus luteum, different corpora lutea at various stages of regression, and several stages of follicular atresia in a section of the entire ovary.

The ovarian surface is covered by a single layer of **germinal epithelium (1)**, under which is the connective tissue layer tunica albuginea. The **cortex (2, 18)** constitutes the greater portion of the ovary, and it contains the **growing follicles (8), primary follicles (12)**, and corpora lutea. The **medulla (7)** occupies the central region of the ovary and contains larger **blood vessels (7)** that supply the cortex (2, 18) of the ovary.

The new **corpus luteum (3)** is a large structure. It is formed after the ovulation of a mature follicle and the collapse of its walls. The **theca lutein cells (4)**, which are formed from the theca interna cells of the follicle, are located on the periphery of the corpus luteum (3) and in the contours of its folds (see Figs. 19-6 and 19-7 for details).

The mass of the corpus luteum wall (3) is formed from **granulosa lutein cells (5)**, which are the hypertrophied granulosa cells of the follicle. The **connective tissue (6)** from the theca externa proliferates in the wall of the corpus luteum. Blood vessels and capillaries fill the former follicular cavity (6).

Also illustrated is a **corpus luteum** in **moderate regression (10)**. The granulosa lutein cells are smaller, the nuclei are **pyknotic (10a)**, and larger **blood vessels (10b)** are growing in from the connective tissue stroma. The theca lutein cells are not visible.

A later stage of **corpus luteum regression (16)** shows shrinkage of lutein cells, **pyknosis** of their nuclei **(16b)**, and a **fibrous center (16a)**. The connective tissue begins to replace the luteal cells as they degenerate, and it forms a **capsule (16c)**. This, however, is not a constant feature. Final replacement by the connective tissue of all the lutein cells leaves a fibrous, hyalinized scar, called the **corpus albicans (15)**.

A **large, mature follicle (17)** exhibits **theca interna (17a)** and **granulosa cells (17b)**. The **cumulus oophorus (17d)** contains a primary **oocyte (17e)**, and the surrounding **antrum (17c)** is filled with follicular fluid.

Numerous follicles undergo atresia before reaching maturity. Atresia in large follicles is gradual. Here, a **follicle** at a **very early** stage of **atresia (14)** is illustrated. The **theca interna (14a)** and the **granulosa cells (14b)** are intact; however, some cells are beginning to slough off into the **antrum (14e)** with **follicular fluid (14d)**. Also, the cumulus oophorus has been disrupted, and the primary oocyte shows degeneration. A **remnant** of this **oocyte (14c)**, which is surrounded by thickened **zona pellucida (14c)**, is visible in the antrum (14e).

A **follicle** in **early atresia (13)** is also illustrated. The **theca interna (13a)** is still visible, but the cells appear hypertrophied. The granulosa cells have sloughed off and resorbed. The basement membrane has thickened and folded and is now called the **hypertrophied glassy membrane (13b)**. Loose **connective tissue (13e)** grows into the **antrum (13d)** and fills the follicular cavity, in which **follicular fluid (13c)** is still present.

With **moderate follicular atresia (9)**, the connective tissue **stroma** replaces the **thecal cells (9a)**. The **hypertrophied glassy membrane (9b)** becomes thicker and more folded. **Loose connective tissue** with small blood vessels fills the **antrum (9c)**. During **late atresia (11)**, the entire follicle is replaced by connective tissue. The **hypertrophied** and folded **glassy membrane (11)** remains for some time as the only indication of a follicle.

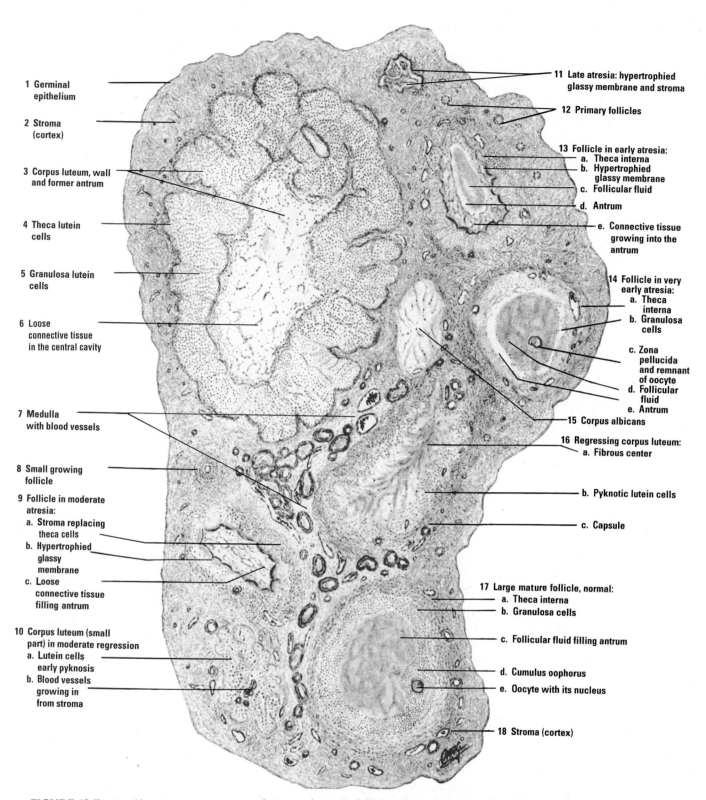

1 Germinal epithelium

2 Stroma (cortex)

3 Corpus luteum, wall and former antrum

4 Theca lutein cells

5 Granulosa lutein cells

6 Loose connective tissue in the central cavity

7 Medulla with blood vessels

8 Small growing follicle

9 Follicle in moderate atresia:
a. Stroma replacing theca cells
b. Hypertrophied glassy membrane
c. Loose connective tissue filling antrum

10 Corpus luteum (small part) in moderate regression
a. Lutein cells early pyknosis
b. Blood vessels growing in from stroma

11 Late atresia: hypertrophied glassy membrane and stroma

12 Primary follicles

13 Follicle in early atresia:
a. Theca interna
b. Hypertrophied glassy membrane
c. Follicular fluid
d. Antrum
e. Connective tissue growing into the antrum

14 Follicle in very early atresia:
a. Theca interna
b. Granulosa cells
c. Zona pellucida and remnant of oocyte
d. Follicular fluid
e. Antrum

15 Corpus albicans

16 Regressing corpus luteum:
a. Fibrous center
b. Pyknotic lutein cells
c. Capsule

17 Large mature follicle, normal:
a. Theca interna
b. Granulosa cells
c. Follicular fluid filling antrum
d. Cumulus oophorus
e. Oocyte with its nucleus

18 Stroma (cortex)

FIGURE 19.5 ■ Human ovary: corpora lutea and atretic follicles. Stain: hematoxylin and eosin. Low magnification.

FIGURE 19.6 ■ Corpus Luteum (Panoramic View)

At a higher magnification, the corpus luteum is a collapsed and folded mass of glandular epithelium that primarily consists of **theca lutein cells (5)** and **granulosa lutein cells (6).** Theca lutein cells (5) extend along the **connective tissue septa (3)** into the folds of the corpus luteum.

The **theca externa (2)** cells form a poorly defined capsule around the corpus luteum. This capsule also extends inward with the connective tissue septa (3) into the folds.

The center of the corpus luteum or **former follicular cavity (9)** contains remnants of follicular fluid, serum, blood cells, and loose **connective tissue** with **blood vessels (7)** from the theca externa that has proliferated and extended into the layers of the glandular epithelium. The connective tissue (7) also covers the inner surface of the granulosa luteal cells (6) and then spreads throughout the core of the corpus luteum. Some corpora lutea may contain a postovulatory **blood clot (8)** in the former follicular cavity (9).

The **connective tissue** of the **cortex (1)** that surrounds the corpus luteum contains numerous **blood vessels (4).**

FIGURE 19.7 ■ Corpus Luteum: Theca Lutein Cells and Granulosa Lutein Cells

The **granulosa lutein cells (6)** represent the hypertrophied former granulosa cells of the mature follicle, and they constitute the highly folded mass of the corpus luteum. The granulosa lutein cells (6) are large, have large vesicular nuclei, and stain lightly because of lipid inclusions. The **theca lutein cells (1, 7)** (i.e., the former theca interna cells) are external to the granulosa lutein cells (6), on the periphery of the glandular epithelium. The theca lutein cells (1, 7) are smaller than the granulosa lutein cells (6), and their cytoplasm stains darker. Also, the nuclei of theca lutein cells (1, 7) are smaller and darker.

The **theca externa (2)** with numerous blood vessels, such as **venules** and **arterioles (4),** and **capillaries (5)** invades granulosa lutein cells (6) and theca lutein cells (7). A fine **connective tissue septum** with **fibrocytes (3)** penetrates the theca lutein cells (7). The fibrocytes (3) in the septum between the theca lutein cells (7) can be identified by their elongated and flattened appearance.

FUNCTIONAL CORRELATIONS

Corpus Luteum

After the ovulation of a mature follicle and the liberation of an oocyte, the wall of the ruptured follicle collapses and becomes highly folded. At this time, the ovary enters the **luteal phase.** During this phase, LH secretion induces hypertrophy and transformation of the granulosa cells and theca interna cells of the ovulated follicle into **granulosa lutein cells** and **theca lutein cells,** respectively. These changes transform the ovulated follicle into the corpus luteum. Then, LH stimulates the cells of the corpus luteum to secrete estrogen and large amounts of progesterone. High levels of estrogen and progesterone further stimulate development of the uterus and mammary glands in anticipation of the implantation of a fertilized egg and pregnancy.

Rising levels of estrogen and progesterone, produced by the corpus luteum, inhibit further release of FSH and LH, influencing both the neurons in the hypothalamus and the gonadotrophs in the adenohypophysis. This effect prevents further ovulation.

If the ovulated oocyte is not fertilized, the corpus luteum eventually regresses into a nonfunctional scar tissue, called the **corpus albicans.** Estrogen and progesterone levels then decline, resulting in the shedding of the stratum functionalis in the uterus, followed by menstruation. With regression of the corpus luteum, the inhibitory effects of estrogen and progesterone on the hypothalamus and pituitary gland cells are removed. As a result, FSH is again released from the adenohypophysis, initiating of a new ovarian cycle of follicular development.

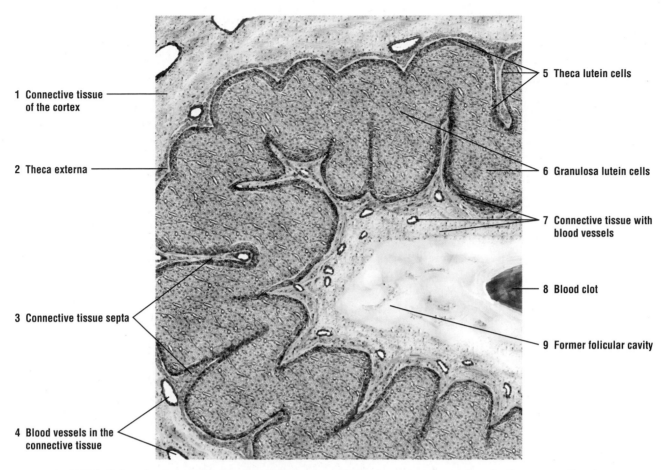

1 Connective tissue of the cortex

2 Theca externa

3 Connective tissue septa

4 Blood vessels in the connective tissue

5 Theca lutein cells

6 Granulosa lutein cells

7 Connective tissue with blood vessels

8 Blood clot

9 Former folicular cavity

FIGURE 19.6 ■ Corpus luteum (panoramic view). Stain: hematoxylin and eosin. Low magnification.

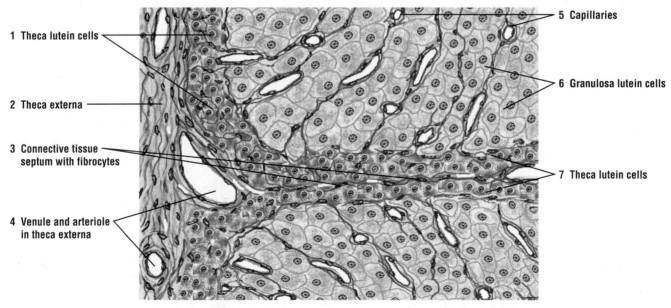

1 Theca lutein cells

2 Theca externa

3 Connective tissue septum with fibrocytes

4 Venule and arteriole in theca externa

5 Capillaries

6 Granulosa lutein cells

7 Theca lutein cells

FIGURE 19.7 ■ Corpus luteum: theca lutein cells and granulosa lutein cells. Stain: hematoxylin and eosin. High magnification.

FIGURE 19.8 ■ Uterine Tube: Ampulla (Panoramic View, Transverse Section)

The extensive **mucosal folds (9)** form an irregular lumen in the uterine (i.e., fallopian) tube. The lumen of the uterine tube extends between the mucosal folds (9) and forms deep grooves. The lining **epithelium (10)** of the uterine tube is simple columnar overlying the vascularized and loose connective tissue **lamina propria (8).**

The muscularis consists of two smooth muscle layers, an inner layer of **circular muscle fibers (1)** and an outer layer of **longitudinal muscle fibers (6).** The **interstitial connective tissue (2)** is abundant, and as a result, the smooth muscle layers—especially the outer layer—are not distinct. Numerous **venules (3, 4)** and an **arteriole (5)** are seen in the interstitial connective tissue (2). The **serosa (7)** forms the outermost layer on the uterine tube.

FIGURE 19.9 ■ Uterine Tube: Mucosal Folds (Early Proliferative Phase)

A higher-magnification view of the uterine tube shows that the lining epithelium consists of **ciliated cells (1)** and nonciliated peg (i.e., secretory) cells. During the early proliferative phase of the menstrual cycle and estrogen influence, the ciliated cells undergo hypertrophy, exhibit cilia growth, and become predominant. In addition, the secretory activity of the nonciliated peg cells increases. The epithelium of the uterine tube shows cyclic changes, and the proportion of ciliated and nonciliated cells varies with the stages of the menstrual cycle.

The **lamina propria (2)** is a cellular, loose connective tissue with fine collagen and reticular fibers.

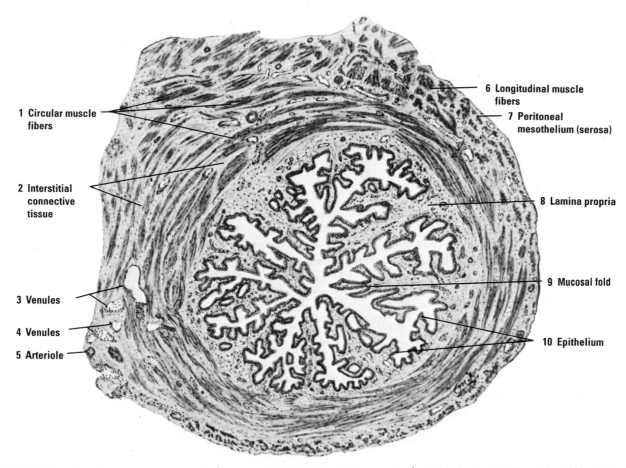

1 Circular muscle fibers
2 Interstitial connective tissue
3 Venules
4 Venules
5 Arteriole
6 Longitudinal muscle fibers
7 Peritoneal mesothelium (serosa)
8 Lamina propria
9 Mucosal fold
10 Epithelium

FIGURE 19.8 ■ Uterine tube: ampulla (panoramic view, transverse section). Stain: hematoxylin and eosin. Low magnification.

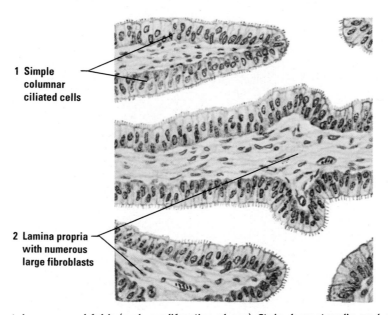

1 Simple columnar ciliated cells
2 Lamina propria with numerous large fibroblasts

FIGURE 19.9 ■ Uterine tube: mucosal folds (early proliferative phase). Stain: hematoxylin and eosin. High magnification.

FIGURE 19.10 ■ Uterine Tube: Mucosal Folds (Early Pregnancy)

During the secretory (i.e., luteal) phase of the menstrual cycle and early pregnancy, the **peg cells** (**secretory cells**) (**2**) predominate in the uterine tube epithelium. These cells are slender, with elongated nuclei and apices that protrude into the tubular lumina. The peg cells (**2**) intermix with **ciliated cells** (**3**) in epithelium of the uterine tube. A prominent **lamina propria** (**1**) supports the epithelium.

FIGURE 19.11 ■ Uterine Tube: Lining Epithelium

A higher-magnification photomicrograph illustrates a section of the wall of the uterine tube with complex mucosal folds that are lined by a **simple columnar epithelium** (**2**).

The luminal epithelium consists of two cell types, the **ciliated cells** (**5**) and the nonciliated **peg cells** (**6**) with apical bulges that extend above the cilia. A thin **basement membrane** (**1**) separates the luminal epithelium (**2**) from the underlying vascularized **connective tissue** (**4**) that forms the core of the mucosal folds. A portion of the **inner circular smooth muscle** (**3**) layer that surrounds the uterine tube is visible in the periphery on the left side of the illustration.

FUNCTIONAL CORRELATIONS

Uterine Tubes

The uterine tubes perform several important reproductive functions. Just before ovulation and rupture of the mature follicle, the finger-like **fimbriae** of the infundibulum sweep the surface of the ovary to capture the released oocyte. This function is accomplished by a gentle, peristaltic action of smooth muscles in the uterine wall and fimbriae. In addition, the heavily ciliated cells on the fimbriae surface create a current that guides the oocyte into the infundibulum of the uterine tube. The cilia action and the muscular contractions in the wall of the uterine tube transport the captured oocyte or fertilized egg through the remaining regions of the uterine tube toward the uterus.

The uterine tubes also serve as the site of oocyte **fertilization,** which normally occurs in the upper region of the **ampulla.** The nonciliated peg cells in the uterine tube are secretory and contribute important nutritive material for the initial development of the fertilized ovum and embryo. The uterine secretions also maintain the viability of sperm in the uterine tubes and allow them to undergo **capacitation,** which is a biochemical process that activates the sperm and enables them to fertilize the released oocyte.

The epithelium in the uterine tubes exhibits changes that are associated with the ovarian cycle. The height of the uterine tube epithelium is at its maximum during the follicular phase, when the ovarian follicles are maturing and circulating levels of estrogen are high.

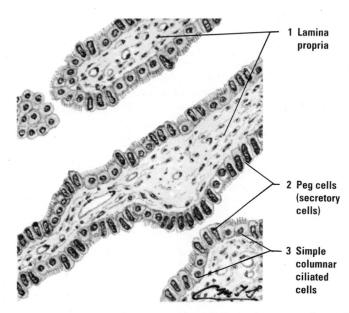

1 Lamina
propria

2 Peg cells
(secretory
cells)

3 Simple
columnar
ciliated
cells

FIGURE 19.10 ■ Uterine tube: mucosal folds (early pregnancy). Stain: hematoxylin and eosin. High magnification.

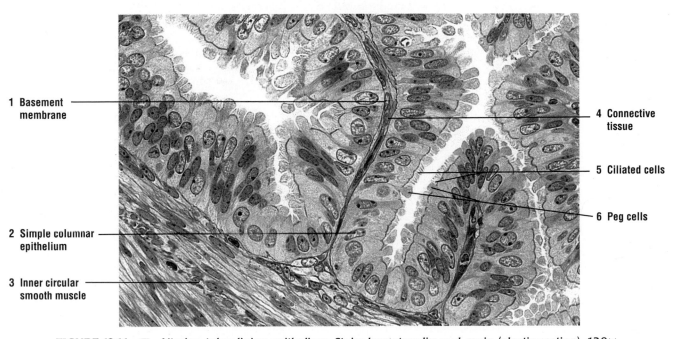

1 Basement
membrane

2 Simple columnar
epithelium

3 Inner circular
smooth muscle

4 Connective
tissue

5 Ciliated cells

6 Peg cells

FIGURE 19.11 ■ Uterine tube: lining epithelium. Stain: hematoxylin and eosin (plastic section). 130×

FIGURE 19.12 ■ Uterus: Proliferative (Follicular) Phase

The surface of the endometrium is lined with a simple columnar **lining epithelium (1)** overlaying the thick **lamina propria (2).** The lining epithelium (1) extends down into the connective tissue of the lamina propria (2) and forms long, tubular **uterine glands (4).** In the proliferative phase, the uterine glands (4) usually are straight in the superficial portion of the endometrium, but they may exhibit branching in the deeper regions near the myometrium. As a result, numerous uterine glands (4) are seen in cross-section.

The wall of the uterus consists of three layers: the inner **endometrium (1, 2, 3, 4),** a middle layer of smooth muscle **myometrium (5, 6),** and the outer serous membrane perimetrium (not illustrated). The endometrium is further subdivided into two zones or layers, a narrow, deep **basalis layer (8)** adjacent to the myometrium (5) and the **functionalis layer (7)** and a wider, superficial layer above the basalis layer (8) that extends to the lumen of the uterus.

During the menstrual cycle, the endometrium exhibits morphological changes that directly correlate with ovarian function. The cyclic changes in a nonpregnant uterus are divided into three distinct phases: the proliferative (follicular) phase, the secretory (luteal) phase, and the menstrual phase.

During the proliferative phase of the cycle and under the influence of ovarian estrogen, the stratum functionalis (7) increases in thickness, and the uterine glands (4) elongate and follow a straight course to the surface. Also, the **coiled** (spiral) **arteries (3)** (in cross-section) are seen primarily in the deeper regions of the endometrium. The lamina propria (2) in the upper regions of the endometrium is cellular and resembles mesenchymal tissue. The connective tissue in the basalis layer (8) is more compact and appears darker. The endometrium continues to develop during the proliferative phase because of the increasing levels of estrogen secreted by the developing ovarian follicles.

The endometrium is situated above the myometrium (5, 6) that consists of compact bundles of **smooth muscle (5, 6)** that are separated by thin strands of **interstitial connective tissue (9)** with numerous **blood vessels (10).** As a result, the muscle bundles are seen in cross, oblique, and longitudinal sections.

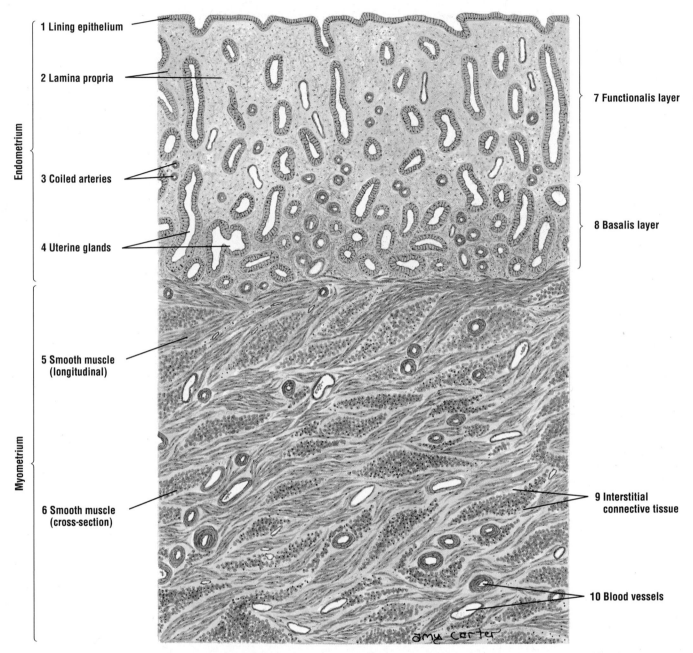

1 Lining epithelium

2 Lamina propria

Endometrium

3 Coiled arteries

4 Uterine glands

7 Functionalis layer

8 Basalis layer

Myometrium

5 Smooth muscle (longitudinal)

6 Smooth muscle (cross-section)

9 Interstitial connective tissue

10 Blood vessels

amy carter

FIGURE 19.12 ■ Uterus: proliferative (follicular) phase. Stain: hematoxylin and eosin. Low magnification.

FIGURE 19.13 ■ Uterus: Secretory (Luteal) Phase

The secretory (luteal) phase of the menstrual cycle is initiated after ovulation of the mature follicle. The additional changes in the endometrium result from the influence of both estrogen and progesterone secreted by the functioning corpus luteum. As a result, the **functionalis layer (1)** and the **basalis layer (2)** of the endometrium become thicker as a result of increased glandular **secretion (5)** and edema in the **lamina propria (6).**

The epithelium of the **uterine glands (5, 8)** undergo hypertrophy (i.e., enlarges) because of increased accumulation of the secretory product (5, 8). The uterine glands (5, 8) also become highly coiled (i.e., tortuous), and their lumina become dilated with nutritive secretory material (5) that is rich in carbohydrates. The **coiled arteries (7)** continue to extend into the upper portion of the endometrium (functionalis layer) (1) and become prominent because of their thicker walls.

The alterations in the surface **columnar epithelium (4),** uterine glands (5), and lamina propria (6) characterize the functionalis layer (1) of the endometrium during the secretory or luteal phase of the menstrual cycle. The basalis layer (2) exhibits minimal changes. Below the basalis layer is the **myometrium (3)** with **smooth muscle bundles (10),** which are sectioned in both longitudinal and transverse planes, and **blood vessels (9).**

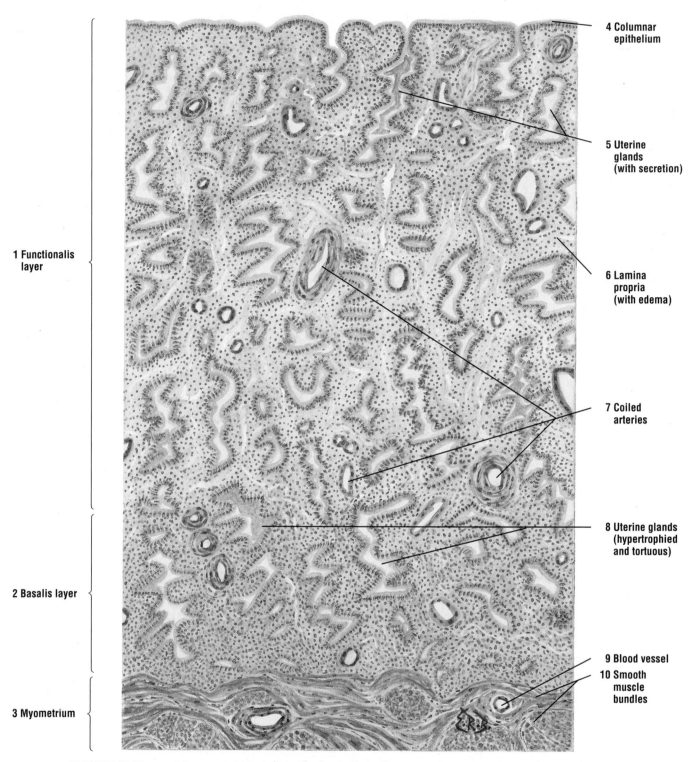

1 Functionalis layer

2 Basalis layer

3 Myometrium

4 Columnar epithelium

5 Uterine glands (with secretion)

6 Lamina propria (with edema)

7 Coiled arteries

8 Uterine glands (hypertrophied and tortuous)

9 Blood vessel

10 Smooth muscle bundles

FIGURE 19.13 ■ Uterus: secretory (luteal) phase. Stain: hematoxylin and eosin. Low magnification.

FIGURE 19.14 ■ Uterine Wall (Endometrium): Secretory (Luteal) Phase

A low-power photomicrograph illustrates a section of the endometrium during the secretory (luteal) phase of the menstrual cycle. The thick and lighter area of the endometrium is the **stratum functionalis (1).** The darker and deeper endometrium is the **stratum basalis (2).** During the secretory phase, the **uterine glands (3)** are coiled (tortuous) and secrete glycogen-rich nutrients into their lumina.

Surrounding the uterine glands (3) is the highly cellular **connective tissue (4).** The light, empty spaces in the connective tissue (4) layer result from increased edema in the endometrium. Below the stratum basalis (2) is the smooth muscle layer **myometrium (5)** of the uterine wall.

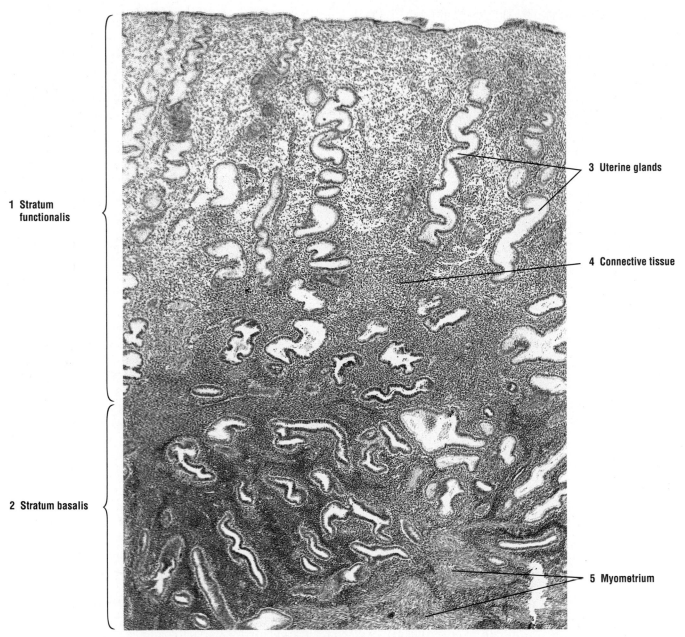

FIGURE 19.14 ■ Uterine wall (endometrium): secretory (luteal) phase. Stain: hematoxylin and eosin. 10×

FIGURE 19.15 ■ Uterus: Menstrual Phase

If fertilization of the ovum and implantation of the embryo do not occur, the uterus enters the menstrual phase, and much of the preparatory changes that have been made for implantation in the endometrium are lost. During the menstrual phase, the **endometrium (1)** in the functionalis layer degenerates and is shed. The shed endometrium contains **fragments of disintegrated stroma (6)**, **blood clots (7)**, and uterine glands. Some of the intact **uterine glands (2)** are filled with blood. In the deeper layers of the endometrium, the **basalis layer (4)**, the **bases of the uterine glands (9)** remain intact during the shedding of functionalis layer and the menstrual flow.

The endometrial stroma of most of the functionalis layer contains aggregations of **erythrocytes (8)** that have been extruded from the torn and disintegrating blood vessels. In addition, the endometrial stroma (6) exhibits infiltration of lymphocytes and neutrophils.

The basalis layer (4) of the endometrium remains unaffected during this phase. The distal (i.e., superficial) portions of the **coiled arteries (3)** become necrotic, whereas the deeper parts of these vessels remain intact.

FUNCTIONAL CORRELATIONS

Uterus

During pregnancy, the uterus provides the site for **implantation** of the embryo and formation of the placenta as well as a suitable environment for development of the embryo and fetus. The endometrium also exhibits cyclic changes in its structure and function in response to the ovarian hormones **estrogen** and **progesterone.** The uterine changes are associated with impending implantation and nourishment of the developing organism. If fertilization of the oocyte and implantation of the embryo do not occur, blood vessels in the endometrium deteriorate and rupture, and the **functionalis layer** of the endometrium is shed as part of the menstrual flow or discharge. With each menstrual cycle, the endometrium passes through three phases, with each phase gradually passing into the next.

The **preovulatory (proliferative, follicular) phase** is characterized by rapid growth and development of the endometrium. This phase starts at the end of the menstrual phase, or on approximately day 5, and it continues to approximately day 14 of the cycle. Increased mitotic activity of the **lamina propria** and in remnants of the **uterine glands** in the **basalis layer** of the endometrium produce cells that begin to cover the raw surface of the uterine mucosa that was denuded or shed during menstruation. The resurfacing of the mucosa produces a new functionalis layer of the endometrium. As the functionalis layer thickens, the uterine glands proliferate, lengthen, and become closely packed. The **spiral arteries** begin to grow toward the endometrial surface and to show light coiling. The resurfacing and growth of the endometrium during the proliferative phase closely coincides with the rapid growth of **ovarian follicles** and their increased production of **estrogen.**

The **postovulatory (secretory, luteal) phase** begins shortly after ovulation, on approximately day 15, and it continues to approximately day 28 of the cycle. This phase is dependent on the secretion of **progesterone** (primarily by granulosa lutein cells) and **estrogen** (by theca lutein cells) of the functional corpus luteum that was formed after ovulation. During the postovulatory phase, the endometrium thickens, accumulates fluid, and becomes **edematous.** In addition, the uterine glands undergo hypertrophy and become tortuous, and their lumina become filled with secretions that are rich in **nutrients,** especially **glycogen.** The spiral arteries in the endometrium also lengthen, become more coiled, and extend almost to the surface of the endometrium.

The **menstrual (menses) phase** of the cycle begins when the oocyte is not fertilized and the embryo does not implant in the uterus. Reduced levels of circulating progesterone and estrogen, resulting from regression of the corpus luteum, initiate this phase. Decreased levels of these hormones cause intermittent constrictions of the spiral arteries and interruption of blood flow to the functionalis layer of the endometrium, whereas the blood flow to the basalis layer remains uninterrupted. These constrictions deprive the functionalis layer of oxygenated blood and produce transitory **ischemia,** causing necrosis (i.e., death) of cells in the walls of blood vessels and degeneration of the functionalis layer in the endometrium. After extended periods of

1 Superficial
endometrium
without epithelium

2 Uterine gland
lumen filled
with blood

3 Coiled arteries

4 Interglandular
lamina propria
of the basalis layer

5 Smooth muscle
fibers (myometrium)

6 Fragments of
disintegrated stroma

7 Blood clots

8 Erythrocytes in
lamina propria

9 Intact bases of the
uterine glands

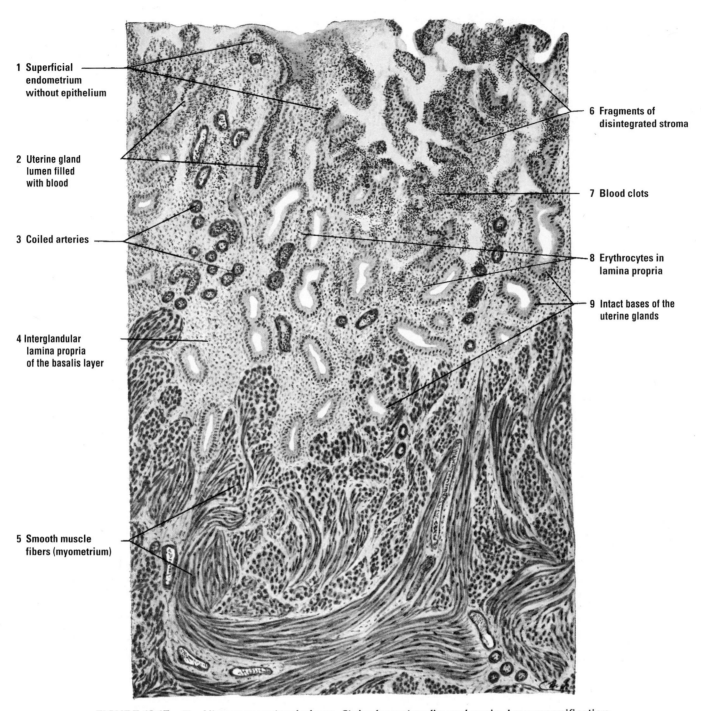

FIGURE 19.15 ■ Uterus: menstrual phase. Stain: hematoxylin and eosin. Low magnification.

vascular constriction, the spiral arteries dilate, resulting in the rupture of their necrotic walls and hemorrhage (i.e., bleeding) into the stroma. The necrotic functionalis layer then detaches from the rest of the endometrium, and blood, uterine fluid, stromal cells, secretory material, and epithelial cells from the functionalis layer mix to form the **menstrual flow.**

The shedding of the functionalis layer of the endometrium continues until only the raw surface of the basalis layer is left. The remnants of the uterine glands in the basalis layer serve as the source of cells for regenerating the next functionalis layer. Rapid proliferation of cells in the glands of the basalis layer, under the influence of rising estrogen levels, resurface and restore the lost endometrial layer and start the next phase of the menstrual cycle.

SECTION 2 ■ Cervix, Vagina, Placenta, and Mammary Glands

Cervix and Vagina

The cervix is located in the lower part of the uterus that projects into the vaginal canal as the **portio vaginalis.** A narrow **cervical canal** passes through the cervix. The opening of the cervical canal that directly communicates with the uterus is called the **internal os** and, with the vagina, the **external os.** Unlike the functionalis layer of the uterine endometrium, the cervical mucosa undergoes only minimal changes during the menstrual cycle and is not shed during menstruation. The cervix contains numerous branched **cervical glands** that exhibit altered secretory activities during the different phases of the menstrual cycle. The amount and type of mucus secreted by the cervical glands change during the menstrual cycle because of different levels of ovarian hormones.

The **vagina** is a fibromuscular structure that extends from the cervix to the vestibule of the external genitalia. Its wall has numerous folds and consists of an inner **mucosa,** a middle **muscular layer,** and an outer connective tissue **adventitia.** The vagina does not have any glands in its wall. The vaginal lumen is lined by **stratified squamous epithelium** and is lubricated using mucus produced by cells in the **cervical glands.** Loose fibroelastic connective tissue and rich vasculature comprise the lamina propria that overlies the smooth muscle layers of the organ. Like the cervical epithelium, the vaginal lining is not shed during the menstrual flow.

Placenta

During pregnancy, the fertilized ovum implants in the endometrium of the uterus and forms a **placenta.** The placenta consists of a **fetal portion,** which is formed by the **chorionic plate** and its **branching chorionic villi,** and a **maternal portion,** which is formed by the **decidua basalis** of the endometrium. Fetal and maternal blood come into close proximity in the villi of the placenta. Exchange of nutrients, electrolytes, hormones, antibodies, gaseous products, and waste metabolites takes place as the blood passes over the villi. Fetal blood enters the placenta through a pair of **umbilical arteries,** passes into the villi, and returns through a single **umbilical vein.**

Mammary Glands

The adult mammary gland is a compound **tubuloalveolar gland** that consists of approximately 20 lobes. All lobes are connected to **lactiferous ducts** that open at the **nipple.** The lobes are separated by connective tissue partitions and adipose tissue.

The resting or inactive mammary glands are small, consist primarily of **ducts,** and do not exhibit any developed or secretory alveoli. Inactive mammary glands also exhibit slight cyclic alterations during the course of the menstrual cycle. Under estrogenic stimulation, the secretory cells increase in height, lumina appear in the ducts, and a small amount of secretory material is accumulated.

FIGURE 19.16   ■   Cervix, Cervical Canal, and Vaginal Fornix (Longitudinal Section)

The cervix is the lower part of the uterus. This figure illustrates a longitudinal section through the cervix, the endocervix or **cervical canal (5)**, a portion of the **vaginal fornix (8)**, and the **vaginal wall (10)**.

The cervical canal (5) is lined with tall, mucus-secreting columnar **epithelium (2)** that is continuous with the uterine epithelium. The cervical epithelium also lines the highly branched and tubular **cervical glands (3)** that extend at an oblique angle to the cervical canal (5) into the **lamina propria (12)**. Some cervical glands may become occluded and develop into small **glandular cysts (4)**. The connective tissue in the lamina propria (12) of the cervix is more fibrous than in the uterus. Blood vessels, nerves, and occasional **lymphatic nodules (11)** may be seen.

The lower end of the cervix, called the **os cervix (6)**, bulges into the lumen of the **vaginal canal (13)**. The columnar epithelium (2) of the cervical canal (5) abruptly changes to nonkeratinized stratified squamous epithelium to line the vaginal portion of the cervix, called the **portio vaginalis (7)**, and the external surface of the vaginal fornix (8). At the base of the fornix, the **epithelium (7)** of the vaginal cervix reflects back to become the **vaginal epithelium (9)** of the vaginal wall (10).

The smooth muscles of the **muscularis (1)** extend into the cervix but are not as compact as the muscles in the body of the uterus.

FUNCTIONAL CORRELATIONS

Cervix

During the **proliferative phase** of the menstrual cycle, the secretion of cervical glands is thin and watery. This type of secretion allows easier passage of sperm through the cervical canal into the uterus. During the luteal phase of the menstrual cycle and pregnancy, the cervical gland secretions change and become highly viscous, forming a **mucus plug** in the cervical canal. The mucus plug is a protective measure that hinders the passage of sperm and/or microorganisms from the vagina into the body of the uterus. The increased viscosity of cervical secretions depends primarily on higher levels of progesterone in the plasma.

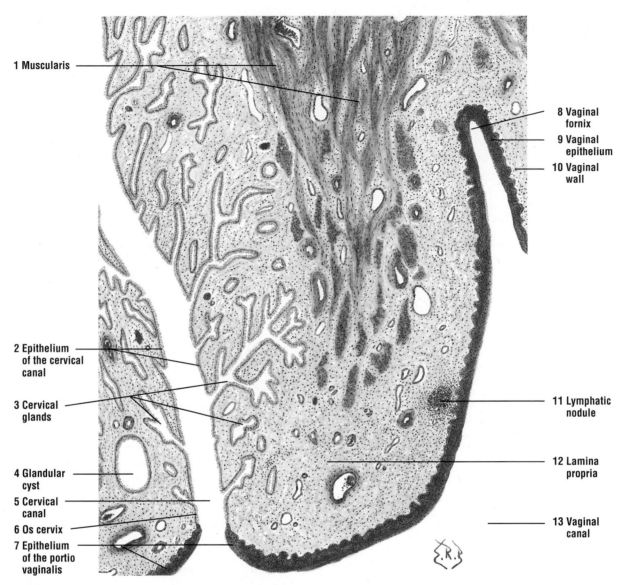

1 Muscularis

8 Vaginal fornix

9 Vaginal epithelium

10 Vaginal wall

2 Epithelium of the cervical canal

3 Cervical glands

11 Lymphatic nodule

4 Glandular cyst

5 Cervical canal

6 Os cervix

7 Epithelium of the portio vaginalis

12 Lamina propria

13 Vaginal canal

FIGURE 19.16 ■ Cervix, cervical canal, and vaginal fornix (longitudinal section). Stain: hematoxylin and eosin. Low magnification.

FIGURE 19.17 ■ Vagina (Longitudinal Section)

The vaginal mucosa is irregular and shows **mucosal folds (1)**. The surface epithelium of the vaginal canal is noncornified **stratified squamous (2)**. The underlying **connective tissue papillae (3)** are prominent and indent the epithelium.

The **lamina propria (7)** contains dense irregular connective tissue with elastic fibers that extend into the muscularis layer as **interstitial connective tissue (10)**. Diffuse **lymphatic tissue (8)**, **lymphatic nodules (4)**, and small **blood vessels (9)** are in the lamina propria (7).

The muscularis of the vaginal wall consists predominantly of **longitudinal bundles (5a)** and oblique bundles of **smooth muscle (5)**. The **transverse bundles (5b)** of the smooth muscle are more frequently found in the inner layers. The interstitial connective tissue (10) is rich in elastic fibers. **Blood vessels (11)** and nerve bundles are abundant in the **adventitia (6, 12)**.

FIGURE 19.18 ■ Glycogen in Human Vaginal Epithelium

Glycogen is a prominent component of the vaginal epithelium, except in the deepest layers, where it is minimal or absent. During the follicular phase of the menstrual cycle, glycogen accumulates in the vaginal epithelium and reaches its maximum level before ovulation. Glycogen can be demonstrated by iodine vapor or iodine solution in mineral oil (Mancini's method); glycogen stains a reddish purple.

The vaginal specimens in illustrations (A) and (B) were fixed in absolute alcohol and formaldehyde. The amount of glycogen in the vaginal epithelium is illustrated during the **interfollicular phase (A)**. During the **follicular phase (B)**, glycogen content increases in the intermediate and superficial cell layers.

The tissue sample in illustration (C) is from the same specimen as that in (B) but was fixed by the Altmann-Gersch method (freezing and drying in a vacuum). This method produces less tissue shrinkage and illustrates more glycogen and its diffuse distribution in the vaginal epithelium during the **follicular phase (C)**.

FUNCTIONAL CORRELATIONS

Vagina

The wall of the vagina consists of mucosa, a smooth muscle layer, and an adventitia. No glands are found in the vaginal mucosa. The surface of the vaginal canal is kept moist and lubricated by secretions from cervical glands.

The vaginal epithelium exhibits minimal changes during each menstrual cycle. During the follicular phase of the menstrual cycle and because of increased estrogen stimulation, the vaginal epithelium increases in thickness. In addition, estrogen stimulates the vaginal cells to synthesize and accumulate increased amounts of **glycogen** as these cells migrate toward the vaginal lumen, into which they are shed or desquamated. Bacterial flora in the vagina metabolize glycogen into **lactic acid.** Increased acidity in the vaginal canal protects it against microorganisms or pathogenic invasion.

Microscopic examination of cells collected (i.e., scraped) from the vaginal and cervical mucosae, called a **Pap smear,** provides highly valuable diagnostic information of clinical importance. Cervicovaginal Pap smears are routinely examined for early detection of pathological changes in the epithelium of these organs that may lead to cervical cancer.

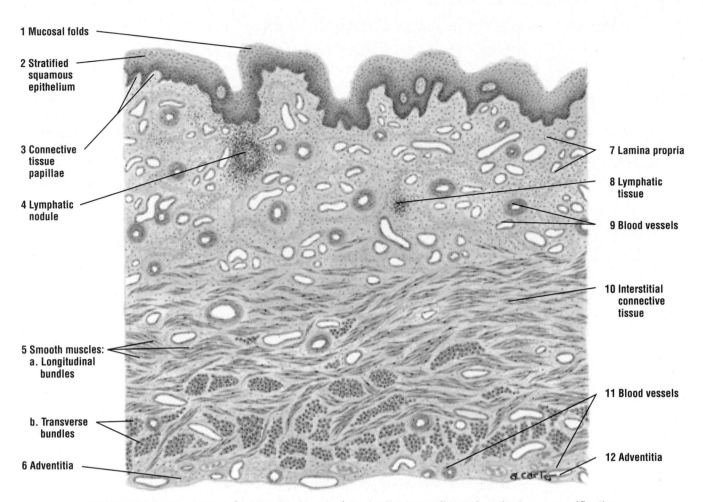

1 Mucosal folds

2 Stratified squamous epithelium

3 Connective tissue papillae

4 Lymphatic nodule

5 Smooth muscles:
a. Longitudinal bundles

b. Transverse bundles

6 Adventitia

7 Lamina propria

8 Lymphatic tissue

9 Blood vessels

10 Interstitial connective tissue

11 Blood vessels

12 Adventitia

FIGURE 19.17 ■ Vagina (longitudinal section). Stain: hematoxylin and eosin. Low magnification.

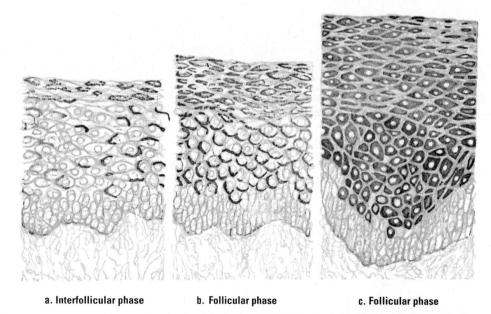

a. Interfollicular phase   b. Follicular phase   c. Follicular phase

FIGURE 19.18 ■ Glycogen in human vaginal epithelium. Stain: Mancini's iodine technique. Medium magnification.

FIGURE 19.19 ■ Vaginal Smears During Various Reproductive Phases

This figure illustrates cells in vaginal smears obtained during the menstrual cycle, early pregnancy, and menopause. The Shorr's trichrome stain (Bierbrich scarlet, orange G, and fast green) plus Harris' hematoxylin facilitates the recognition of different cell types.

Figure A illustrates a vaginal smear collected during the **postmenstrual phase** (fifth day of the menstrual cycle). The **intermediate cells (1)** are predominant. In addition, a few **superficial cells (acidophilic and basophilic) (2)** and leukocytes are present.

Figure B represents a vaginal smear collected during the **ovulatory phase** (14th day of the menstrual cycle) of the menstrual cycle. The large **superficial acidophilic cells (8),** the scarcity of **superficial basophilic cells (10)** and **intermediate cells (9),** and the absence of leukocytes characterize this phase. This smear is characteristic of the high estrogenic stimulation that normally is observed before ovulation and is called the follicular smear. The superficial cells (8) "mature" with increased estrogen levels and become acidophilic. A similar type of smear can be obtained from a menopausal woman treated with high doses of estrogen.

Figure C represents a vaginal smear collected during the **luteal** (secretory) **phase** (21st day of the menstrual cycle). This phase shows the effects of increased levels of progesterone. The large **intermediate cells (3)** from the intermediate layers (precornified superficial cells) with folded borders aggregate into clumps and are predominant. **Superficial acidophilic cells (4), superficial basophilic cells (5),** and leukocytes are scarce.

Figure D represents a vaginal smear taken during the **premenstrual phase** (28th day of the menstrual cycle). This stage is characterized by a predominance of grouped **intermediate cells (13, 14)** with **folded borders (13),** an increase in the number of **neutrophilic cells (12),** a scarcity of the **superficial acidophilic cells (11),** and an abundance of mucus.

Figure E illustrates a vaginal smear taken during the **third month** of **pregnancy.** This smear contains predominantly **intermediate cells** with **folded borders (6).** These cells form dense groups, or **conglomerations (7).** Cells from superficial layers and neutrophilic cells are scarce.

The vaginal smear during menopause in Figure F differs from those of all other phases. Here, the predominant cells are the oval **basal cells (17).** The **intermediate cells (15)** are scarce, whereas the **neutrophilic cells (16)** are abundant. Menopausal smears vary depending on the stage of menopause and the estrogen levels.

Figure G illustrates individual cell types that are observed in a normal vaginal smear. The **superficial acidophilic cell (a)** of the vaginal epithelium appears flat and irregular in outline, measures from 35 to 65 μm in diameter, exhibits a small nucleus, and contains cytoplasm that stains light orange. The similar **superficial basophilic cell (b)** exhibits blue-green cytoplasm. The **intermediate cell (c),** like the superficial cell, is flat but smaller, measuring from 20 to 40 μm in diameter, and shows a basophilic blue-green cytoplasm. The nucleus is somewhat larger than that of the superficial cells and is often vesicular. Also depicted are **intermediate cells** in **profile (d).** These cells are characterized by an elongated form with folded borders and an elongated, eccentric nucleus. The larger **basal cells (e)** are from the basal layers of the vaginal epithelium. The smaller **parabasal cells (e)** are from the more superficial portion of the basal layers. All basal cells are oval, measure from 12 to 15 m in diameter, and exhibit a large nucleus with prominent chromatin. Most of these cells exhibit basophilic staining.

Vaginal exfoliate cytology (i.e., vaginal smear) is correlated with the ovarian cycle and permits recognition of the follicular activity during normal menstrual phases or after hormonal therapy. Also, exfoliate cytology together with cells from the endocervix provides a very important source of information for detecting cervical/vaginal cancers.

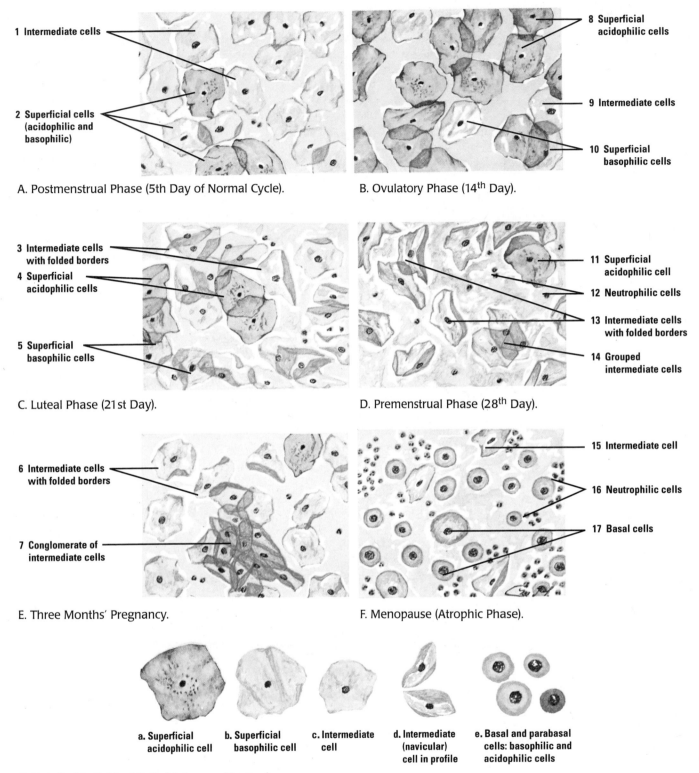

1 Intermediate cells

2 Superficial cells (acidophilic and basophilic)

A. Postmenstrual Phase (5th Day of Normal Cycle).

8 Superficial acidophilic cells

9 Intermediate cells

10 Superficial basophilic cells

B. Ovulatory Phase (14th Day).

3 Intermediate cells with folded borders
4 Superficial acidophilic cells
5 Superficial basophilic cells

C. Luteal Phase (21st Day).

11 Superficial acidophilic cell
12 Neutrophilic cells
13 Intermediate cells with folded borders
14 Grouped intermediate cells

D. Premenstrual Phase (28th Day).

6 Intermediate cells with folded borders
7 Conglomerate of intermediate cells

E. Three Months' Pregnancy.

15 Intermediate cell
16 Neutrophilic cells
17 Basal cells

F. Menopause (Atrophic Phase).

a. Superficial acidophilic cell
b. Superficial basophilic cell
c. Intermediate cell
d. Intermediate (navicular) cell in profile
e. Basal and parabasal cells: basophilic and acidophilic cells

G. Detail of Individual Cells (high magnification).

FIGURE 19.19 ■ Vaginal smears during various reproductive phases. Stain: Shorr's trichrome. Medium magnification.

FIGURE 19.20 ■ Vagina: Surface Epithelium

This higher-magnification photomicrograph illustrates the vaginal epithelium and the underlying connective tissue. The surface **epithelium** is **stratified squamous nonkeratinized (1)**. Most of the superficial cells in the vaginal epithelium appear empty because of increased accumulation of glycogen in their cytoplasm. During the histologic preparation of the organ, the glycogen was extracted by chemicals.

The **lamina propria (2)** contains dense irregular connective tissue. The lamina propria lacks glands but does have numerous **blood vessels (4)** and **lymphocytes (3)**.

FIGURE 19.21 ■ Placenta at 5 Months (Panoramic View)

The upper region of the figure illustrates the fetal portion of the placenta. This includes the **chorionic plate (10)**, **chorion frondosum (11)**, and both **anchoring villi (4, 7)** and **floating villi (5)**. The maternal placenta is the **decidua basalis (8)** and includes the functionalis layer of the endometrium, including **fibrin deposits (12)**, **blood vessels opening** into the **intervillous space (13)**, and **uterine glands (14)**, that lies directly beneath the fetal placenta (10, 11). Below this region is the basalis layer of the endometrium with the **basal uterine glands (15)**. The basalis layer of the endometrium is not shed during parturition. A portion of the **myometrium (17)** of the uterus is visible in the lower right.

The **amnion (1)** is lined by a squamous **epithelium (1)**, below which is the merged **connective tissue (2)** of the amnion (1) and chorion (10). Inferior to the connective tissue (2) layer is the **trophoblast (3)** of the chorion (10). The trophoblast (3, 10) and the underlying connective tissue (2) form the chorionic plate (10).

The anchoring villi (4, 7) arise from the chorionic plate (10), extend to the uterine wall, and embed in the decidua basalis (8). Numerous floating villi (5) of the chorion frondosum (11), sectioned in various planes, extend in all directions from the anchoring villi (7). These villi "float" in the **intervillous blood spaces (6)** that are bathed in maternal blood.

The maternal portion of the placenta, the decidua basalis (8), contains anchoring villi (7), large **decidual cells (8)**, and typical connective tissue stroma. The decidua basalis (8) also contains the distal portions of the uterine glands (14) in various stages of regression. The **maternal blood vessels (9)** in the decidua basalis (8) are recognized by their size or by the presence of blood cells in their lumina. Here, a maternal blood vessel opening into an intervillous space (13) is visible.

The **coiled arteries (16)** and the basal uterine glands (15) are located deep in the endometrium. Fibrin deposits (12) of fine fibers appear on the surface of the decidua basalis (8) and increase in volume and extent as the pregnancy continues.

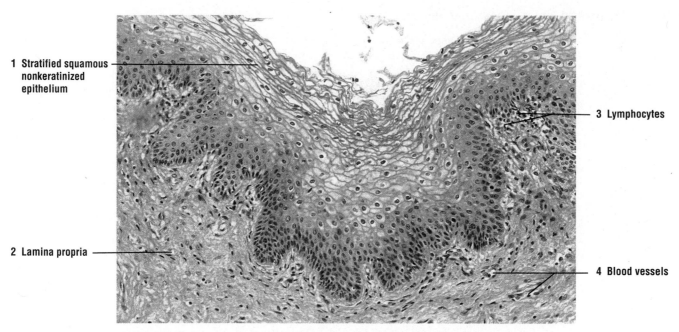

1 Stratified squamous nonkeratinized epithelium

2 Lamina propria

3 Lymphocytes

4 Blood vessels

FIGURE 19.20 ■ Vagina: surface epithelium. Stain: hematoxylin and eosin. 50×

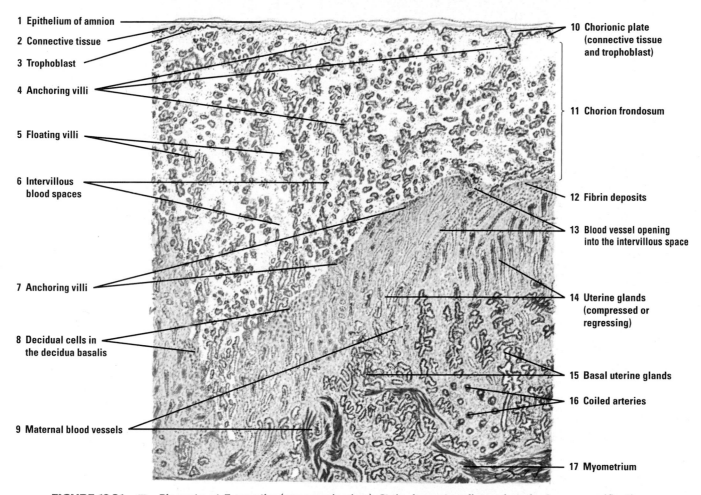

1 Epithelium of amnion
2 Connective tissue
3 Trophoblast
4 Anchoring villi
5 Floating villi
6 Intervillous blood spaces
7 Anchoring villi
8 Decidual cells in the decidua basalis
9 Maternal blood vessels

10 Chorionic plate (connective tissue and trophoblast)
11 Chorion frondosum
12 Fibrin deposits
13 Blood vessel opening into the intervillous space
14 Uterine glands (compressed or regressing)
15 Basal uterine glands
16 Coiled arteries
17 Myometrium

FIGURE 19.21 ■ Placenta at 5 months (panoramic view). Stain: hematoxylin and eosin. Low magnification.

FIGURE 19.22 ■ Chorionic Villi: Placenta During Early Pregnancy

The **chorionic villi (6)** from a placenta during early pregnancy are illustrated at a high magnification. The trophoblast cells of the embryo give rise to the embryonic portion of the placenta. The chorionic villi (6) arise from the chorionic plate and become surrounded by the trophoblast epithelium, which consists of an outer layer of darker-staining **syncytiotrophoblasts (1, 10)** and an inner layer of lighter-staining **cytotrophoblasts (2, 9).**

The core of each chorionic villus (6) contains mesenchyme or embryonic connective tissue and two cell types, the fusiform **mesenchymal cells (8)** and the darker-staining **macrophage (Hofbauer cell) (4).** The **fetal blood vessels (3, 7),** which are branches of the umbilical arteries and veins, are located in the core of the chorionic villi (6) and contain fetal nucleated erythroblasts, although nonnucleated cells can also be seen. The **intervillous space (11)** is bathed by **maternal blood cells (5)** and nonnucleated erythrocytes.

FIGURE 19.23 ■ Chorionic Villi: Placenta at Term

The chorionic villi are illustrated from a placenta at term. In contrast to the chorionic villi in the placenta during pregnancy, the chorionic epithelium in the placenta at term is reduced to a thin layer of **syncytiotrophoblasts (1).** The connective tissue in the villi is differentiated, with more fibers and **fibroblasts (4),** and it contains large, round **macrophages (Hofbauer cells) (5).** The villi also contain mature blood cells in the **fetal blood vessels (2),** which have increased in complexity during pregnancy. The **intervillous space (6)** is surrounded by **maternal blood cells (3).**

FUNCTIONAL CORRELATIONS

Placenta

The placenta performs an important function in regulating the **exchange** of different substances between the maternal circulation and the fetal circulation. Metabolic waste products, carbon dioxide, hormones, and water are passed from the fetal circulation to the maternal circulation. Oxygen, nutrients, vitamins, electrolytes, hormones, immunoglobulins (i.e., antibodies), metabolites, and other substances pass in the opposite direction.

The placenta also serves as a temporary—yet major—**endocrine organ** that produces essential hormones for the maintenance of pregnancy. **Placental cells (syncytial trophoblasts)** secrete the hormone **chorionic gonadotropin** shortly after implantation of the fertilized ovum. Chorionic gonadotropin is similar to LH in both structure and function, and it maintains the **corpus luteum** in the maternal ovary during the early stages of pregnancy. Chorionic gonadotropin also stimulates the corpus luteum to produce estrogen and progesterone, the two hormones that are essential for maintaining pregnancy. The placenta also secretes **chorionic somatomammotropin,** a glycoprotein hormone that exhibits both **lactogenic** and **growth-promoting** functions.

As the pregnancy proceeds, the placenta takes over the production of estrogen and progesterone from the corpus luteum, and it produces sufficient amounts of progesterone to maintain the pregnancy until birth. The placenta also produces **relaxin,** which is a hormone that softens the fibrocartilage in the pubic symphysis to widen the pelvic canal for impending birth. In some mammals, the placenta also secretes **placental lactogen,** which is a hormone that promotes growth and development of the maternal mammary glands.

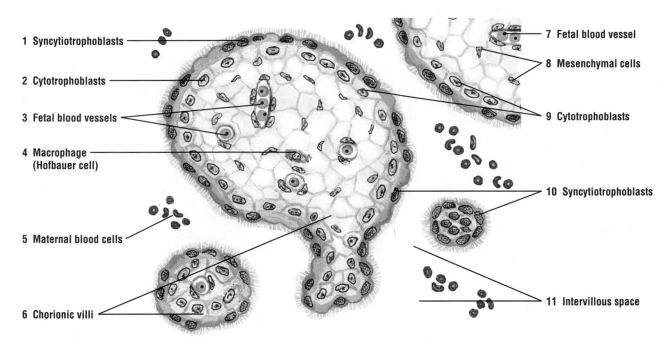

1 Syncytiotrophoblasts

2 Cytotrophoblasts

3 Fetal blood vessels

4 Macrophage (Hofbauer cell)

5 Maternal blood cells

6 Chorionic villi

7 Fetal blood vessel

8 Mesenchymal cells

9 Cytotrophoblasts

10 Syncytiotrophoblasts

11 Intervillous space

FIGURE 19.22 ■ Chorionic villi: placenta during early pregnancy. Stain: hematoxylin and eosin. High magnification.

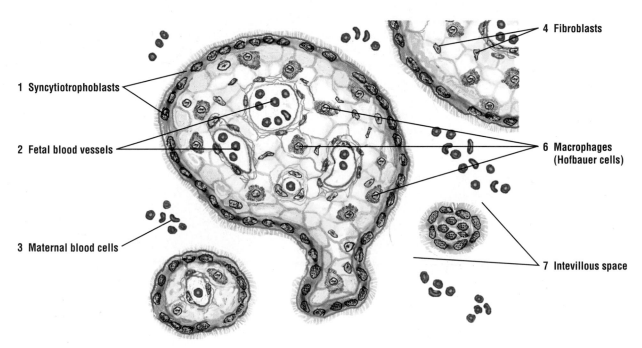

1 Syncytiotrophoblasts

2 Fetal blood vessels

3 Maternal blood cells

4 Fibroblasts

6 Macrophages (Hofbauer cells)

7 Intevillous space

FIGURE 19.23 ■ Chorionic villi: placenta at term. Stain: hematoxylin and eosin. High magnification.

FIGURE 19.24 ■ Inactive Mammary Gland

The inactive mammary gland is characterized by an abundance of connective tissue and a scarcity of glandular elements. Some cyclic changes in the mammary gland may be seen during the menstrual cycles.

A glandular **lobule (1)** consists of small tubules or **intralobular ducts (4, 7)** that are lined with a cuboidal or low columnar epithelium. At the base of the epithelium are the contractile **myoepithelial cells (6).** The larger **interlobular ducts (5)** surround the lobules (1) and the intralobular ducts (4, 7).

The intralobular ducts (4, 7) are surrounded by loose **intralobular connective tissue (3, 8)** that contains fibroblasts, lymphocytes, plasma cells, and eosinophils. Surrounding the lobules (1) is a dense **interlobular connective tissue (2, 10)** that contains blood vessels, such as **venules** and **arterioles (9).**

The mammary gland consists of 15 to 25 lobes, each of which is an individual compound tubuloalveolar type of gland. Each lobe is separated by dense interlobar connective tissue. A lactiferous duct independently emerges from each lobe at the surface of the nipple.

FIGURE 19.25 ■ Mammary Gland During Proliferation and Early Pregnancy

In preparation for milk secretion (i.e., lactation), the mammary gland undergoes extensive structural changes. During the first half of pregnancy, the intralobular ducts undergo rapid proliferation and form terminal buds that differentiate into **alveoli (2, 7).** At this stage, most alveoli are empty, and it is difficult to distinguish them from the small **intralobular excretory ducts (10).** The intralobular excretory ducts (10), however, appear more regular, with a more distinct epithelial lining. The intralobular excretory ducts (10) and the alveoli (2, 7) are lined by two layers of cells, the luminal epithelium and a basal layer of flattened **myoepithelial cells (8).**

A loose **intralobular connective tissue (1, 9)** surrounds the alveoli (2, 7) and the intralobular excretory ducts (10). A denser connective tissue with **adipose cells (6)** surrounds the individual lobules and forms **interlobular connective tissue septa (3).** The **interlobular excretory ducts (4, 11),** which are lined with taller columnar cells, course in the interlobular connective tissue septa (3) to join the larger **lactiferous duct (5),** which usually is lined with low pseudostratified columnar epithelium. Each lactiferous duct (5) collects the secretory product from the lobe and transports it to the nipple.

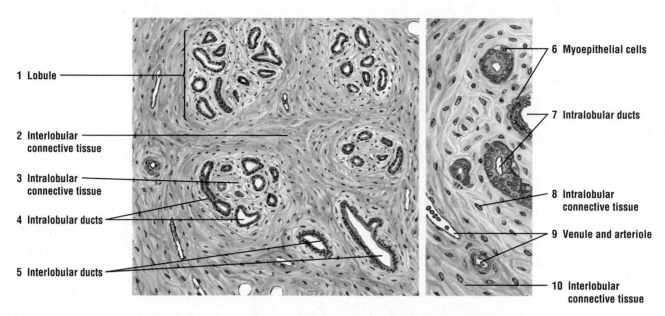

1 Lobule

2 Interlobular connective tissue

3 Intralobular connective tissue

4 Intralobular ducts

5 Interlobular ducts

6 Myoepithelial cells

7 Intralobular ducts

8 Intralobular connective tissue

9 Venule and arteriole

10 Interlobular connective tissue

FIGURE 19.24 ■ Inactive mammary gland. Stain: hematoxylin and eosin. Left side: medium magnification; right side: high magnification.

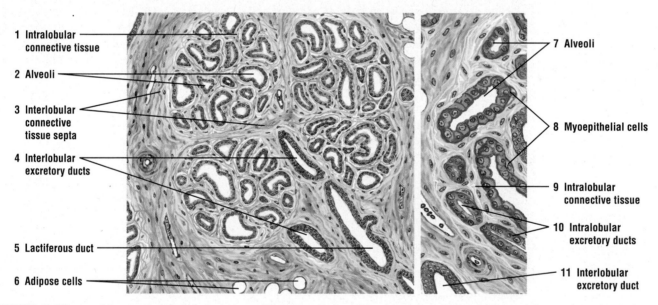

1 Intralobular connective tissue

2 Alveoli

3 Interlobular connective tissue septa

4 Interlobular excretory ducts

5 Lactiferous duct

6 Adipose cells

7 Alveoli

8 Myoepithelial cells

9 Intralobular connective tissue

10 Intralobular excretory ducts

11 Interlobular excretory duct

FIGURE 19.25 ■ Mammary gland during proliferation and early pregnancy. Stain: hematoxylin and eosin. Left side: medium magnification; right side: high magnification.

FIGURE 19.26 ■ Mammary Gland During Late Pregnancy

A small section of a mammary gland with lobules, connective tissue, and excretory ducts is illustrated at lower (left) and higher (right) magnification. During pregnancy, the glandular epithelium is prepared for lactation. The alveolar cells become secretory, and the **alveoli (2, 8)** and the **ducts (1, 7, 13)** enlarge. Some of the alveoli (2) contain a secretory product (2, upper leader). Secretion of milk by the mammary gland, however, does not begin until after parturition (birth). Because the **intralobular excretory ducts (1)** of the mammary gland also contain secretory material, distinguishing between alveoli and ducts is difficult.

As pregnancy progresses, the amount of **intralobular connective tissue (4, 11)** decreases, whereas the amount of **interlobular connective tissue (3, 9)** increases due to enlargement of the glandular tissue. Surrounding the alveoli are the flattened **myoepithelial cells (10, 12)** that are more visible in the higher-magnification view on the right. Located in the interlobular connective tissue (3, 9) are the **interlobular excretory ducts (7, 13)**, **lactiferous ducts (14)** with secretory product in their lumina, various types of **blood vessels (5)**, and **adipose cells (6)**.

FIGURE 19.27 ■ Mammary Gland During Lactation

This illustration depicts a section of a lactating mammary gland at low (left) and high (right) magnification.

The lactating mammary gland contains a large number of distended **alveoli** filled with **secretions** and **vacuoles (2, 9)**. The alveoli (2, 9) show irregular **branching** patterns **(3).** Because of the increased size of the glandular epithelium (alveoli), the **interlobular connective tissue (4)** is reduced.

During lactation, the histology of individual alveoli varies. Not all alveoli exhibit secretory activity. The **active alveoli (2, 9)** are lined with low epithelium and filled with milk that appears as eosinophilic (pink) material with large vacuoles of dissolved fat droplets. Some alveoli accumulate secretory product in their **cytoplasm (8)**, and their apices appear vacuolated because of the removal of fat during tissue preparation. Other alveoli appear **inactive (6, 11)**, with empty lumina that are lined by a taller epithelium.

In the mammary gland, the myoepithelial cells (not illustrated) are present between the alveolar cells and the basal lamina. The contraction of myoepithelial cells expels milk from the alveoli into the excretory ducts. The **interlobular excretory ducts (5, 7)** are embedded in the connective tissue septa that contain **adipose cells (1, 12).**

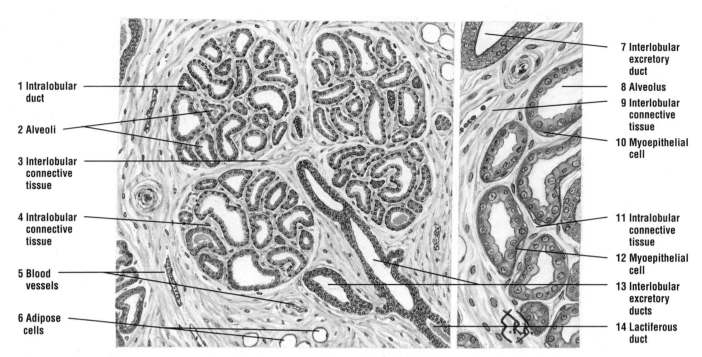

1 Intralobular duct
2 Alveoli
3 Interlobular connective tissue
4 Intralobular connective tissue
5 Blood vessels
6 Adipose cells

7 Interlobular excretory duct
8 Alveolus
9 Interlobular connective tissue
10 Myoepithelial cell
11 Intralobular connective tissue
12 Myoepithelial cell
13 Interlobular excretory ducts
14 Lactiferous duct

FIGURE 19.26 ■ Mammary gland during late pregnancy. Stain: hematoxylin and eosin. Left side: low magnification; right side: high magnification.

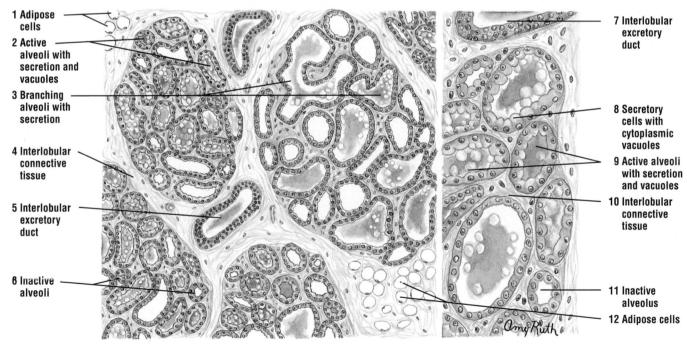

1 Adipose cells
2 Active alveoli with secretion and vacuoles
3 Branching alveoli with secretion
4 Interlobular connective tissue
5 Interlobular excretory duct
6 Inactive alveoli

7 Interlobular excretory duct
8 Secretory cells with cytoplasmic vacuoles
9 Active alveoli with secretion and vacuoles
10 Interlobular connective tissue
11 Inactive alveolus
12 Adipose cells

FIGURE 19.27 ■ Mammary gland during lactation. Stain: hematoxylin and eosin. Left side: low magnification; right side: high magnification.

FIGURE 19.28 ■ Mammary Gland During Lactation

This photomicrograph illustrates a lobule of a lactating mammary gland that is separated from the adjacent lactating lobule by a thin layer of **connective tissue (3).** The lactating mammary gland contains **alveoli (1)** with the **secretory product (4),** or milk; the alveoli are separated by thin **connective tissue (3)** septa. Some of the alveoli (1) are single, whereas others are **branching alveoli (2).** All the alveoli eventually drain into larger excretory ducts, which in turn eventually deliver the milk to the lactiferous ducts in the nipple.

FUNCTIONAL CORRELATIONS

Mammary Glands

Before puberty, the mammary glands are undeveloped and consist primarily of branched **lactiferous ducts** that open at the nipple. In males, the mammary glands remain undeveloped. In females, mammary glands enlarge during puberty because of stimulation by estrogen. As a result, adipose tissue and connective tissue accumulate and grow, and branching of the lactiferous ducts in the mammary glands increase.

During pregnancy, the mammary glands undergo increased growth because of the continuous and prolonged stimulatory actions of estrogen and progesterone. Initially, these hormones are produced by the corpus luteum of the ovary; later, they are produced by cells in the placenta. In addition, further growth of mammary glands depends on the pituitary hormone **prolactin, placental lactogen,** and **adrenal corticoids.** These hormones stimulate the intralobular ducts of the mammary glands to rapidly proliferate, branch, and form numerous **alveoli.** The alveoli then undergo hypertrophy and become active sites of **milk production** during the lactation period. All alveoli become surrounded by contractile **myoepithelial cells.**

At the end of pregnancy, the alveoli initially produce a fluid, called **colostrum,** that is rich in proteins, vitamins, minerals, and antibodies. Unlike milk, however, colostrum contains little lipid. Milk is not produced until a few days after parturition (i.e., birth). The hormones estrogen and progesterone from the corpus luteum and placenta suppress milk production.

After parturition and elimination of the placenta, the hormones that inhibited milk secretion are eliminated, and the mammary glands begin the active secretion of milk. As the pituitary hormone prolactin activates milk secretion, the production of colostrum ceases. During nursing of the newborn, tactile stimulation of the nipple by the suckling infant promotes further release of prolactin and prolonged milk production.

In addition, tactile stimulation of the nipple initiates the **milk ejection reflex,** which causes release of the hormone **oxytocin** from the neurohypophysis of the pituitary gland. Oxytocin causes the contraction of myoepithelial cells around the secretory alveoli and excretory ducts in the mammary glands, resulting in milk ejection from the mammary glands toward the nipple.

Decreased nursing and suckling by the infant soon results in the cessation of milk production and eventual regression of the mammary glands to an inactive state.

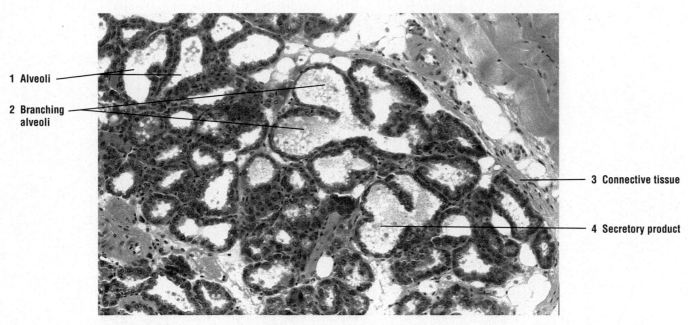

1 Alveoli

2 Branching alveoli

3 Connective tissue

4 Secretory product

FIGURE 19.28 ■ Mammary gland during lactation. Stain: hematoxylin and eosin. 50×

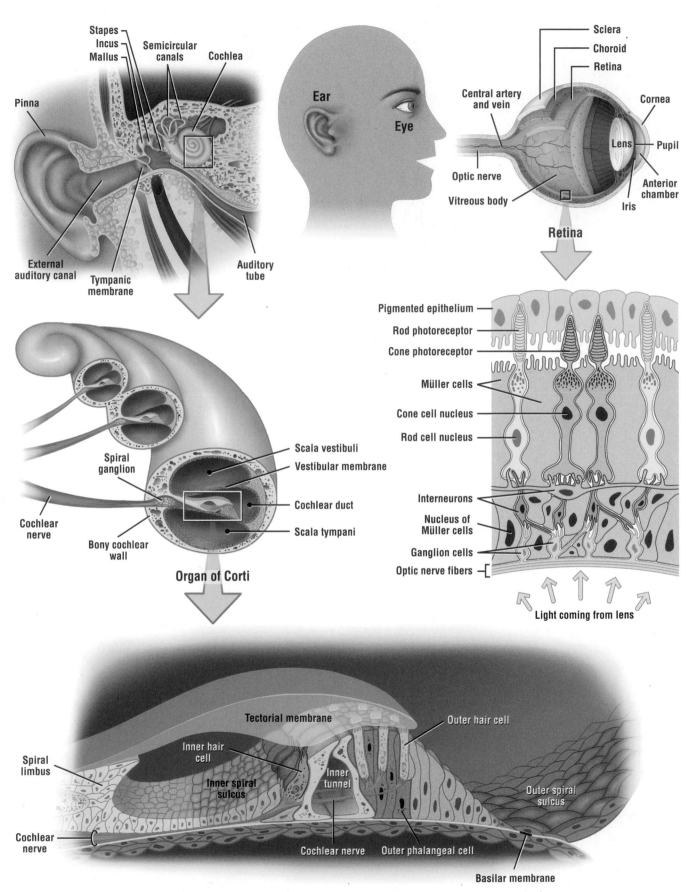

OVERVIEW FIGURE ■ Internal structures of the eye and the ear, with emphasis on cells that constitute the photosensitive retina and the hearing organ of corti.

CHAPTER 20

Organs of Special Senses

Eye Structure

The eye is a highly specialized organ for the perception of form, light, and color. The eyes are located in protective cavities within the skull, called **orbits.** Each eye contains a protective cover to maintain its shape, a lens for focusing, photosensitive cells that respond to light stimuli, numerous cells that process visual information, and nerves that conduct the information to the brain (see overview figure).

Layers in the Eye

Each eyeball is surrounded by three distinct layers: the sclera, the vascular layer (uvea), and the retina.

Sclera. The outer layer in the eye is the **sclera,** which is an opaque layer of dense connective tissue. Anteriorly, the sclera is modified into a transparent **cornea,** through which light rays enter the eye.

Vascular Layer (Uvea). Internal to the sclera is the middle or vascular layer (**uvea**). This layer consists of three parts: a densely pigmented layer, called the **choroid;** a **ciliary body;** and an **iris.** Located in the choroid are numerous blood vessels that nourish the photoreceptor cells in the retina and structures of the eyeball.

Retina. The innermost lining of the most posterior chamber of the eye is the **retina.** The posterior three-quarters of the retina are **photosensitive.** In this region, cells are stimulated by and respond to light. The photosensitive retina terminates in the region of the eye called the **ora serrata.** Anterior to the ora serrata is the **nonphotosensitive** part of the retina. This nonphotosensitive region continues forward in the eye to line the inner part of the ciliary body and posterior region of iris.

Chambers in the Eye

The eye also contains three chambers: the anterior, posterior, and vitreous.

The anterior and posterior chambers are filled with a watery fluid, called the **aqueous humor.** This fluid is continually produced by the **ciliary process** behind the iris. Aqueous humor circulates from the posterior to the anterior chamber, where it is drained by veins.

Anterior Chamber. The **anterior chamber** is situated between the cornea and the iris.

Posterior Chamber. The **posterior chamber** is situated between the iris and the lens.

Vitreous Chamber. The **vitreous chamber** is a larger, posterior chamber in the eye that is situated between the lens and the retina. This chamber contains the gelatinous **vitreous body.**

Cells in the Eye

The retina contains numerous cell types that are organized into numerous cell layers. The layer that is sensitive to light contains **photoreceptor cells,** called **rods** and **cones.** These cells are stimulated by light rays that pass through the lens. Leaving the retina are **afferent** (sensory) **axons** (nerve fibers) that conduct light impulses from the retina via the **optic nerve** to the brain for visual interpretation.

417

The posterior region of the eye also contains a yellowish-pigmented spot, called the **macula lutea.** In the center of the macula lutea is a depression, called the **fovea.** The fovea is devoid of photoreceptive rods and blood vessels. Instead, it contains a dense concentration of photosensitive cones.

Ear Structure

The ear is a specialized organ for hearing, balance, and maintenance of equilibrium.

The Auditory System

The **auditory system** consists of three major parts: the external ear, the middle ear, and the inner ear (including the cochlea) (see overview figure).

External Ear. The auricle, or **pinna,** of the **external ear** gathers sound waves and directs them through the **external auditory canal** interiorly to the eardrum, or **tympanic membrane.**

Middle Ear. The **middle ear** is a small, air-filled cavity,.called the **tympanic cavity.** It is located in and protected by the temporal bone of the skull. The tympanic membrane separates the external auditory canal from the middle ear. Located in the middle ear are three very small bones, called the **auditory ossicles,** that consist of the **stapes, incus,** and **malleus;** also in the middle ear is the **auditory (eustachian) tube.** The cavity of the middle ear communicates with the nasopharyngeal region of the head via the auditory tube. The auditory tube allows for equalization of air pressure on both sides of the tympanic membrane while swallowing or blowing the nose.

Inner Ear. The inner ear lies deep in the temporal bone. It consists of small, communicating cavities and canals of different shapes. These cavities, which consist of the **semicircular canals, vestibule,** and **cochlea,** are collectively called the **bony labyrinth.** Located within the bony labyrinth is the **membranous labyrinth,** which consists of a series of interconnected, thin-walled compartments that are filled with fluid.

Cochlea. The organ that is specialized for receiving and transmitting sound (i.e., hearing) is found in the inner ear in the structure called the cochlea. It is a spiral, bony canal that resembles a snail's shell. The cochlea makes three turns on itself around a central bony pillar, called the **modiolus.**

Interiorly, the cochlea is partitioned into three channels: the **scala vestibuli,** the **scala tympani,** and the **cochlear duct** (i.e., scala media). Within the cochlear duct on the **basilar membrane** is the hearing **organ of Corti.** This organ consists of numerous auditory receptor cells, or **hair cells,** and several supporting cells. The auditory stimuli (i.e., sounds) are carried away from the receptor cells via afferent axons of the **cochlear nerve** to the brain for interpretation.

Vestibular Functions

The organ of vestibular functions that is responsible for **balance** and **equilibrium** is found in the **utricle, saccule,** and three **semicircular canals.**

FIGURE 20.1 ■ Eyelid (Sagittal Section)

The exterior layer of the eyelid is composed of thin skin (left side). The **epidermis (4)** consists of stratified squamous epithelium with papillae. In the **dermis (6)** are **hair follicles (1, 3)** with associated **sebaceous glands (3)** and **sweat glands (5).**

The interior layer of the eyelid is a mucous membrane, called the **palpebral conjunctiva (15).** It lies adjacent to the eyeball. The lining epithelium of the palpebral conjunctiva (15) is low stratified columnar, with a few goblet cells. The stratified squamous epithelium (4) of the thin skin continues over the margin of the eyelid and then merges into the stratified columnar of the palpebral conjunctiva (15).

The thin lamina propria of the palpebral conjunctiva (15) contains both elastic and collagen fibers. Beneath the lamina propria is a plate of dense, collagenous connective tissue, called the **tarsus (16),** in which are found large, specialized sebaceous glands, called the **tarsal (meibomian) glands (17).** The secretory acini of the tarsal glands (17) open into a **central duct (19)** that runs parallel to the palpebral conjunctiva (15) and, in turn, opens at the margin of the eyelid.

The free end of the eyelid contains **eyelashes (10)** that arise from large, long **hair follicles (9).** Associated with the eyelashes (10) are small **sebaceous glands (11).** Between the hair follicles (9) of the eyelashes (10) are large **sweat glands (of Moll) (18).**

The eyelid contains three sets of muscles: the palpebral portion of the skeletal muscle, called the **orbicularis oculi (8);** the skeletal **ciliary muscle (of Roilan) (20)** in the region of the hair follicles (9), eyelashes (10), and tarsal glands (17); and the smooth muscle, called the **superior tarsal muscle (of Müller) (12)** in the upper eyelid.

The **connective tissue (7)** of the eyelid contains **adipose cells (2), blood vessels (14),** and **lymphatic tissue (13).**

FUNCTIONAL CORRELATIONS

Lacrimal Secretions (Tears)

Each eyeball is covered on its anterior surface with thin **eyelids** and fine hairs, called **eyelashes,** on the margins of eyelids. Eyelids and eyelashes protect the eyes from foreign objects and excessive light. Above each eye is a secretory **lacrimal gland** that continually produces **lacrimal secretions,** or **tears.** Blinking spreads the lacrimal secretion across the outer surface of the eyeball and the inner surface of the eyelid. The lacrimal secretion contains mucus, salts, and the antibacterial enzyme **lysozyme.** Lacrimal secretions clean, protect, moisten, and lubricate the surface of the eye (i.e., conjunctiva and cornea).

Aqueous Humor

Aqueous humor is the product of the **ciliary epithelium** of the eye. This watery fluid flows into the anterior and posterior chambers of the eye between the cornea and lens. Aqueous humor bathes the nonvascular **cornea** and **lens.** It also supplies the cornea and lens with nutrients and oxygen.

Vitreous Body

The vitreous chamber of the eye is located behind the lens and contains a gelatinous substance, called the vitreous body. The vitreous body is a transparent, colorless gel that consists mainly of water. In addition, the vitreous body contains hyaluronic acid, very thin collagen fibers, and some proteins. The vitreous body transmits incoming light, is nonrefractive with respect to the lens, contributes to the intraocular pressure of the eyeball, and holds the retina in place against the pigmented layer of the eyeball.

Retina

The photosensitive retina contains three types of neurons that are distributed in different layers: photoreceptive **rods** and **cones, bipolar cells,** and **ganglion cells.** The rods and cones are receptor neurons that are essential for vision. They synapse with the bipolar cells, which then connect the receptor neurons with the ganglion cells. The afferent axons that leave the ganglion cells converge posteriorly in the eye at the **optic papilla** (i.e., optic disk) and leave the eye as the

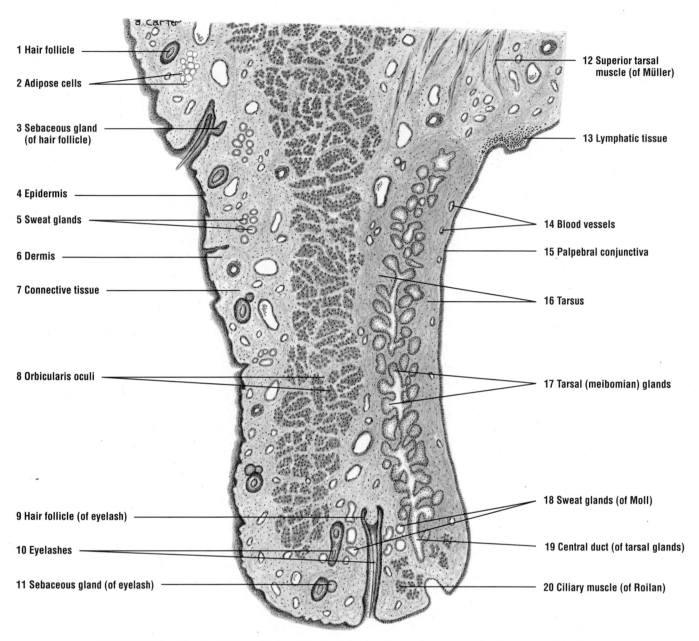

1 Hair follicle

2 Adipose cells

3 Sebaceous gland
(of hair follicle)

4 Epidermis

5 Sweat glands

6 Dermis

7 Connective tissue

8 Orbicularis oculi

9 Hair follicle (of eyelash)

10 Eyelashes

11 Sebaceous gland (of eyelash)

12 Superior tarsal
muscle (of Müller)

13 Lymphatic tissue

14 Blood vessels

15 Palpebral conjunctiva

16 Tarsus

17 Tarsal (meibomian) glands

18 Sweat glands (of Moll)

19 Central duct (of tarsal glands)

20 Ciliary muscle (of Roilan)

FIGURE 20.1 ▪ Eyelid (sagittal section). Stain: hematoxylin and eosin. Low magnification.

optic nerve. The optic papilla is also called the **blind spot,** because this area lacks photoreceptor cells and only contains axons.

Because the rods and cones are situated adjacent to the **choroid layer** of the retina, light rays must first pass through the ganglion and bipolar cell layers to reach and activate the photosensitive rods and cones. The **pigmented layer** of the choroid next to the retina absorbs light rays and prevents them from reflecting back through the retina.

Rods and Cones

The rods are highly sensitive to light, and they function best in dim or **low light,** such as at dusk or at night. In the dark, a visual pigment, called **rhodopsin,** is synthesized and accumulates in the rods. In contrast, the cones are less sensitive to low light; the cones respond best to **bright light.** Cones are also essential for high visual acuity and **color vision** (red, green, or blue). The cones contain the visual pigment **iodopsin.** Absorption and interaction of light rays with these pigments cause transformations in the pigment molecules. This action excites the rods or cones and produces a nerve impulse for vision.

At the posterior region of the eye is a shallow depression in the retina. This thin region is called the **fovea,** and in its center, only cones are found. The visual axis of the eye passes through the fovea. As a result, light rays fall directly on and stimulate the tightly packed cones. For this reason, the fovea in the eye produces the greatest **visual acuity** and the sharpest **color discrimination.**

FIGURE 20.2 ■ Lacrimal Gland

The lacrimal gland consists of several lobes that are separated into separate lobules by the **connective tissue (2)** septa that contain **nerves (4), adipose cells (6),** and **blood vessels (9).** The lacrimal gland is a serous compound gland, which resembles the salivary glands in lobular structure, and includes **tubuloalveolar acini (8)** that vary in size and shape. The well-developed **myoepithelial cells (1, 5)** surround the individual secretory acini (8) of the gland.

A small **intralobular excretory duct (7),** which is lined with simple cuboidal or columnar epithelium, is located between the tubuloalveolar acini (8). The larger **interlobular excretory duct (3)** is lined with two layers of low columnar cells or pseudostratified epithelium.

FIGURE 20.3 ■ Cornea (Transverse Section)

The cornea is a thick, transparent, nonvascular structure of the eye. The anterior surface of the cornea is covered with a **stratified squamous corneal epithelium (1)** that is nonkeratinized and consists of five or more cell layers. The basal cell layer is columnar and rests on a thin basement membrane that, in turn, is supported by a thick, homogeneous **anterior limiting (Bowman's) membrane (4).** The underlying **corneal stroma (substantia propria) (2)** forms the body of the cornea; it consists of parallel bundles of **collagen fibers (5)** and layers of flat **fibroblasts (6).**

The **posterior limiting (Descemet's) membrane (4)** is a thick basement membrane located at the posterior portion of the corneal stroma (2). The posterior surface of the cornea that faces the anterior chamber of the eye is covered with a simple squamous epithelium, called the **posterior epithelium (3),** which is also the corneal endothelium.

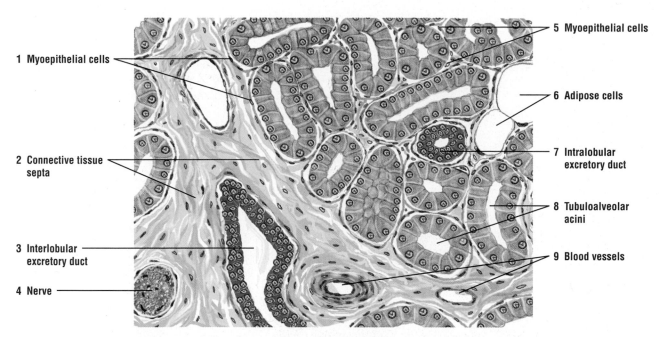

1 Myoepithelial cells

2 Connective tissue
  septa

3 Interlobular
  excretory duct

4 Nerve

5 Myoepithelial cells

6 Adipose cells

7 Intralobular
  excretory duct

8 Tubuloalveolar
  acini

9 Blood vessels

FIGURE 20.2 ■ Lacrimal gland. Stain: hematoxylin and eosin. Medium magnification.

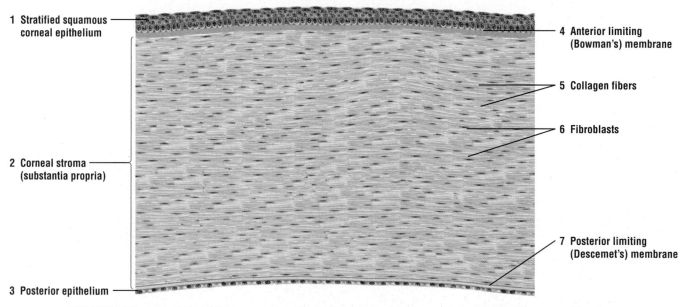

1 Stratified squamous
  corneal epithelium

2 Corneal stroma
  (substantia propria)

3 Posterior epithelium

4 Anterior limiting
  (Bowman's) membrane

5 Collagen fibers

6 Fibroblasts

7 Posterior limiting
  (Descemet's) membrane

FIGURE 20.3 ■ Cornea (transverse section). Stain: hematoxylin and eosin. Medium magnification.

FIGURE 20.4   ■   Whole Eye (Sagittal Section)

The eyeball is surrounded by three major concentric layers: an outer, tough fibrous tissue layer, which is composed of the **sclera (18)** and **cornea (1)**; a middle layer, or uvea, which is composed of the highly vascular, pigmented **choroid (7)**, the ciliary body (consisting of **ciliary processes [4, 15]** and **ciliary muscle [14]**), and the **iris (13)**; and the innermost layer, which is composed of the photosensitive **retina (8)**.

The sclera (18) is a white, opaque, and tough connective tissue layer that is composed of densely woven collagen fibers. The sclera (18) maintains the rigidity of the eyeball and appears as the "white" of the eye. The junction between the cornea and the sclera occurs at a transition area called the **limbus (12)**, which is located in the anterior region of the eye. In the posterior region of the eye, where the **optic nerve (10)** emerges from the ocular capsule, is the transition site between the sclera (18) of the eyeball and the connective tissue **dura mater (23)** of the central nervous system.

The choroid (7) and the ciliary body (4, 14, 15) are adjacent to the sclera (18). In a sagittal section of the eyeball, the ciliary body (4, 14, 15) appears triangular in shape and is composed of the smooth ciliary muscle (14) and the ciliary processes (4, 15). The fibers in the ciliary muscle (14) exhibit longitudinal, circular, and radial arrangement. The folded and highly vascular extensions of the ciliary body constitute the ciliary processes (4, 15) that attach to the equator of the **lens (16)** by the **zonular fibers (suspensory ligament) (5)**, of the lens. Contraction of the ciliary muscle (14) reduces the tension on the zonular fibers (5) and allows the lens (16) to assume a convex shape.

The iris (13) partially covers the lens and is the colored portion of the eye. The circular and radial smooth muscle fibers form an opening in the iris, called the **pupil (11)**.

The interior portion of the eye in front of the lens is subdivided into two compartments, the **anterior chamber (2)** between the iris (13) and the cornea (1), and the **posterior chamber (3)** between the iris (13) and the lens (16). Both the anterior (2) and posterior (3) chambers are filled with a watery fluid, called the aqueous humor. The large posterior compartment in the eyeball behind the lens, called the **vitreous body (19)**, is filled with a gelatinous material (the transparent vitreous humor).

Behind the ciliary body (4, 14, 15) is the **ora serrata (6, 17)**, which is the sharp, anteriormost boundary of the photosensitive portion of the retina (8). The retina (8) consists of numerous cell layers, one of which contains the light-sensitive cells, the rods and cones. Anterior to the ora serrata (6, 17) lies the nonphotosensitive portion of the retina, which continues forward in the eyeball to form the inner lining of the ciliary body (4, 14, 15) and the posterior part of the iris (13). The histology of the retina is presented in greater detail in Figures 20-5, 20-6, and 20-7.

In the posterior wall of the eye is the **macula lutea (20)** and the **optic papilla (9)**, or the optic disk. The macula lutea (20) is a small, yellow-pigmented spot with a shallow, central depression, called the **fovea (20)**. The macula lutea (20) is the area of greatest visual acuity in the eye. The center of the fovea (20) is devoid of rod cells and blood vessels; this region contains only cone cells.

The optic papilla (9) is the region where the optic nerve (10) leaves the eyeball. The optic papilla (9) lacks both rods and cones, and constitutes the "blind spot" of the eye.

The outer sclera (18) is adjacent to the orbital tissue and contains loose connective tissue, **adipose cells** of the **orbital fatty tissue (21)**, nerve fibers, **blood vessels (22)**, lymphatics, and glands.

FIGURE 20.5   ■   Retina, Choroid, and Sclera (Panoramic View)

The wall of the eyeball is composed of three layers: the **sclera (1)**, the **choroid (2)**, and the **retina (3)**. The retina (3) contains the photosensitive rods and cones. In this figure, only the deeper portion of the sclera is illustrated.

The sclera (1) is composed of dense **collagen fibers (4)** that course parallel to the surface of the eyeball. Between the collagen bundles is a network of elastic fibers. Flattened fibroblasts are present throughout the sclera (1), whereas the **melanocytes (5)** are located in the deepest layer.

Structures in the retina labeled **6** through **16** are discussed in Figure 20-6, where they are shown at higher magnification.

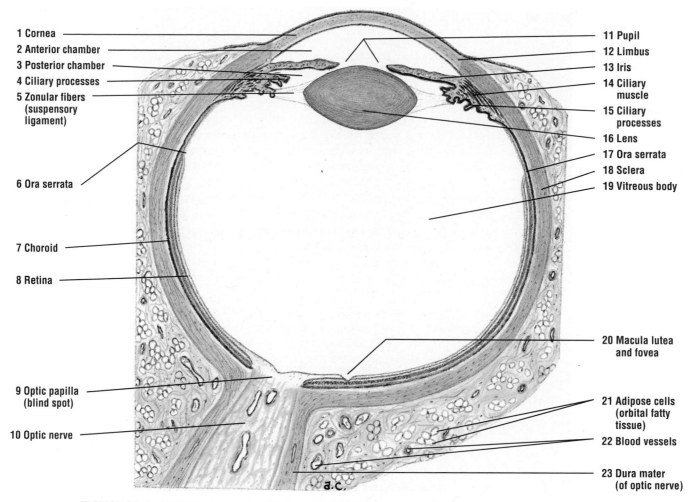

1 Cornea
2 Anterior chamber
3 Posterior chamber
4 Ciliary processes
5 Zonular fibers (suspensory ligament)

6 Ora serrata

7 Choroid

8 Retina

9 Optic papilla (blind spot)

10 Optic nerve

11 Pupil
12 Limbus
13 Iris
14 Ciliary muscle
15 Ciliary processes
16 Lens
17 Ora serrata
18 Sclera
19 Vitreous body

20 Macula lutea and fovea

21 Adipose cells (orbital fatty tissue)
22 Blood vessels

23 Dura mater (of optic nerve)

FIGURE 20.4 ■ Whole eye (sagittal section). Stain: hematoxylin and eosin. Low magnification.

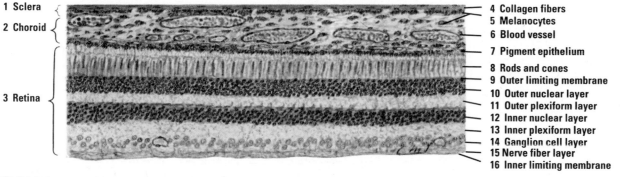

1 Sclera
2 Choroid
3 Retina

4 Collagen fibers
5 Melanocytes
6 Blood vessel
7 Pigment epithelium
8 Rods and cones
9 Outer limiting membrane
10 Outer nuclear layer
11 Outer plexiform layer
12 Inner nuclear layer
13 Inner plexiform layer
14 Ganglion cell layer
15 Nerve fiber layer
16 Inner limiting membrane

FIGURE 20.5 ■ Retina, choroid, and sclera (panoramic view). Stain: hematoxylin and eosin. Medium magnification.

FIGURE 20.6 ■ Layers of the Choroid and Retina (Detail)

The choroid is subdivided into several layers: the **suprachoroid lamina** with **melanocytes (17)**, the **vascular layer (18)**, the **choriocapillary layer (19)**, and the transparent limiting membrane, or glassy membrane (Bruch's membrane).

The suprachoroid lamina (17) consists of fine collagen fibers, a network of elastic fibers, fibroblasts, and numerous melanocytes. The vascular layer (18) contains medium-sized and large **blood vessels (1)**. In the loose connective tissue between the blood vessels (1) are large, flat **melanocytes (2)** that impart a dark color to this layer. The choriocapillary layer (19) contains a network of capillaries with large lumina. The innermost layer of the choroid, the glassy membrane, lies adjacent to the **pigment cells** of the **retina (3)** and separates the choroid and retina.

The outermost layer of the retina contains the pigment cells (epithelium) (3). The basement membrane of the pigment cells (3) forms the innermost layer of the glassy membrane of the choroid. The cuboidal pigment cells (3) contain melanin (i.e., pigment) granules in apices of their cytoplasm, whereas their cytoplasmic **processes (20)** with pigment granules extend between the **rods (22)** and **cones (22)** of the retina.

Adjacent to the pigment cells (3) is a photosensitive layer of slender **rods (4, 22)** and thicker **cones (5, 21)**. These cells are situated next to the **outer limiting membrane (6, 23)** that is formed by the processes of neuroglial cells, called **Müller's cells (30)**.

The **outer nuclear layer (7, 8)** contains **nuclei** of the **rods (8, 25)** and **cones (7, 24)** and the **outer processes** of **Müller's cells (26)**. In the **outer plexiform layer (9)**, the axons of the rods (22) and cones (21) synapse with the dendrites of **bipolar cells (28)** and **horizontal cells (27)**. The **inner nuclear layer (10)** contains the nuclei of **bipolar (29)**, horizontal, **amacrine (31)**, and neuroglial Müller's cells (30). The horizontal and amacrine cells are association cells. In the **inner plexiform layer (11)**, the axons of bipolar cells (29) synapse with the dendrites of the ganglion and amacrine cells.

The **ganglion cell layer (12)** contains the cell bodies of **ganglion cells (33)** and neuroglial cells. The dendrites from the ganglion cells synapse in the inner plexiform layer (11, 32, 33).

The **optic nerve fiber layer (13, 14, 15)** contains the **axons** of the **ganglion cells (14)** and the **inner fibers** of **Müller's cells (13, 37)**. **Axons** of **ganglion cells (14, 33)** converge toward the optic disk and form the **fibers** of the **optic nerve (34)**. The terminations of the inner fibers of Müller's cells (13, 37) expand to form the **inner limiting membrane (15, 36)** of the retina.

Blood vessels of the retina course in the optic nerve fiber layer (13, 14, 15) and penetrate as far as the **inner nuclear layer (10)**. Sections in various planes of some of the vessels can be seen in this layer (unlabeled).

FIGURE 20.7 ■ Eye: Layers of Retina and Choroid

A high-power photomicrograph illustrates the layers of the photosensitive retina. The **choroid (1)** is a vascular outer layer with loose connective tissue and pigmented melanocytes. The choroid (1) layer is adjacent to the outermost retinal layer, which is the single, **pigment epithelium (2)** layer. The light-sensitive **rods** and **cones (3)** form the next layer, which is separated from the dense **outer nuclear layer (4)** by a thin **outer limiting membrane (5)**. Deep to the outer nuclear layer (4) is a clear area of synaptic connections, called the **outer plexiform layer (6)**.

The dense layer of cell bodies of the integrating neurons form the **inner nuclear layer (7)**, which is adjacent to the clear **inner plexiform layer (8)**. In the inner plexiform layer (8), the axons of the integrating neurons form synaptic connections with the axons of the neurons that form the optic tract. The cell bodies of the optic tract neurons form the **ganglion cell layer (9)**, and their afferent axons form the light-staining **optic nerve fiber layer (10)**. The innermost layer of the retina is the **inner limiting membrane (11)** that separates the retina from the vitreous body of the eyeball.

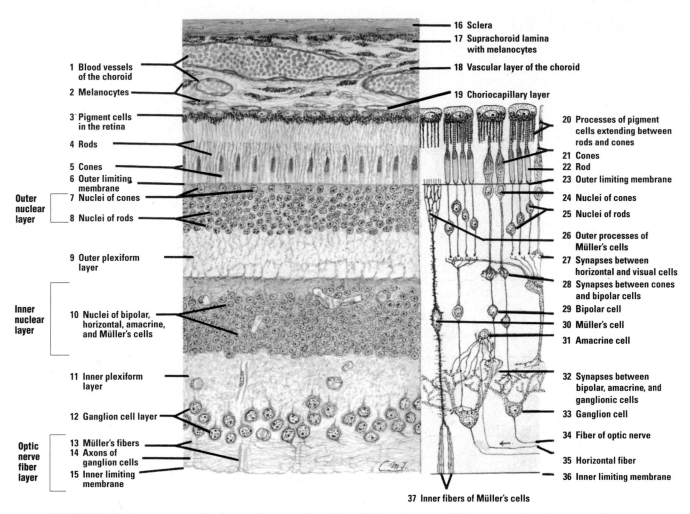

1 Blood vessels of the choroid
2 Melanocytes
3 Pigment cells in the retina
4 Rods
5 Cones
6 Outer limiting membrane
Outer nuclear layer
7 Nuclei of cones
8 Nuclei of rods
9 Outer plexiform layer
Inner nuclear layer
10 Nuclei of bipolar, horizontal, amacrine, and Müller's cells
11 Inner plexiform layer
12 Ganglion cell layer
Optic nerve fiber layer
13 Müller's fibers
14 Axons of ganglion cells
15 Inner limiting membrane

16 Sclera
17 Suprachoroid lamina with melanocytes
18 Vascular layer of the choroid
19 Choriocapillary layer
20 Processes of pigment cells extending between rods and cones
21 Cones
22 Rod
23 Outer limiting membrane
24 Nuclei of cones
25 Nuclei of rods
26 Outer processes of Müller's cells
27 Synapses between horizontal and visual cells
28 Synapses between cones and bipolar cells
29 Bipolar cell
30 Müller's cell
31 Amacrine cell
32 Synapses between bipolar, amacrine, and ganglionic cells
33 Ganglion cell
34 Fiber of optic nerve
35 Horizontal fiber
36 Inner limiting membrane
37 Inner fibers of Müller's cells

FIGURE 20.6 ■ Layers of the choroid and retina (detail). Stain: hematoxylin and eosin. High magnification.

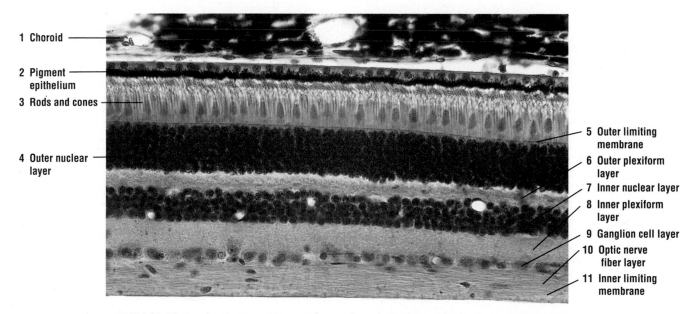

1 Choroid
2 Pigment epithelium
3 Rods and cones
4 Outer nuclear layer

5 Outer limiting membrane
6 Outer plexiform layer
7 Inner nuclear layer
8 Inner plexiform layer
9 Ganglion cell layer
10 Optic nerve fiber layer
11 Inner limiting membrane

FIGURE 20.7 ■ Layers of the retina and choroid. Stain: Masson's trichrome. 100×

FIGURE 20.8 ▪ Inner Ear: Cochlea (Vertical Section)

The **osseous** (bony) **labyrinth** of the **cochlea (16, 18)** spirals around a central axis of a spongy bone, called the **modiolus (17).** Embedded within the modiolus (17) is the **spiral ganglion (14),** which is composed of bipolar afferent neurons. The axons from the bipolar cells join to form the **cochlear nerve (9),** whereas the dendrites innervate the hair cells in the hearing apparatus called the **organ of Corti (13).**

The bony labyrinth of the inner ear is divided into two major cavities by the **osseous spiral lamina (8)** and the **basilar membrane (7).** The osseous spiral lamina (8) projects from the modiolus (17) approximately halfway into the lumen of the cochlear canal. The basilar membrane (7) continues from the osseous spiral lamina (8) to the **spiral ligament (6, 15),** which is a thickening of the periosteum on the **outer bony wall (5)** of the cochlear canal.

The cochlear canal is subdivided into two large compartments, the lower **scala tympani (4)** and the upper **scala vestibuli (2).** The separate scala tympani (4) and scala vestibuli (2) continue in a spiral course to the apex of the cochlea, where they communicate through a small opening, called the **helicotrema (1).**

The **vestibular (Reissner's) membrane (10)** separates the scala vestibuli (2) from the **cochlear duct (scala media) (3)** and forms the roof of the cochlear duct (3). The vestibular membrane (10) attaches to the **spiral ligament (11).** The sensory cells for sound detection are located in the organ of Corti (13) that rests on the basilar membrane (7) of the cochlear duct (3). A **tectorial membrane (12)** overlies the cells in the organ of Corti (13).

FIGURE 20.9 ▪ Inner Ear: Cochlear Duct (Scala Media)

This illustration shows the **cochlear duct (9),** the **organ of Corti (12),** and associated cells at higher magnification.

The outer wall of the cochlear duct (9) is formed by a vascular area, called the **stria vascularis (16).** The stratified epithelium covering the stria vascularis (16) contains an intraepithelial capillary network that is formed from the vessels of the connective tissue in the **spiral ligament (17).** The lamina propria in this region is the **spiral ligament (17, 19),** which consists of collagen fibers, pigmented fibroblasts, and numerous blood vessels.

The roof of the cochlear duct (9) is formed by the **vestibular (Reissner's) membrane (6),** which separates the cochlear duct (9) from the **scala vestibuli (7).** The vestibular membrane (6) extends from the spiral ligament (17) of the outer wall of the cochlea, the **attachment (16)** of which is located at the upper extent of the stria vascularis (16), to the thickened **periosteum** of the **osseous spiral lamina (4)** near the **spiral limbus (5).**

The spiral limbus (5) forms part of the floor of the cochlear duct (9). The limbus (5) is a thickened mass of periosteal connective tissue (4) of the **osseous spiral lamina (1)** that extends into the cochlear duct (9). It is supported by a lateral extension of the osseous spiral lamina (1). The limbus (5) is covered by an epithelium, which appears columnar. The lateral extracellular extension of the epithelium beyond the limbus forms the **tectorial membrane (10).** The tectorial membrane (10) overlies the **internal spiral sulcus (8)** and a portion of the organ of Corti (12), including its **hair cells (11).**

The **basilar membrane (13)** is a vascularized connective tissue under the thinner plate of the basilar fibers. The organ of Corti (12) rests on the basilar fibers. The organ of Corti (12) consists of the sensory hair cells (11), supporting cells, and associated spaces and tunnels.

The **peripheral** (afferent) **processes** of the **ganglion cells (2)** from the bipolar **cells** in the **spiral ganglion (3)** course through the osseous spiral lamina (1) and synapse with hair cells (11) in the organ of Corti (12).

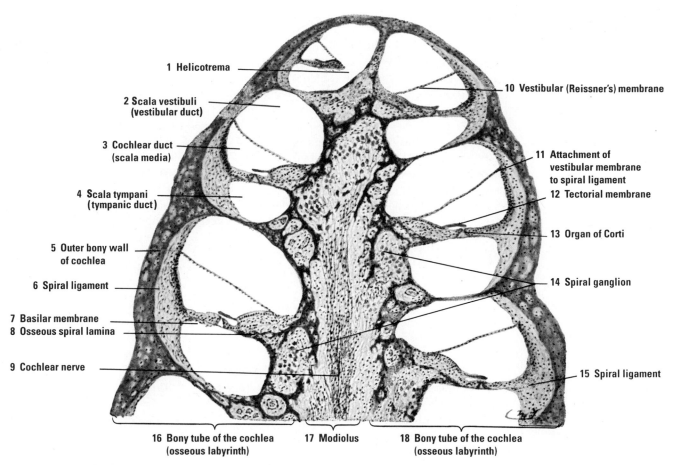

1 Helicotrema
2 Scala vestibuli
(vestibular duct)
3 Cochlear duct
(scala media)
4 Scala tympani
(tympanic duct)
5 Outer bony wall
of cochlea
6 Spiral ligament
7 Basilar membrane
8 Osseous spiral lamina
9 Cochlear nerve

10 Vestibular (Reissner's) membrane
11 Attachment of
vestibular membrane
to spiral ligament
12 Tectorial membrane
13 Organ of Corti
14 Spiral ganglion
15 Spiral ligament

16 Bony tube of the cochlea
(osseous labyrinth)
17 Modiolus
18 Bony tube of the cochlea
(osseous labyrinth)

FIGURE 20.8 ■ Inner ear: cochlea (vertical section). Stain: hematoxylin and eosin. Low magnification.

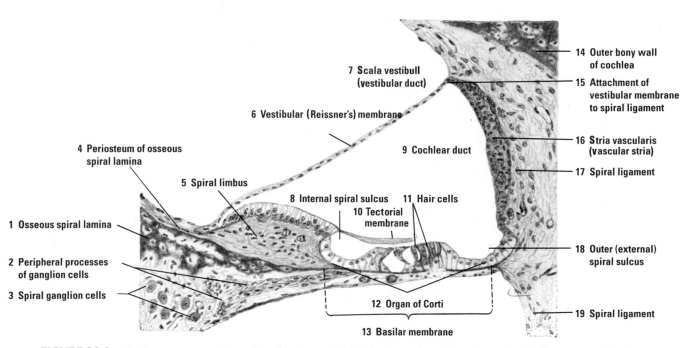

4 Periosteum of osseous
spiral lamina
5 Spiral limbus
1 Osseous spiral lamina
2 Peripheral processes
of ganglion cells
3 Spiral ganglion cells

7 Scala vestibuli
(vestibular duct)
6 Vestibular (Reissner's) membrane
9 Cochlear duct
8 Internal spiral sulcus
10 Tectorial
membrane
11 Hair cells
12 Organ of Corti
13 Basilar membrane

14 Outer bony wall
of cochlea
15 Attachment of
vestibular membrane
to spiral ligament
16 Stria vascularis
(vascular stria)
17 Spiral ligament
18 Outer (external)
spiral sulcus
19 Spiral ligament

FIGURE 20.9 ■ Inner ear: cochlear duct (scala media). Stain: hematoxylin and eosin. Medium magnification.

FIGURE 20.10 ■ Inner Ear: Cochlear Duct and the Organ of Corti

A higher-magnification photomicrograph illustrates the inner ear with the cochlear canal and the hearing **organ of Corti (8)** in the **bony cochlea (1, 9).** The cochlear canal is subdivided into the **scala vestibuli (10),** the **cochlear duct** (scala media) **(3),** and the **scala tympani (14).** A thin **vestibular membrane (2)** separates the cochlear duct (3) from the scala vestibuli (10). A thicker **basilar membrane (7)** separates the cochlear duct (3) from the scala tympani (14).

The basilar membrane (7) extends from the connective tissue **spiral ligament (6)** to a thickened **spiral limbus (11).** The basilar membrane (7) supports the organ of Corti (8) with its sensory **hair cells (5)** and supportive cells. Extending from the spiral limbus (11) is the **tectorial membrane (4),** which covers a portion of the organ of Corti (8) and the hair cells (5). The sensory bipolar **spiral ganglion cells (13)** are located in the bony cochlea (1, 9). The afferent axons from the spiral ganglion cells (13) pass through the **osseous spiral lamina (12)** to the organ of Corti (8), where their dendrites synapse with the hair cells (5) in the organ of Corti (8).

FUNCTIONAL CORRELATIONS

Cochlea

The cochlea of the inner ear contains the auditory **organ of Corti.** Sound waves that enter the ear and pass through the **external auditory canal** vibrate the **tympanic membrane.** The vibrations activate the three bony **ossicles** (stapes, incus, and malleus) in the middle ear, which then transmit these vibrations across the air-filled **middle ear,** or **tympanic cavity,** to the fluid-filled **inner ear.** The sounds vibrate the **basilar membrane** on which the **organ of Corti** is located. The vibrations stimulate sensitive **hair cells** in the organ of Corti, which convert the mechanical vibrations into **nerve impulses.**

Impulses for sound pass along the afferent axons of bipolar **ganglion cells** in the **spiral ganglia** of the inner ear. The axons from the spiral ganglia join and form the **auditory,** or **cochlear, nerve,** which carries the impulses from the sensitive cells in the organ of Corti to the brain for sound interpretation.

Vestibular Apparatus

The vestibular apparatus consists of the **utricle, saccule,** and **semicircular canals.** These sensitive organs respond to linear and/or angular accelerations or movements of the head. Sensory inputs from the vestibular apparatus initiate the very complex neural pathways that activate specific skeletal muscles that correct balance and equilibrium and restore the body to its normal position.

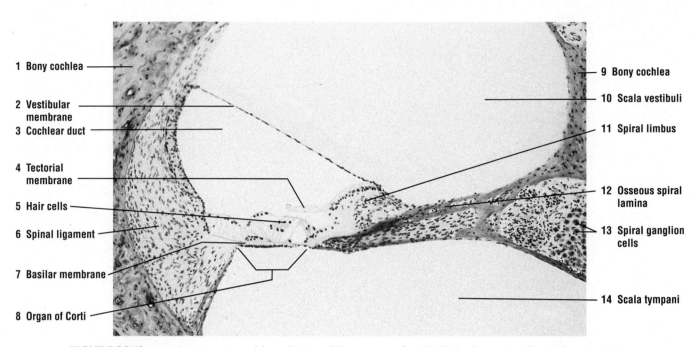

1 Bony cochlea

2 Vestibular membrane

3 Cochlear duct

4 Tectorial membrane

5 Hair cells

6 Spinal ligament

7 Basilar membrane

8 Organ of Corti

9 Bony cochlea

10 Scala vestibuli

11 Spiral limbus

12 Osseous spiral lamina

13 Spiral ganglion cells

14 Scala tympani

FIGURE 20.10 ■ Inner ear: cochlear duct and the organ of corti. Stain: hematoxylin and eosin. 30×

Page numbers in *italics* designate illustrations